Progress in
Cancer Research and Therapy
Volume 32

MOLECULAR BIOLOGY OF
TUMOR CELLS

Progress in Cancer Research and Therapy

Vol. 32: Molecular Biology of Tumor Cells
Britta Wahren, Göran Holm, Sten Hammarström, and Peter Perlmann, editors, 1985

Vol. 31: Hormones and Cancer 2: Proceedings of the Second International Congress
Francesco Bresciani, Roger J. B. King, Marc E. Lippman, Moïse Namer, and Jean-Pierre Raynaud, editors, 1984

Vol. 30: Gene Transfer and Cancer
Mark L. Pearson and Nat L. Sternberg, editors, 1984

Vol. 29: Markers of Colonic Cell Differentiation
Sandra R. Wolman and Anthony J. Mastromarino, editors, 1984

Vol. 28: The Development of Target-Oriented Anticancer Drugs
Yung-Chi Cheng, Barry Goz, and Mimi Minkoff, editors, 1983

Vol. 27: Environmental Influences in the Pathogenesis of Leukemias and Lymphomas
Ian T. Magrath, Gregory T. O'Conor, and Bracha Ramot, editors, 1984

Vol. 26: Radiation Carcinogenesis: Epidemiology and Biological Significance
John D. Boice, Jr. and Joseph F. Fraumeni, editors, 1983

Vol. 25: Steroids and Endometrial Cancer
Valerio Maria Jasonno, Italo Nenci, and Carlo Flamigni, editors, 1983

Vol. 24: Recent Clinical Developments in Gynecologic Oncology
C. Paul Morrow, John Bonnar, Timothy J. O'Brien, and William E. Gibbons, editors, 1983

Vol. 23: Maturation Factors and Cancer
Malcolm A. S. Moore, editor, 1982

Vol. 22: The Potential Role of T Cells in Cancer Therapy
Alexander Fefer and Allen L. Goldstein, editors, 1982

Vol. 21: Hybridomas in Cancer Diagnosis and Treatment
Malcolm S. Mitchell and Herbert F. Oettgen, editors, 1982

Vol. 20: Lymphokines and Thymic Hormones: Their Potential Utilization in Cancer Therapeutics
Allen L. Goldstein and Michael A. Chirigos, editors, 1982

Vol. 19: Mediation of Cellular Immunity in Cancer by Immune Modifiers
Michael A. Chirigos, Malcolm S. Mitchell, and Michael J. Mastrangelo, editors, 1982

Vol. 18: Carcinoma of the Bladder
John G. Connolly, editor, 1981

Vol. 17: Nutrition and Cancer: Etiology and Treatment
Guy R. Newell and Neil M. Ellison, editors, 1981

Vol. 16: Augmenting Agents in Cancer Therapy
E. M. Hersch, M. A. Chirigos, and M. J. Mastrangelo, editors, 1981

Vol. 15: Role of Medroxyprogesterone in Endocrine-Related Tumors
Stefano Iacobelli and Aurelio Di Marco, editors, 1980

Vol. 14: Hormones and Cancer
Stefano Iacobelli, R. J. B. King, Hans R. Lindner, and Marc E. Lippman, editors, 1980

Vol. 13: Colorectal Cancer: Prevention, Epidemiology, and Screening
Sidney J. Winawer, David Schottenfeld, and Paul Sherlock, editors, 1980

Vol. 12:   Advances in Neuroblastoma Research
Audrey E. Evans, editor, 1980

Vol. 11:   Treatment of Lung Cancer
Marcel Rozencweig and Franco Muggia, editors, 1978

Vol. 10:   Hormones, Receptors, and Breast Cancer
William L. McGuire, editor, 1978

Vol. 9:   Endocrine Control in Neoplasia
R. K. Sharma and W. E. Criss, editors, 1978

Vol. 8:   Polyamines as Biochemical Markers of Normal and Malignant Growth
D. H. Russell and B. G. M. Durie, editors, 1978

Vol. 7:   Immune Modulation and Control of Neoplasia by Adjuvant Therapy
Michael A. Chirigos, editor, 1978

Vol. 6:   Immunotherapy of Cancer: Present Status of Trials in Man
William D. Terry and Dorothy Windhorst, editors, 1978

Vol. 5:   Cancer Invasion and Metastasis: Biologic Mechanisms and Therapy
Stacey B. Day, W. P. Laird Myers, Philip Stansly, Silvio Garattini, and Martin G. Lewis, editors, 1977

Vol. 4:   Progesterone Receptors in Neoplastic Tissues
William L. McGuire, Jean-Pierre Raynaud, and Etienne-Emile Baulieu, editors, 1977

Vol. 3:   Genetics of Human Cancer
John J. Mulvihill, Robert W. Miller, and Joseph F. Fraumeni, Jr., editors, 1977

Vol. 2:   Control of Neoplasia by Modulation of the Immune System
Michael A. Chirigos, editor, 1977

Vol. 1:   Control Mechanisms in Cancer
Wayne E. Criss, Tetsuo Ono, and John R. Sabine, editors, 1976

Progress in
Cancer Research and Therapy
Volume 32

Molecular Biology of
Tumor Cells

Editors

Britta Wahren, M.D., Ph.D.
Department of Virology
National Bacteriological Laboratory
and Karolinska Institute
Stockholm, Sweden

Göran Holm, M.D., Ph.D.
Department of Clinical Immunology
Huddinge Hospital
at Karolinska Institute
Huddinge, Sweden

Sten Hammarström Ph.D.
Department of Immunology
University of Stockholm
Stockholm, Sweden

Peter Perlmann, Ph.D.
Department of Immunology
University of Stockholm
Stockholm, Sweden

Raven Press ■ New York

Raven Press, 1140 Avenue of the Americas, New York, New York 10036

Made in the United States of America

Library of Congress Cataloging in Publication Data
Main entry under title:

Molecular biology of tumor cells.

(Progress in cancer research and therapy ; v. 32)
Includes index.
1. Cancer cells.   2. Molecular biology.   I. Wahren,
Britta.   II. Series.   [DNLM: 1. Cell Transformation,
Neoplastic—congresses.   2. Molecular Biology—congresses.
3. Oncogenes—congresses.   W1 PR667M v.32 /
QZ 202 M7183 1984]
RC267.M65 1985   616.99'4071   84-23786
ISBN 0-88167-066-9

Papers or parts thereof have been used as camera-ready copy as submitted by the authors whenever possible; when retyped, they have been edited by the editorial staff only to the extent considered necessary for the assistance of an international readership. The views expressed and the general style adopted remain, however, the responsibility of the named authors. Great care has been taken to maintain the accuracy of the information contained in the volume. However, neither Raven Press nor the editors can be held responsible for errors or for any consequences arising from the use of information contained herein.

The use in this book of particular designations of countries or territories does not imply any judgment by the publisher or editors as to the legal status of such countries or territories, of their authorities or institutions or of the delimitation of their boundaries.

Some of the names of products referred to in this book may be registered trademarks or proprietary names, although specific reference to this fact may not be made: however, the use of a name with designation is not to be construed as a representation by the publisher or editors that it is in the public domain. In addition, the mention of specific companies or of their products or proprietary names does not imply any endorsement or recommendation on the part of the publisher or editors.

Authors were themselves responsible for obtaining the necessary permission to reproduce copyright material from other sources. With respect to the publisher's copyright, material appearing in this book prepared by individuals as part of their official duties as government employees is only covered by this copyright to the extent permitted by the appropriate national regulations.

Materials appearing in this book prepared by individuals as part of their official duties as U.S. Government employees are not covered by the above-mentioned copyright.

Preface

The aim of this volume is to disseminate the latest findings and stimulate interdisciplinary discussions on various aspects of cancer cell biochemistry and biology.

Rapid progress in biotechnology is helping to clarify carcinogenetic mechanisms. Descriptions are given of the startling developments in the oncogene field. The modes of cellular and viral onc gene functions in carcinogenesis are indicated by a variety of experiments by the authors. A number of onc genes may be activated in neoplasms. The functional importance of activating the ras and myc genes is discussed in terms of morphologic alteration and transformation of cells.

There are chapters on the interaction between malignant cell products and cellular receptors for growth factors. It seems that the onc gene sis codes for a transforming protein homologous to platelet derived growth factor, and that erb codes for a truncated receptor for epidermal growth factor. Thus, transformed cells may be independent of exogenous growth factors. Unregulated tumor growth may depend instead on the endogenous synthesis of growth factor-like substances or receptors for these.

The surface of tumor cells interacts with the environment and is also susceptible to immune and growth regulating interactions from the host. Changes associated with the membrane include uncommon phosphorylating enzymes, transferrin-like molecules, carbohydrate and protein moieties of unknown structures. Tumor cells can be killed with monoclonal antibodies to structures exposed in large amounts on tumor cells. These reagents also can be used as diagnostic reagents. Leukemias and lymphomas have been much studied in this respect, as have melanomas and colo-rectal adenocarcinomas. As a consequence of the genomic rearrangements in carcinogenesis, absolute tumor specificity is not found except in cases of tumors caused by exogenous viruses. This appears to be the case with the retroviruses inducing T-cell leukemia. Blood cells are frequently used to study normal and malignant differentiation. The endogenous and exogenous factors that influence the differentiation process are described.

This volume will be of interest to a wide audience, from postgraduate students of biology to specialized scientists, and from those mainly interested in basic science to those concerned with the development of clinical medicine.

Britta Wahren

Acknowledgments

The chapters in this volume are based on papers presented at the 8th Nobel Conference of the Karolinska Institute, held on June 3 to 6, 1984 at Skogshem, Lidingö, Sweden.

The conference was sponsored by The Nobel Assembly at the Karolinska Institute, Astra Läkemedel, Abbott Diagnostics Division, Bristol Laboratories, Cancerföreningen i Stockholm, Farmitalia Carlo Erba, Fortia, Leo AB, National Bacteriological Laboratory, Scandinavian Airlines System, Stockholm Site and Development Company, Swedish Society for Cancer Research, and University of Stockholm.

Contents

Activated Genes and Oncogenes

1   Molecular and Functional Analysis of *ras* and *Blym*
    Transforming Genes
    Geoffrey M. Cooper

11 Activation of the c-myc Oncogene in Murine Plasmacytomas
    K. B. Marcu, J. O. Yang, L. W. Stanton, J. F. Mushinski,
    P. D. Fahrlander, L. W. Eckhardt, and B. K. Birshtein

29 Disrupted Expression of the c-myc Oncogene in Burkitt's
    Lymphoma
    T. H. Rabbitts, R. Baer, A. Forster, and P. H. Rabbitts

39 Interacting Oncogenes
    Alan Schechter, David F. Stern, Lalitha Vaidyanathan,
    Hartmut Land, Luis F. Parada, and Robert A. Weinberg

45 Pathogenetic and Clinical Significance of Chromosomal
    Aberrations in B-Cell Chronic Lymphocytic Leukemia
    G. Gahrton, G. Juliusson, K.-H. Robèrt, K. Friberg, and
    L. Zech

Promotors and Growth Factors for Induction of Cancer

55 Molecular Mechanisms of Multistage Chemical Carcinogenesis
    I. Bernard Weinstein, John Arcoleo, Michael Lambert,
    Wendy Hsiao, Sebastiano Gattoni-Celli, Alan M. Jeffrey,
    and Paul Kirschmeier

71 Subversion of Growth Factor Signal Transduction by
    Oncogenes
    M. D. Waterfield

87 Platelet-Derived Growth Factor: Comments on the Structural
    and Functional Relationship with the Transforming Protein
    of Simian Sarcoma Virus
    Bengt Westermark, Ann Johnsson, Christer Betsholtz,
    Åke Wasteson, and Carl-Henrik Heldin

xi

Cell Surface Changes in Neoplastic Transformation and Transformation-Associated Proteins

95 Phosphorylation-Dephosphorylation Events in Cells Transformed by Rous Sarcoma Virus
R. L. Erikson, John Blenis, Jordan G. Spivack, and Y. Sugimoto

107 Retroviral *onc* Gene Proteins: Intracellular Localization and Studies on Transformation Mechanisms
L. R. Rohrschneider, V. M. Rothwell, L. M. Najita, C. H. Ooi, and R. L. Manger

123 Human Tumor Antigens
Hilary Koprowski and Meenhard Herlyn

139 Glycosphingolipids as Differentiation and Tumor Markers and as Regulators of Cell Proliferation
Sen-itiroh Hakomori

157 Isolation of a cDNA Clone for Human Melanoma-Associated Antigen p97
Joseph P. Brown, Timothy M. Rose, John W. Forstrom, Ingegerd Hellström, and Karl Erik Hellström

169 Molecular and Biological Profiles of Two Unique Antigens Associated with Human Melanoma
Ralph A. Reisfeld, Gregor Schulz, David A. Cheresh, and John R. Harper

Differentiation of Normal and Malignant Cells

183 Human Leukemia Viruses: The HTLV "Family" and Their Role in Human Malignancies and Immune Deficiency Disease
R. C. Gallo, F. Wong-Staal, P. D. Markham, M. Popovic, and M. G. Sarngadharan

215 Role of the Colony Stimulating Factors in the Emergence and Suppression of Myeloid Leukemia Populations
Donald Metcalf and Nicos A. Nicola

233 Phorbol Ester (TPA)-Induced Differentiation of B-Type Chronic Lymphocytic Leukemia Cells
Kenneth Nilsson, Thomas Tötterman, Antero Danersund, Klas Forsbeck, Lars Hellman, and Ulf Pettersson

243 Change in Expression of Oncogenes (*sis, ras, myc,* and *abl*) During *In Vitro* Differentiation of L6 Rat Myoblasts
Thomas Sejersen, J. Pedro Wahrmann, Janos Sümegi, and Nils R. Ringertz

251 Activation and Differentiation *In Vitro* of Human Lymphoma Cells: A New Method for the Cytological Evaluation of the Lymphoma Patient
Karl-Henrik Robèrt, Gunnar Juliusson, Gösta Gahrton, and Peter Biberfeld

257 Regulators of Growth, Differentiation, and the Reversion of Malignancy: Normal Hematopoiesis and Leukemia
Leo Sachs

281 Subject Index

Contributors

John Arcoleo
Division of Environmental Sciences and
    Cancer Center
Institute of Cancer Research
Columbia University
New York, New York 10032

R. Baer
Memorial Sloan Kettering Cancer Center
1275 York Avenue
New York, New York 10021

Christer Betsholtz
Department of Pathology
University of Uppsala
Akademiska Hospital
S-751 85 Uppsala, Sweden

Peter Biberfeld
Department of Pathology
Karolinska Hospital
Box 60500
S-104 01 Stockholm, Sweden

B. K. Birshtein
Department of Cell Biology
Albert Einstein College of Medicine
Bronx, New York 10462

John Blenis
Department of Cellular and
    Developmental Biology
Harvard University
Cambridge, Massachusetts 02138

Joseph P. Brown
Program in Tumor Immunology
Fred Hutchinson Cancer Research Center
Seattle, Washington 98104;
and Department of Pathology
University of Washington
Seattle, Washington 98195

David A. Cheresh
Department of Immunology
Scripps Clinic and Research Foundation
10666 North Torrey Pines Road
La Jolla, California 92037

Geoffrey M. Cooper
Dana-Farber Cancer Institute, and
    Department of Pathology
Harvard Medical School
Boston, Massachusetts 02115

Antero Danersund
Department of Pathology
University of Uppsala
Akademiska Hospital
S-751 85 Uppsala, Sweden

L. W. Eckhardt
Department of Biological Sciences
Columbia University
New York, New York 10027;
and Department of Cell Biology
Albert Einstein College of Medicine
Bronx, New York 10462

Raymond L. Erikson
Department of Cellular and
    Developmental Biology
Harvard University
Cambridge, Massachusetts 02138

P. D. Fahrlander
Biochemistry Department
State University of New York
    at Stony Brook
Stony Brook, New York 11794

Klas Forsbeck
Department of Pathology
University of Uppsala
Akademiska Hospital
S-751 85 Uppsala, Sweden

xv

A. Forster
MRC Laboratory of Molecular Biology
Hills Road
Cambridge CB2 2QH, United Kingdom

John W. Forstrom
Program in Tumor Immunology
Fred Hutchinson Cancer Research Center
Seattle, Washington 98104

Kristina Friberg
Institute of Medical Cell Genetics
Medical Nobel Institute
Karolinska Institute
Box 60400
S-104 01 Stockholm, Sweden

Gösta Gahrton
Division of Clinical Hematology and
  Oncology
Department of Medicine
Huddinge Hospital and Karolinska
  Institute
S-141 86 Huddinge, Sweden

Robert C. Gallo
National Institutes of Health
National Cancer Institute
Building 37, Room 6A09
9000 Rockville Pike
Bethesda, Maryland 20205

Sebastiano Gattoni-Celli
Division of Environmental Sciences and
  Cancer Center
Institute of Cancer Research
Columbia University
New York, New York 10032

Sen-itiroh Hakomori
Program of Biochemical Oncology/
  Membrane Research
Fred Hutchinson Cancer Research Center
1124 Columbia Street
Seattle, Washington 98104

John R. Harper
Department of Immunology
Scripps Clinic and Research Foundation
10666 North Torrey Pines Road
La Jolla, California 92037

Carl-Henrik Heldin
Department of Medical and Physiological
  Chemistry
University of Uppsala
Akademiska Hospital
S-751 85 Uppsala, Sweden

Lars Hellman
Department of Medical Genetics
University of Uppsala
Akademiska Hospital
S-751 85 Uppsala, Sweden

Ingegerd Hellström
Program in Tumor Immunology
Fred Hutchinson Cancer Research Center
Seattle, Washington 98104;
and Department of Microbiology/
  Immunology
University of Washington
Seattle, Washington 98195

Karl Erik Hellström
Program in Tumor Immunology
Fred Hutchinson Cancer Research Center
Seattle, Washington 98104;
and Department of Pathology
University of Washington
Seattle, Washington 98195

Meenhard Herlyn
The Wistar Institute of Anatomy and
  Biology
36th Street at Spruce
Philadelphia, Pennsylvania 19104

Wendy Hsiao
Division of Environmental Sciences and
  Cancer Center
Institute of Cancer Research
Columbia University
New York, New York 10032

Alan M. Jeffrey
Division of Environmental Sciences and
  Cancer Center
Institute of Cancer Research
Columbia University
New York, New York 10032

Ann Johnsson
Department of Medical and Physiological
Chemistry
University of Uppsala
Akademiska Hospital
S-751 85 Uppsala, Sweden

Gunnar Juliusson
Division of Clinical Hematology and
Oncology
Department of Medicine
Huddinge Hospital and Karolinska
Institute
S-141 86 Huddinge, Sweden

Paul Kirschmeier
Division of Environmental Sciences and
Cancer Center
Institute of Cancer Research
Columbia University
New York, New York 10032

Hilary Koprowski
The Wistar Institute of Anatomy and
Biology
36th Street at Spruce
Philadelphia, Pennsylvania 19104

Michael Lambert
Division of Environmental Sciences and
Cancer Center
Institute of Cancer Research
Columbia University
New York, New York 10032

Hartmut Land
Center for Cancer Research
Massachusetts Institute of Technology
and Whitehead Institute for Biomedical
Research
Cambridge, Massachusetts 02139

R. L. Manger
Fred Hutchinson Cancer Research Center
1124 Columbia Street
Seattle, Washington 98104

Kenneth B. Marcu
Biochemistry Department
State University of New York at Stony
Brook
Stony Brook, New York 11794

P. D. Markham
National Institutes of Health
National Cancer Institute
Building 37, Room 6A09
9000 Rockville Pike
Bethesda, Maryland 20205

Donald Metcalf
Cancer Research Unit
The Walter and Eliza Hall Institute of
Medical Research
Royal Melbourne Hospital
Post Office 3050
Victoria, Australia

J. F. Mushinski
Laboratory of Genetics
National Cancer Institute
Bethesda, Maryland 20205

L. M. Najita
Fred Hutchinson Cancer Research Center
1124 Columbia Street
Seattle, Washington 98104

Nicos A. Nicola
Cancer Research Unit
The Walter and Eliza Hall Institute of
Medical Research
Royal Melbourne Hospital
Post Office 3050
Victoria, Australia

Kenneth Nilsson
Department of Pathology
University of Uppsala
Akademiska Hospital
S-751 85 Uppsala, Sweden

C. H. Ooi
Fred Hutchinson Cancer Research Center
1124 Columbia Street
Seattle, Washington 98104

Luis F. Parada
Center for Cancer Research
Massachusetts Institute of Technology
and Whitehead Institute for Biomedical
Research
Cambridge, Massachusetts 02139

Ulf Pettersson
Department of Medical Genetics
University of Uppsala
Akademiska Hospital
S-751 85 Uppsala, Sweden

Mikulas Popovic
National Institutes of Health
National Cancer Institute
Building 37, Room 6A09
9000 Rockville Pike
Bethesda, Maryland 20205

P. H. Rabbitts
Ludwig Institute for Cancer Research
MRC Centre
Hills Road
Cambridge CB2 2QH, United Kingdom

Terence H. Rabbitts
MRC Laboratory of Molecular Biology
Hills Road
Cambridge CB2 2QH, United Kingdom

Ralph A. Reisfeld
Department of Immunology
Scripps Clinic and Research Foundation
10666 North Torrey Pines Road
La Jolla, California 92037

Nils R. Ringertz
Department of Medical Cell Genetics
Medical Nobel Institute
Karolinska Institute
Box 60400
S-104 01 Stockholm, Sweden

Karl-Henrik Robèrt
Division of Clinical Hematology and
    Oncology
Department of Medicine
Huddinge Hospital and Karolinska
    Institute
S-141 86 Huddinge, Sweden

Larry R. Rohrschneider
Fred Hutchinson Cancer Research Center
1124 Columbia Street
Seattle, Washington 98104

Timothy M. Rose
Program in Tumor Immunology
Fred Hutchinson Cancer Research Center
Seattle, Washington 98104

V. M. Rothwell
Fred Hutchinson Cancer Research Center
1i24 Columbia Street
Seattle, Washington 98104

Leo Sachs
Department of Genetics
Weizmann Institute of Science
P.O.B. 26
Rehovot 76100, Israel

Mangalasseril Sarngadharan
National Institutes of Health
National Cancer Institute
Building 37, Room 6A09
9000 Rockville Pike
Bethesda, Maryland 20205

Alan Schechter
Center for Cancer Research
Massachusetts Institute of Technology
and Whitehead Institute for Biomedical
    Research
Cambridge, Massachusetts 02139

Gregor Schulz
Department of Immunology
Scripps Clinic and Research Foundation
10666 North Torrey Pines Road
La Jolla, California 92037

Thomas Sejersen
Department of Medical Cell Genetics
Medical Nobel Institute
Karolinska Institute
Box 60400
S-104 01 Stockholm, Sweden

Jordan G. Spivack
Department of Cellular and
    Developmental Biology
Harvard University
Cambridge, Massachusetts 02138

L. W. Stanton
Biochemistry Department
State University of New York
  at Stony Brook
Stony Brook, New York 11794

David F. Stern
Center for Cancer Research
Massachusetts Institute of Technology
and Whitehead Institute for Biomedical
  Research
Cambridge, Massachusetts 02139

Y. Sugimoto
Department of Cellular and
  Developmental Biology
Harvard University
Cambridge, Massachusetts 02138

Janos Sümegi
Department of Tumor Biology
Karolinska Institute
Box 60400
S-104 01 Stockholm, Sweden

Thomas Tötterman
Department of Pathology
University of Uppsala
Akademiska Hospital
S-751 85 Uppsala, Sweden

Lalitha Vaidyanathan
Center for Cancer Research
Massachusetts Institute of Technology
and Whitehead Institute for Biomedical
  Research
Cambridge, Massachusetts 02139

J. Pedro Wahrmann
Institut de Pathologie Moléculaire
24, rue du Faubourg Saint Jacques
F-75214 Paris, France

Åke Wasteson
Department of Medical and Physiological
  Chemistry
University of Uppsala
Akademiska Hospital
S-751 85 Uppsala, Sweden

Michael D. Waterfield
Protein Chemistry Laboratory
Imperial Cancer Research Fund
Lincoln's Inn Fields
London WC2A 3PX, United Kingdom

Robert A. Weinberg
Center for Cancer Research
Massachusetts Institute of Technology
77 Massachusetts Avenue
Cambridge, Massachusetts 02139

I. Bernard Weinstein
Division of Environmental Sciences and
  Cancer Center
Institute of Cancer Research
Columbia University
New York, New York 10032

Bengt Westermark
Department of Pathology
University of Uppsala
Akademiska Hospital
S-751 85 Uppsala, Sweden

Flossie Wong-Staal
National Institutes of Health
National Cancer Institute
Building 37, Room 6A09
9000 Rockville Pike
Bethesda, Maryland 20205

J. O. Yang
Biochemistry Department
State University of New York at Stony
  Brook
Stony Brook, New York 11794

Lore Zech
Institute of Medical Cell Genetics
Medical Nobel Institute
Karolinska Institute
Box 60400
S-104 01 Stockholm, Sweden

Molecular Biology of Tumor Cells, edited by
B. Wahren et al. Raven Press, New York © 1985.

Molecular and Functional Analysis of *ras* and *Blym* Transforming Genes

Geoffrey M. Cooper

Dana-Farber Cancer Institute, and Department of Pathology, Harvard Medical School, Boston, Massachusetts 02115

A variety of different types of neoplasms contain activated transforming genes which have been detected by transfection. These neoplasm DNAs induce transformation of NIH 3T3 cells with high efficiencies. In contrast, DNAs of normal cells lack efficient transforming activity, including normal DNAs of the same individual animals or patients whose tumor DNAs induce transformation. These findings imply that the development of many neoplasms involves dominant genetic alterations leading to the activation of transforming genes which are then detectable by their biological activity in this gene transfer assay.

At least eleven different neoplasm transforming genes have now been identified via the transfection assay (Table 1). Three of these genes (ras^H, ras^K, and ras^N), which are activated in neoplasms of many different cell types, are cellular homologs of the transforming genes of Harvey and Kirsten sarcoma viruses (11, 20, 29, 32, 37). In contrast, the other neoplasm transforming genes identified by transfection are unrelated to those of retroviruses. These include Blym-1, which is discussed below, and Tlym-I, which is related to class I MHC genes (25). Four additional genes (designated tx-1 through tx-4) can be distinguished from ras, Blym-1, Tlym-I and each other by cleavage with restriction endonucleases (22,24). However, since these genes have not yet been isolated as molecular clones, it is possible that they are members of a gene family defined by one of the already characterized transforming genes. Two additional novel transforming genes, hos and pro, have also been recently identified in other laboratories (5,6).

The frequent activation of such transforming genes in a variety of tumors suggests that they play a significant role in neoplasm development. I will discuss here recent work dealing with functional analysis of the ras and Blym genes.

1

Table 1. Neoplasm Transforming Genes Detected by Transfection

	Human	Avian or Rodent
ras^H	bladder and lung carcinoma	epithelial and mammary carcinomas
ras^K	lung, colon, bladder, pancreatic, gall bladder and ovarian carcinomas rhabdomyosarcoma T cell ALL	sarcomas, T cell lymphomas
ras^N	neuroblastoma, fibrosarcomas, promyelocytic leukemia, acute myelogenous leukemia, Burkitt's lymphoma, T cell ALL, colon carcinoma, melanoma, teratocarcinoma	T cell lymphomas
Blym-1	Burkitt's lymphomas	B cell lymphomas
Tlym-1	T cell lymphomas	T cell lymphomas
tx-1	pre B cell neoplasms	pre B cell neoplasms
tx-2	myelomas	plasmacytomas
tx-3	mature T cell neoplasm	mature T cell neoplasms
tx-4	mammary carcinoma	mammary carcinomas
hos	chemically - transformed	--------------
pro	---------------------	promoter-responsive epidermal cells

ras GENE ACTIVATION AND FUNCTION

The ras genes all encode closely related proteins of approximately 21,000 daltons which are designated p21s. Experimental manipulations of the normal human ras^H gene have shown that over-expression of the normal gene product is sufficient to induce cell transformation (4). However, activation of ras genes in human tumors is commonly a consequence of structural, rather than regulatory, mutations (2, 3, 12, 31, 36, 38, 39, 40, 44). The mutations in tumors which have been analyzed to date alter either codon 12 or codon 61. At either of these positions, substitution of multiple different amino acids is sufficient to endow p21 with transforming activity. In addition, most activating mutations appear to induce conformational alterations in p21 which are detectable by abnormal electophoretic mobilities (12, 38, 44).

Studies of viral ras proteins have indicated that they are localized to the inner face of the plasma membrane (17,43) and modified by acylation (34). The only established biochemical activity common to all viral ras transforming proteins is guanine nucleotide binding (17, 33).

To attempt to elucidate the biochemical basis for the transforming activity of mutant p21s in human tumors, we have compared

the biochemical properties of p21s encoded by normal and activated human ras genes. These experiments indicated that both
normal and transforming human p21s were localized to the plasma
membrane and were modified to similar extents by post-translational acylation (16). Neither normal nor activated p21s were glycosylated or phosphorylated (12,16). Thus the subcellular localization and posttranslational processing of human p21s were not
altered by ras gene activation.

Since guanine nucleotide binding represented the only known
biochemical activity of p21, we investigated the possibility
that the affinity or specificity of p21 for nucleotides was
altered as a consequence of mutational activation. However,
the GTP binding affinities of both normal and activated human
p21s were indistinguishable (K_D's of 1-2 x 10^{-8}M) and both
the normal and activated proteins were specific for GTP and GDP
binding (16). Thus mutational activation of p21 does not directly affect its intrinsic nucleotide binding properties.

In order to investigate the physiologic function of ras proteins, we have attempted to identify other cellular proteins
with which p21 might interact (15). Immunoprecipitation of extracts of human carcinoma cell lines with anti-p21 monoclonal
antibodies revealed the co-precipitation of a second protein of
approximately 90,000 daltons. This coprecipitated protein was
identified as the transferrin receptor by three criteria:
1) comigration in both reducing and non-reducing gels 2) immunological reactivity with monoclonal antibody raised against
transferrin receptor and 3) identity of partial proteolysis
maps of the 90,000 dalton coprecipitated protein and transferrin
receptor. Co-precipitation of transferrin receptor was detected
with three different ras monoclonal antibodies and was dependent
on the presence of ras proteins in cell extracts, indicating
that p21 and transferrin receptor form a molecular complex. This
complex was dissociated by addition of transferrin to cell
extracts, suggesting that transferrin binding induced a conformational change in the receptor which led to the dissociation
of ras proteins. Preliminary experiments further indicate that
the transferrin binding stimulates a GTPase activity of ras
proteins (Finkel and Cooper, unpublished observations).

Transferrin is an iron-binding protein which is required for
the growth of most cells in culture. Expression of transferrin
receptor is closely correlated with cell proliferation. Furthermore, monoclonal antibodies against transferrin receptor inhibit
cell growth, in some cases even if iron is supplied in an alter-
nate form. Transferrin and its receptor thus appear to play
a fundamental role in the growth of many differentiated cell
types. The findings of interaction between ras proteins and
transferrin receptor therefore suggest that p21 may function
in conjunction with this cell surface receptor in regulation of
cell growth, perhaps by transducing growth signals mediated by
transferrin binding. It is possible that the role of p21 in this
respect is analogous to other membrane guanine nucleotide binding

proteins, such as the adenyl cyclase G proteins and transducin (18).

BLYM TRANSFORMING GENES

The Blym-1 transforming gene was initially identified in DNAs of chicken B cell lymphomas (7) and was isolated as a molecular clone by sib-selection (19). The cloned chicken Blym-1 gene was unusually small (only about 600 nucleotides) and its nucleotide sequence indicated that it encoded a small protein of 65 amino acids (19). Comparison of the predicted chicken Blym-1 amino acid sequence with sequences of known cellular proteins revealed partial homology (36%) between the chicken Blym-1 protein and the amino-terminal region of transferrin family proteins (19). This homology was concentrated in regions which were conserved between different members of the transferrin family, suggesting a common ancestry for chicken Blym-1 and a region of the transferrins, as well as stimulating the speculation that this homology might also suggest a functional relationship.

Blot hybridization analysis indicated that the chicken Blym-1 gene was a member of a small family of related genes which were present in human as well as chicken DNA. We therefore investigated the possibility that the transforming gene detected by transfection of Burkitt's lymphoma DNAs might be a member of the human gene family defined by homology to chicken Blym-1. A genomic library of DNA from a Burkitt's lymphoma was screened using chicken Blym-1 probe and a biologically active human transforming gene, designated human Blym-1, was isolated (13). This human homolog of chicken Blym-1 was found to represent the transforming gene detected by transfection of six out of six Burkitt's lymphoma DNAs studied.

Restriction mapping and nucleotide sequencing indicate that human Blym-1, like chicken Blym-1, is quite small (approximately 700 nucleotides) (13,14). Also like chicken Blym-1, the sequence of human Blym-1 predicts a small protein (58 amino acids) which consists of two exons and is rich in lysine and arginine.Alignment of the human and chicken Blym-1 amino acid sequences indicates 33% amino acid identities. The human and chicken Blym-1 proteins are therefore clearly related (p<0.005), but significant divergence between the two sequences has occurred. This divergence suggests the possibility that the chicken and human genes may represent relatively distant members of the Blym family.

In spite of the divergence between the chicken and human Blym-1 genes, the human Blym-1 sequence also displays significant homology (20%) to the amino-terminal region of transferrins. Significantly, amino acids which are conserved between the chicken and human Blym-1 genes also tend to be conserved between members of the transferrin family. It is unlikely that such

divergent sequences as chicken and human Blym-1 have maintained
homology to transferrin by chance. Rather, the conservation of
transferrin homology in these Blym transforming genes suggests
that this homology reflects some functional property of the
Blym transforming proteins. In view of the molecular interaction between ras proteins and transferrin receptor, these
findings suggest the hypothesis that the Blym transforming
genes may also affect cell proliferation via a pathway related
to transferrin and its surface receptor.

TRANSFORMING GENE ACTIVATION AND PATHOGENESIS OF NEOPLASMS

The development of neoplasms in vivo clearly involves progressive pre-neoplastic and neoplastic stages rather than oc-
curing as a single-step conversion of a normal cell to a fully
neoplastic cell. Therefore we have regarded the transforming
genes detected by transfection of tumor DNAs as representing
only one event in neoplasm development. In fact, many neoplasms
involve activation of at least two distinct oncogenes, suggesting that different oncogenes may function at different stages
of neoplasm development.
    In chicken B cell lymphomas, the Blym-1 gene is detected
by the transfection assay (7). However, a different gene
(myc) is activated in the same tumors by adjacent integration
of viral DNA (21). Blym-1 and myc are unrelated to each other
and are not closely linked in cellular DNA (8). Thus, their
co-activation in these neoplasms represent two distinct events.
Since both genes are reproducibly activated in the vast majority
(90%) of individual lymphomas, both appear to play important
roles in the disease process.
    Human myc and Blym-1 genes are also both activated in Bur-
kitt's lymphomas. In this disease, human myc is translocated
from chromosome 8 to an immunoglobulin locus (10,41). In the
same tumors, human Blym-1, which is located on chromosome 1 (26),
is detected as an active transforming gene in the transfection
assay (13). Thus the same two oncogenes are involved in B cell
lymphomas of both chicken and man. The reproducible activation
of both myc and Blym in this disease in two different species
presents a strong argument for the causal role of both genes in
the disease process.
    The initial stage in the pathogenesis of B cell lymphomas
in the chicken is the outgrowth of pre-neoplastic transformed
lymphoid follicles (27). Approximately 10-100 such hyper-
proliferative lesions are observed out of approximately 10^5 lymphocyte follicles in the bursa. These pre-neoplastic follicles
retain the organization of normal lymphoid follicles and the
majority appear to regress under the normal physiological
controls which mediate regression of the bursa. However, a
small fraction (<5%) of these pre-neoplastic follicles are
instead thought to progress to clonal neoplasms (27).
    Activation of both myc and Blym-1 has occurred in the

earliest detectable clonal bursal neoplasms (7). Since the
disease process is inititated by infection with a virus which
activates myc, it is attractive to speculate that activation
of myc is directly responsible for pre-neoplastic follicle
proliferation but is insufficient to induce the full neoplastic
phenotype. Activation of Blym within some pre-neoplastic lymphocytes would then represent a second event responsible for
progression to neoplasia.

Recent evidence in support of this hypothesis has come
from experiments in which the biological effects of an
activated myc gene on bursal lymphocytes have been investigated
(Neiman et al, manuscript submitted). Activated myc was
introduced into bursal lymphocytes by infection with the retrovirus HB1, which contains a myc gene recovered by recombination
from chicken DNA (1). Infected lymphocytes were then transplanted into recipient chicken embryos which had been treated
with cyclophosphamide to ablate their endogenous bursal
lymphocyte population. Histologic examination of the bursas
of these transplanted embryos indicated that the HB1 myc gene
acutely induced formation of pre-neoplastic follicles. DNAs
from these pre-neoplastic follicles did not induce transformation
of NIH 3T3 cells, indicating that Blym-1 was not activated.
These results indicate that myc alone can induce the initial
pre-neoplastic stage of lymphomagenesis and suggest that
activation of Blym-1 is associated with further progression
to neoplasia.

In addition to myc and Blym-1 activation in B cell lymphomas,
pairs of transforming genes are similarly implicated in several
other types of neoplasms. Mouse plasmacytomas involve activation
of myc by chromosomal translocation (9,35) as well as activation
of a distinct transforming gene (tx-2) detected by transfection
(24). Abelson virus induced mouse pre-B cell lymphomas
involve the viral abl gene as well as a distinct and unlinked
NIH 3T3 transforming gene (tx-1) (23). Murine leukemia
virus-induced T cell lymphomas and mouse mammary tumor virus-
induced carcinomas involve activation of genes by virus integration (MLVI and MMTVint) (28, 30, 42) and of unrelated transforming genes detected by transfection (Tlym-I and tx-4) (22.25).
The activation of two distinct transforming genes in neoplasms
thus appears to be a common occurrence. By analogy to the myc
and Blym-1 combination, these genes may function at distinct
stages of tumor development.

REFERENCES

1. Bister, K., Jansen, H.W., Graf, T., Enrietto, P.J. and
   Hayman, M.J. (1983): J. Virol. 46, 337-356.

2. Capon, D.J. Chen, E.Y., Levinson, A.D., Seeburg, P.H.,
   Goeddel, D.V. (1983a): Nature 302, 33-37.

3. Capon, D.J., Seeburg, P.H., McGrath, J.P., Hayflick, J.S., Edman, U., Levinson, A.D. and Goeddel, D.V. (1983b): Nature 304, 507-513.

4. Chang, E.H., Furth, M.E., Scolnick, E.M. and Lowy, D.R. (1982): Nature 297, 497-483.

5. Colburn, N.H., Talmadge, C.B. and Gindhart, T.D. (1983): Mol. Cell. Biol. 3, 1182-1186.

6. Cooper, C.S., Blair, D.G. Oskarsson, M.A., Tainsky, M.A., Eader, L.A. and Vande Woude, G.F. (1984): Cancer Res. 44, 1-10.

7. Cooper, G.M. and Neiman, P.E. (1980): Nature 287, 656-658.

8. Cooper, G.M. and Neiman, P.E. (1981): Nature 292, 857-858.

9. Crews, S., Barth, R., Hood, L., Prehn, J. and Calame, K. (1982): Science 218, 1319-1321.

10. Dalla-Favera, R., Bregni, M., Erikson, J., Patterson, D., Gallo, R.C. and Croce, C.M. (1982): Proc. Natl. Acad. Sci. USA 79, 7824-7827.

11. Der, C.J., Krontiris, T.G. and Cooper, G.M. (1982): Proc. Natl. Acad. Sci. USA 79, 3637-3640.

12. Der, C.J. and Cooper, G.M. (1983): Cell 32, 201-208.

13. Diamond, A.D., Cooper, G.M., Ritz, J. and Lane, M.A. (1983): Nature 305, 112-116.

14. Diamond, A.D., Devine, J. and Cooper, G.M. (1984): Science, in press.

15. Finkel, T. and Cooper, G.M. (1984): Cell 36, 1115-1121.

16. Finkel, T., Der, C.J. and Cooper, G.M. (1984): Cell 37, 151-158.

17. Furth, M.E., Davis, L.J., Fleurdelys, B. and Scolnick. E.M. (1982): J. Virol. 43, 294-304.

18. Gilman, A.G. (1984): Cell 36, 577-579.

19. Goubin, G., Goldman, D.S., Luce, J., Neiman, P.E. and Cooper, G.M. (1983): Nature 302, 114-119.

20. Hall, A., Marshall, C.J., Spurr, N.K. and Weiss, R.A. (1983): Nature 303, 396-400.

21. Hayward, W.S., Neel, B.G. and Astrin, S.M. (1981): Nature 290, 475-480.

22. Lane, M.-A., Sainten, A. and Cooper, G.M. (1981): Proc. Natl. Acad. Sci. USA 78, 5185-5189.

23. Lane, M.-A., Neary, D. and Cooper, G.M. (1982a) Nature 300, 659-661.

24. Lane, M.-A., Sainten, A. and Cooper, G.M. (1982b): Cell 28, 873-880.

25. Lane, M.-A., Sainten, A., Doherty, K.M. and Cooper, G.M. (1984): Proc. Natl. Acad. Sci USA 81, 2227-2231.

26. Morton, C.C., Taub, R., Diamond, A., Lane, M.-A., Cooper, G.M. and Leder, P. (1984): Science 223, 173-175.

27. Neiman, P.E., Jordan. L., Weiss, R.A. and Payne, L.N. (1980): Cold Spring Harbor Conf. on Cell Proliferation 7, 519-528.

28. Nusse, R. and Varmus, H.E. (1982). Cell 31, 99-109.

29. Parada, L.F., Tabin, C.J., Shih, C. and Weinberg, R.A. (1982): Nature: 297, 474-478.

30. Peters, G., Brookes, S., Smith, R. and Dickson, C. (1983): Cell 33, 369-377.

31. Reddy, E.P., Reynolds, R.K., Santos, E. and Barbacid, M. (1982): Nature 300, 149-152.

32. Santos, E., Tronick, S.R., Aaronson, S.A., Pulciani, S. and Barbacid, M. (1982): Nature 298, 343-347.

33. Scolnick, E.M., Papageorge, A.G. and Shih, T.Y. (1979): Proc. Natl. Acad. Sci. USA 76, 5355-5359.

34. Sefton, B.M., Trowbridge, I.S., Cooper, J.A. and Scolnick, E.M. (1982): Cell 31, 465-474.

35. Shen-Ong, G.L.C., Keath, E.J., Piccoli, S.P. and Cole, M.D. (1982): Cell 31, 443-452

36. Shimizu, K., Birnbaum, D., Ruley, M.A., Fasano, O., Suard, Y., Edlund, L., Taparowsky, E., Goldfarb, M. and Wigler, M. (1983a): Nature 304, 497-500.

37. Shimizu, K., Goldfarb, M., Perucho, M. and Wigler, M. (1983b): Proc. Natl. Acad. Sci USA 80, 383-387.

38. Tabin, C.J., Bradley, S.M., Bargmann, C.I., Weinberg, R.A., Papageorge, A.G., Scolnick, E.M., Dhar, R., Lowy, D.R. and Chang, E.H. (1982): <u>Nature</u> 300, 143-149.

39. Taparowsky, E., Suard, Y., Fasano, O., Shimizu, K., Goldfarb, M. and Wigler, M. (1982): <u>Nature</u> 300, 762-765.

40. Taparowsky, E., Shimizu, K., Goldfarb, M., and Wigler, M. (1983): Cell 34, 581-586.

41. Taub, R., Kirsch, I., Morton, C., Lenoir, G. Swarz, D., Tronick, S., Aaronson, S. and Leder, P. (1982): <u>Proc. Natl. Acad. Sci.</u> USA 79, 7837-7841.

42. Tsichlis, P.N., Strauss, P.G. and Hu, L.F. (1983): <u>Nature</u> 302, 445-449.

43. Willingham, M.C., Pastan, I., Shih, T.Y. and Scolnick, (1980): <u>Cell</u> 19, 1005-1014.

44. Yuasa, Y., Srivastava, S.K., Dunn, C.Y., Rhim, J.S., Reddy, E.P. and Aaronson, S.A. (1983): <u>Nature</u> 303, 775-779.

Molecular Biology of Tumor Cells, edited by
B. Wahren et al. Raven Press, New York © 1985.

Activation of the c-myc Oncogene in Murine Plasmacytomas

K. B. Marcu, J. O. Yang, L. W. Stanton, *J. F. Mushinski,
P. D. Fahrlander, †, ‡L. W. Eckhardt, and ‡B. K. Birshtein

*Biochemistry Department, State University of New York at Stony Brook, Stony Brook, New York
11794; *Laboratory of Genetics, National Cancer Institute, Bethesda, Maryland 20205;
†Department of Biological Sciences, Columbia University, New York, New York 10027;
‡Department of Cell Biology, Albert Einstein College of Medicine, Bronx, New York 10462*

ABSTRACT

There appear to be at least three discernible modes
for c-myc activation in murine plasmacytoid tumors: 1)
c-myc gene breakage and cryptic intron promoter activation; 2) alterations in normal promoter usage caused by
nearby translocations; 3) alterations in normal promoter
usage caused by myc associated chromosome 15 band deletions. C-myc activation is most likely reflected in the
inappropriate expression of this proto-oncogene in these
differentiated cells. We define myc expression as inappropriate in PC tumors since the normal allele is
transcriptionally silent in rearrangement positive PCs
(1,4,29). Mutational events do not appear to significantly contribute to c-myc activation in PC tumors.
Furthermore, a significant number of translocation positive PC tumors contain no detectable alterations in c-
myc DNA or RNA structure but do express somewhat elevated myc RNA levels (3-5x) compared to normal cells. However, myc RNA levels in this group of PCs are comparable to those found in other lymphoid tumors without
myc associated translocations. The effect on the c-myc
locus could be a subtle one which may only be measur-
able at the chromatin level. Alternatively, alterations
in c-myc expression may not significantly contribute to
cellular transformation in this class of PC tumors. We
consider the later possibility unlikely since essentially all of the PC tumors possess cytogenetic abnor-

11

malities associated with the identical band on chromosome 15 (25).

INTRODUCTION

The cellular myc proto-oncogene is rearranged and
inappropriately expressed in most murine plasmacytomas
(PCs) as a consequence of a reciprocal 12;15 chromosome
translocation (reviewed in 15,19,26). C-myc targets on
chromosome 12 most often reside within the switch (S)
regions of the immunoglobulin heavy chain constant region (C_H) genes (1,2,4-12,14,15,18,19,21,22,26,28-31).
The strong preference for S region targets (especially
S_α) implicates C_H switching enzymes in the translocation mechanism. However, the c-myc locus is not a
pseudo S region since it bears no obvious homology to
S region repetitive sequences. Target loci of high
transcriptional activity do not seem to be essential
since S regions of germ line context provide acceptable
sites for the translocation (9,30). The normal myc
allele in this class of PC tumors is either silent or
expressed at a low level implying that the translocation results in the inappropriate expression of myc
transcripts in these differentiated cells (1,19,29). In
the majority of PCs, the translocation breaks the c-myc
locus, thereby resulting in the activation of normally
silent promoters within the first myc intron which then
produce elevated levels of truncated myc transcripts
(1,2,18,21,29). Myc breakage occurs within a 1 Kb region
spanning a large 5' non-coding exon and the 5' portion
of the first c-myc intron (1,4,6,9,19,30). Breakages
within this region are probably highly selected to allow
for the loss of the normal gene's promoters while re-
taining several cryptic intron promoters. Therefore, the
activation of c-myc in this class of PCs would seem to
result from the loss of normal regulatory sequences and
the production of elevated levels of truncated myc
transcripts (1,18,29). Multiple cryptic promoters appear
to be clustered in different regions within the first
c-myc intron. The initiation codon for the myc polypeptide is located at the 5' end of the first of two coding
exons (4,30).

A significant number of Pristane induced, translocation positive PC tumors possess intact myc genes and in
a number of cases no detectable rearrangements near the
myc locus (11,20,21,25,35). A normal, unrearranged myc
gene is transcribed from two closely spaced promoters
located at the 5' end of a large non-coding exon. In
normal spleen cells, the 3' promoter (P_2) is 2-3x
favoured over the 5' promoter (P_1). P_2 is 2-10x preferred over P_1 in all pre B and mature B lymphoid cell

lines tested. In either 12;15 or 6;15 positive PCs where no myc associated DNA rearrangement is detected, P_2 is also generally 2x favoured over P_1 with a few exceptions. However, in six PCs wherein the translocation breakpoint resides close to the 5' end of c-myc, a dramatic shift is observed in favour of P_1. The level of steady state myc RNAs are 3-5x elevated in most of these lymphoid tumor cells in comparison to normal spleen cells. However, the steady state levels of myc RNAs are independent of the translocation event. S_1 nuclease protection experiments fail to reveal mutations in the vast majority of these murine tumors. We conclude that multiple pathways exist for c-myc activation in these tumors and that some are preferentially selected over others.

PRODUCTS OF C-MYC RECIPROCAL EXCHANGES AND MOLECULAR REQUIREMENTS FOR THE TRANSLOCATION MECHANISM

The 12;15 myc associated chromosome translocation has been shown to be a reciprocal exchange of variable precision by several laboratories (6,8,22,30,31). The products of the reciprocal myc translocation in the MPC-11 tumor are displayed in Figure 1. The target for c-myc in MPC-11 is an unrearranged, $S\gamma_{2a}$ region (30). However, a non-productively rearranged $S\gamma_{2b}$ region resides ~15 Kb 5' of this $S\gamma_{2a}$ target site (16). We conclude that a myc target need not to be transcriptionally active but may possess some degree of transcriptional competence. At the level of restriction enzyme mapping, no differences between the 5' and 3' myc translocation products in MPC-11 are discernible (Figure 1 and ref. 30). As shown in Figure 2, nucleotide sequencing and fine structure restriction enzyme mapping on subcloned DNA fragments reveal that 11 bp of c-myc and ~300 bp of $S\gamma_{2a}$ sequences have been lost as a consequence of the translocation. A recent elegant study performed by Gerondakis et al., on three independent PCs suggests that this translocation is an imprecise reciprocal exchange resulting in either deletions or duplications of c-myc and S region sequences (9). Deletions and duplications at the site of translocation were proposed to result from the fusion of broken chromosome ends mediated by DNA repair enzymes (9). It is important to note that c-myc has directly recombined with a germ line $S\gamma_{2a}$ region in MPC-11 without the apparent involvement of either S_μ or S_α sequences. Gerondakis et al., have also shown that either germ line or rearranged S regions represent acceptable myc targets (9). These observations would imply that c-myc does not initially translocate to the S_μ region

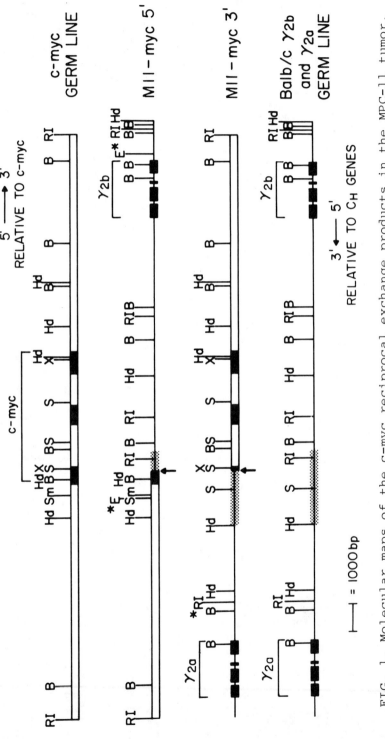

FIG. 1. Molecular maps of the c-myc reciprocal exchange products in the MPC-11 tumor. Restriction sites: RI, EcoRI; B, BamHI; Hd, HindIII; S, Sst I; X, Xho I; Sma I; E, EcoRI*. C γ2a switch region is denoted by a stippled box.

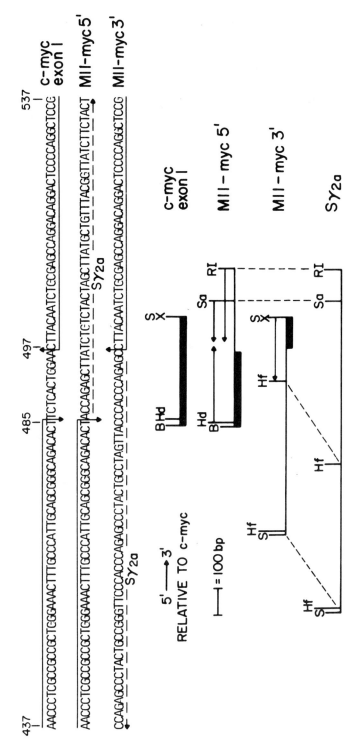

FIG. 2. Nucleotide sequences and restriction maps at the breakpoint of the myc trans-location in the MPC-11 tumor. Nucleotide numbers correspond to those in Figure 6A. Restriction maps have been aligned to indicate loss of $S_{\gamma 2a}$ sequences in recombina-tion.

and subsequently switch downstream to 3' S regions.

We presume that c-myc activation in MPC-11 was selected for by breaking the 5' non-coding myc exon and thereby activating numerous cryptic intron promoters associated with the first c-myc intron 18,19,29). No known transcriptional enhancer elements reside in this region of the C_H locus. In any event the level of myc transcripts in MPC-11 is 10-20x higher than in normal spleen cells (18,29).

A comparison of the myc sequences in the vicinity of seven translocation sites within the c-myc gene are presented in Figure 3. Three of these breakpoints reside in the first exon and four in the first myc intron and they collectively span ~1 Kb of the myc locus. The myc associated translocation is not mediated by homologous recombination (4,6,9,11,29). Even though nucleotide sequences commonly found in S region repeats (GAGCT, GGGGT and YAGGTTG and their analogues; 17,23) are not prevalent in the myc locus (4,8,9,29), some myc breakpoints reside near an S region like sequence (8,9). It is not unreasonable to propose the involvement to C_H switch recombination enzymes in this phenomenon since the precise molecular details for C_H gene switching remain speculative (17). Other structural parameters shared by c-myc and S regions may contribute to the molecular requirements of this reciprocal exchange. As shown in Figure 3, short inverted repeats (4-7 bp in length) are consistantly found 2-35 bp apart, 5' and 3' of each myc breakpoint. These inverted repeats are not conserved between independent breakpoints. In addition, the frequency of short palindromic sequences within the c-myc recombination region is consistant with its high G + C content (60-70%). Interestingly, S region sequences consist of large numbers of tandemly repeated AGCT palindromes. If a higher order secondary structure somehow facilitates c-myc translocation, S region sequences may provide numerous site specific targets for this phenomenon. Normal C_H switch recombinations appear to be more efficient or favoured over 12;15 translocations since myc-S fusions are not present in normal B cells (2,5,11). This could in part be reconciled by the poor S region homology of the c-myc locus. We conclude that c-myc translocations are highly selected for in B cell neoplasia and c-myc-S region fusions probably represent the preferred pathway for c-myc activation in PC tumors. Molecular studies of PCs with either 6;15 variant translocations (24,25) or chromosome 15 band deletions (34) should help to assess the importance of S region like sequences for these myc associated translocations.

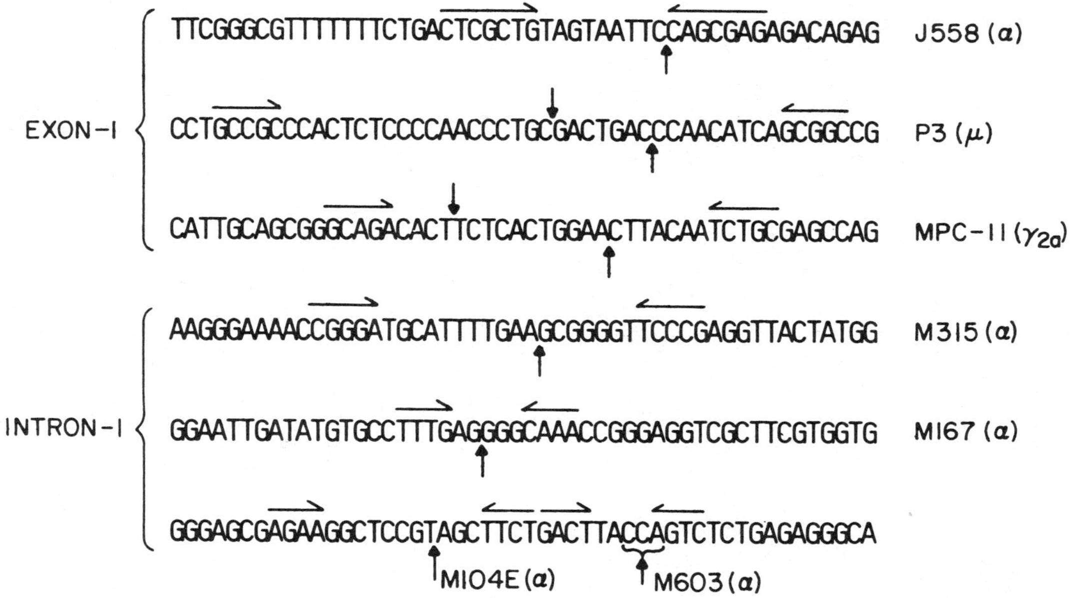

TTCGGGCGTTTTTTCTGACTCGCTGTAGTAATTCCAGGAGAGACAGAG   J558 (α)

CCTGCCGCCCACTCTCCCCAACCCTGCGACTGACCCAACATCAGCGCGCCG   P3 (μ)

CATTGCAGCGGCGGCAGACACTTCTCACTGGAACTTACAATCTGCGAGCCAG   MPC-11 (γ$_{2α}$)

AAGGGAAAACCGGGATGCATTTTGAAGCGGGGTTCCCGAGGTTACTATGG   M315 (α)

GGAATTGATATGTGCCTTTGAGGGGCAAACCGGGAGGTCGCTTCGTGGTG   M167 (α)

GGGAGCGAGAAGGCTCCGTAGCTTCTGACTTACCAGTCTCTGAGAGGGCA   M104E (α)   M603 (α)

EXON-I

INTRON-I

FIG. 3. Comparisons of nucleotide sequences in the vicinity of seven myc recombination sites. Horizontal arrows indicate the location of short inverted repeats. Vertical arrows above and below the sequences indicate 5' and 3' reciprocal breakpoints respectively. C-myc switch region targets are indicated beside each plasmacytoma. J558(16,20), MPC-11(21), P3(17,18,22), MOPC 603 and 167(7), MOPC 104E and 315 (M. Cole, personal communication.

THE TRANSLOCATED C-MYC ALLELE IS INAPPROPRIATELY EXPRESSED IN MOST PCs

C-myc gene breakage results in the expression of elevated levels of truncated myc transcripts which initiate from cryptic promoters within the first c-myc intron (1,18,29). A tabulated summary of Northern blot hybridizations performed with a variety of PC RNA samples and probes of different portions of intron 1 is presented in Figure 4. All 2.0 Kb truncated myc RNAs hybridized to the 3' end of intron 1 (SX-3 probe). Several PC RNAs also displayed hybridization of a 2.0 Kb RNA species to more 5' portions of the first intron (Sl0-20 and BHS-10 probes in Figure 4). We have previously shown that some promoter sites reside within ∼300 bp 5' of exon 2 (29). Transcripts initiated from sites further 5' in intron 1 are spliced to exon 2 sequences (Fahrlander, Yang and Marcu, in preparation). These results collectively suggest that multiple promoters reside in distinct regions of intron 1. Figure 5 shows the results of Northern blots performed with poly(A)$^+$ nuclear RNAs from several PCs. PC 10916 contains no detectable myc rearrangement and possesses a myc RNA processing pattern consistant for a gene with three exons. The size of the initial transcription unit of the unrearranged c-myc gene in PC 10916 is ∼4.85 Kb. The two myc introns are spliced out of the 4.85 Kb transcription unit in a 5'- >3' direction. However, the pattern of myc nuclear RNAs from PCs with rearranged myc genes is considerably more complex. Different PCs appear to possess distinctive myc RNA processing patterns. For instance, PCs 8701 and 8982 contain activated promoters at the 5' end of intron 1 while PCs 3386 and 6684 do not (see BHS 10 blot in Figure 4). These results may either be a consequence of the target site for the myc translocation or the breakpoint within the c-myc gene. In addition, a c-myc exon 1 probe fails to significantly hybridize to the nuclear RNAs of the myc rearrangement positive PCs (see Figure 5). This is additional compelling evidence for the notion that the normal myc allele is transcriptionally silent in most PCs (1,4,29). We conclude that the breakage of the c-myc locus results in the activation of multiple cryptic promoters within intron 1 which contribute to an elevated level of inappropriately expressed myc transcripts in these cells.

TRUNCATED C-MYC TRANSCRIPTS CAN INITIATE FROM MULTIPLE SITES IN C-MYC INTRON 1

PLASMACYTOMAS	CYTO MYC RNA	PROBES: EXON 1 BX-9	INTRON 1 S_{10}-20	INTRON 1 BHS10	INTRON 1 P16	INTRON 1 SX-3	EXON 2 P28
PC 3741	2.4kb	+	-	-	-	-	+
PC 10916	2.4kb	+	-	-	-	-	+
J558	2.0kb	-	-	-	-	+	+
MPC-11	2.0kb	-	-	-	-	+	+
PC 3386	2.0kb	-	-	-	-	+	+
PC8701	2.0kb	-	+	-	-	+	+
PC8982	2.0kb	-	-	-	-	+	+
PC6684	2.0kb	-	+	-	-	+	+
PC6308	2.0kb	-	ND	ND	ND	+	+
PC7210	2.0kb	-	ND	-	-	+	+
PC2960	2.0kb	-	ND	-	-	+	+

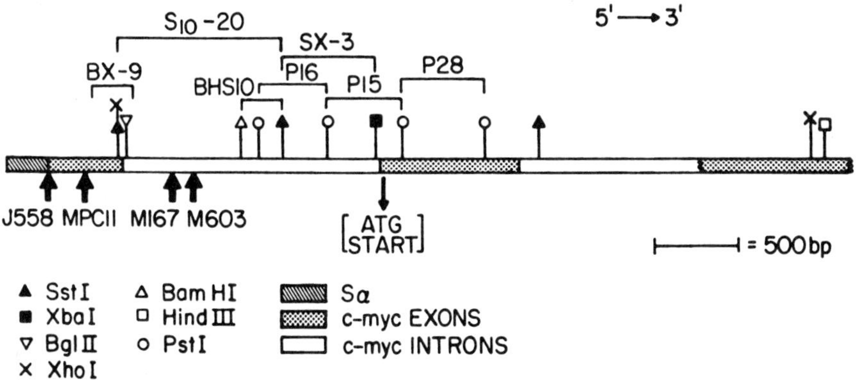

FIG. 4. Analysis of Northern blots performed with PC poly $(A)^+$ cytoplasmic RNAs and single stranded DNA probes derived from the c-myc locus.

C-MYC EXPRESSION IN TRANSLOCATION POSITIVE PC TUMORS WITH INTACT MYC GENES

The nucleotide sequence of the first exon of the

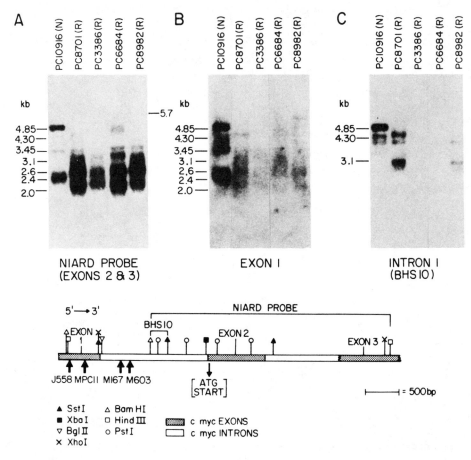

FIG. 5. Northern blots of poly(A)$^+$ nuclear RNAs of five NZB plasmacytomas hybridized to c-myc specific probes. The identical filter was stripped (by treatment with 95°C H₂O) and rehybridized in the following sequence: exons 2 & 3, exon 1 and finally BHS-10. The weak bands in the lanes of myc rearrangement positive PCs, which were probed with exon 1, represent residual signals from the previous blotting experiment (i.e., exons 2 & 3).

c-myc locus, which is lost upon gene breakage is presented in Figure 6. This is an atypically large noncoding sequence of 569 bp with translation termination

codons in all three reading frames and no methionine
initiator codon (4,29,30). Surprisingly, two functional
promoter sites with TATA box motifs reside 155 bp apart
at the 5' end of this large non-coding exon (13,30,35).
The loss of portions or all of this 5' exon upon myc
breakage and its high degree of conservation between
mice and humans (3,4,19,33) implies an important regulatory role in c-myc expression.

We have employed quantitative S_1 nuclease mapping to
measure the relative expression of the two normal myc
promoters in this remaining class of murine plasmacytoid
tumors which possess intact myc genes. Twenty PC tumors
with either 12;15 or 6:15 translocations or other chromosome 15 associated abnormalities were analyzed in this
survey. Figure 7 displays a representative S_1 mapping
experiment of the 5'P_1 and 3'P_2 myc promoters for several of these tumors. A summary of the P_1/P_2 ratios in
the steady state myc RNAs of a variety of tumors and
cell lines is presented in Table 1. The level of myc
RNAs in B lymphoid neoplasias appear to be comparable
and are generally independent of the myc associated
translocation. Furthermore, only 1 in 20 PC tumors
shows any evidence of mutational events within exon 1
(see TEPC 1165 in Table I). This latter result would
imply that qualitative alterations in the c-myc locus
which are analogous to those detected by S_1 mapping of
myc RNAs in human Burkitt lymphomas (27,32) are not
generally observed in the c-myc gene of the translocation positive, murine PC tumors. In agreement with
these findings, we have recently compared the nucleotide sequence of a PC rearranged myc gene to a normal
c-myc cDNA clone derived from BALB/c spleen and found
only a single substitution in the 5' non-coding exon
(Stanton et al., submitted for publication). Mutational
events in the PC c-myc genes do not significantly contribute to myc activation and are therefore not preferentially selected. The absence of such extensive
modifications in the PC myc genes could imply that this
translocation occurs later in B cell development than
the analogous chromosome abnormality in human Burkitt
lymphomas.

Some translocations in PC tumors alter the relative
utilization of the P_1 and P_2 promoters. All five PCs
which contain chromosome breakpoints within 2 Kb 5' of
c-myc possess atypical P_1/P_2 ratios in favour of P_1.
In addition P_2 to P_1 shifts are observed in 4 PCs without a detectable myc rearrangement. Promoter shifts are
also observed in 2 out of 3 translocation negative PCs

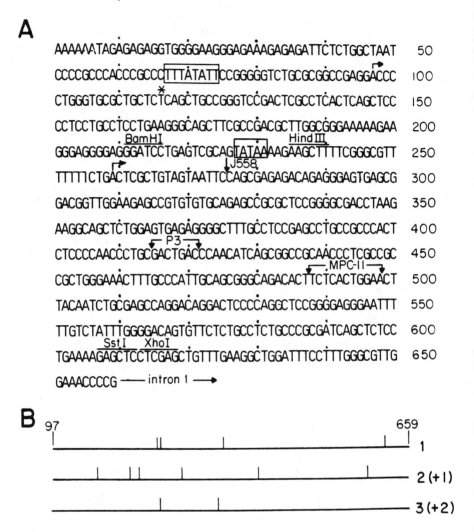

FIG. 6. (A) Nucleotide sequence of c-myc exon 1 and 5'
flanking region. Transcription initiation sites are indicated by horizontal arrows and promoter elements are
boxed. Recombination sites in several PCs are indicated
by vertical arrows. An asterisk indicates the 5' end of
a normal c-myc cDNA clone. (B) Translation termination
codons in each of three reading frames of exon 1 are
indicated by vertical lines.

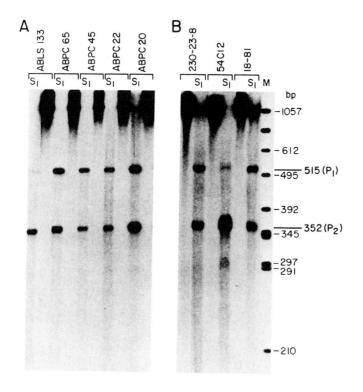

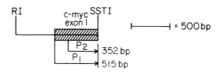

FIG. 7. Relative expression of two normal myc promoters (P1 and P2) in lymphoid tumors and transformed cell lines. Total cytoplasmic and poly(A)+ RNAs were hybridized to a uniformly labeled, single stranded DNA probe encompassing c-myc 5' flanking and exon 1 sequences, exhaustively digested with S nuclease and then analyzed on a 7M urea polyacrulamide gel (25; Yang, J.Q. et al., manuscript in preparation.

TABLE 1. Relative activity of two c-myc promoters in murine lymphoid tumors

		Rearranged c-myc gene[a]	P1/P2[b]
	BALB/c spleen	−	0.43
	BALB/c thymus	−	0.432
	ABPC 47	−	0.42
	ABPC 52	−	0.49
	ABPC 89	−	0.39
	ABPC 60	−	0.85
	ABPC 65		0.54
rcpt (12;15)	ABPC 33	+ (5'c-myc)[f]	1.71
	TEPC 1194	+ (5'c-myc)[f]	1.79
	TEPC 1165	+ (5'c-myc)[f]	2.62[c]
	TEPC 1033	+ (5'c-myc)[f]	1.49
	ABPC 4	−	0.48
	ABPC 20	−	0.38
	ABPC 22	−	0.71
rcpt (6;15)	ABPC 103	−	0.18
	ABPC 105	−	0.50
	ABPC 17	+ (5'c-myc)[f]	2.23
	CBPC 112	−	1.05
del 15	ABPC 45	+ (5'c-myc)[f]	0.75
	ABPC 26	−	0.42
	PC 3741[d]	−	1.07
	PC 7183[d]	−	0.44
Lymphosar-comas	ABLS 133	−	0.09
	ABLS 5	−	0.45
B lymphoma	WEHI 231	−	0.11
Pre B lymphomas	18-81	−	0.35
	230-23-8	−	0.32
	54C12[e]	(25-30 c-myc genes)[e]	0.02[e]

Text for Table 1

(a) Determined by Eco RI digestion: (−) indicates no rearrangement within ~9 Kb 5' of c-myc.

(b) Ratios of densitometric tracings of autoradio-grams of 515 and 352 bp S_1 nuclease protected fragments corresponding to transcripts initiating from promoters 1 and 2 (P_1 & P_2). S_1 probes were uniformly labeled. Corrections have been made due to the larger size of P_1 protected bands.

(c) The sizes of the S_1 nuclease protected fragments were 467 and 331 bp.

(d) NZB plasmacytomas of unknown karyotype.

(e) 54Cl2 is an Abelson murine leukemia virus trans-formed BALB/c fibroblast cell line with an amplified myc locus. Relative level of P_1 + P_2 in 54Cl2 is 4-fold higher than observed in 18-81 or 230-23-8.

(f) Site of DNA rearrangements are within ~2 Kb 5' of c-myc exon 1.

---

which possess a chromosome 15 band deletion (34). How-ever, 10 other translocation positive PCs display P_1/P_2 raties which are comparable to normal cells and other B lymphoid neoplasias (see Table 1). We conclude that a nearby translocation alters c-myc expression by either removing 5' c-myc regulatory sequences or by providing the equivalent of a transcriptional enhancer element which somehow overrides the normal control of c-myc ex-pression. A shift in promoter ratios could conceivably contribute to myc activation in several ways: 1) in-appropriate constitutive expression due to alterations in gene regulation; 2) alterations in RNA structure which could effect steady state myc RNA levels or RNA splicing; and 3) alterations in myc polypeptide struc-ture possibly caused by novel RNA splices resulting from a shift in promoter usage.

ACKNOWLEDGEMENTS

This work was supported by NIH grants GM-26939 and AI-00416 and ACS grants NP-405, RD-178 and MV-167 awar-ded to KBM. KBM is a Research Career Development Awardee of the National Institutes of Health. PDF is a post-doctoral fellow of the American Cancer Society. We gratefully acknowledge the assistance of Ms. Mary Vogelle and Ms. Mary Anne Huntington for their assis-tance in the preparation of this manuscript.

REFERENCES

1. Adams, J., Gerondakis, S., Webb, E., Corcoran, L.M. and Cory, S. (1983): Proc. Natl. Acad. Sci. USA 80:1982-1986
2. Adams, J.M., Gerondakis, S., Webb, E., Mitchell, J., Bernard, O., and Cory S. (1982): Proc. Natl. Acad. Sci. USA 79:6966-6970

3. Battey, J., Moulding, C., Taub, R., Murphy, W., Stewart, T., Potter, H., Lenoir, G., and Leder, P. (1983): Cell 34:787-799
4. Bernard, O., Cory, S., Gerondakis, S., Webb, E., Adams, J.M. (1983): EMBO J 2:2375-2383
5. Calame, K., Kim, S., Lalley, P., Hill, R., Davis, M., and Hood, L. (1982): Proc. Natl. Acad. Sci. USA 79:6994-6998
6. Cory, S., Gerondakis, S., and Adam, J.M. (1983): EMBO J 2:697-703
7. Crews, S., Barth, R., Hood, L., Prehn, J., and Calame, K. (1982): Science 218:1319-1321
8. Dunnick, W., Shell, B.E., and Dery, C. (1983): Proc. Natl. Acad. Sci. USA 80:7269-7273
9. Gerondakis, S., Cory, S., and Adams, J.M. (1984): Cell 36:973-982
10. Harris, L.J., D'Eustachio, P., Ruddle, F.H., and Marcu, K.B. (1982): Proc. Natl. Acad. Sci. USA 79:6622-6626
11. Harris, L.J., Lang, R.B., and Marcu, K.B. (1982): Proc. Natl. Acad. Sci. USA 79:4175-4179
12. Harris, L.J., Remmers, E.F., Brodeur, P., Riblet, R., D'Eustachio, P., and Marcu, K.B. (1983): Nucl. Acids Res. 11:8303-8315
13. Kelly, K., Cochran, B.H., Stiles, C.D., and Leder, P. (1983): Cell 35:603-610
14. Kirsch, I.R., Ravetch, J.V., Kwan, S.P., Max, E.E., Ney, R.L., and Leder, P. (1981): Nature (London) 293:585-587
15. Klein, G. (1983): Cell 32:311-315
16. Lang, R.B., Stanton, L.W., and Marcu, K.B. (1982): Nucl. Acids Res. 10:611-630
17. Marcu, K.B., Lang, R.B., Stanton, L.W., and Harris, L.J. (1982): Nature (London) 299:87-89
18. Marcu, K.B., Harris, L.J., Stanton, L.W., Erikson, J., Watt, R., and Croce, C.M. (1983): Proc. Natl. Acad. Sci. USA 80:519-523
19. Marcu, K.B., Stanton, L.W., Harris, L.J., Watt, R., Yang, J.Q., Eckhardt, L.A., Birshtein, B., Remmers, E.F., Greenberg, R., and Fahrlander, P. (1984): In: Genetic Engineering, edited by J.K. Setlow and A. Hollaender, Vol. VI. Plenum Press, New York (in press)
20. Mushinski, J.F. (1983): In: Mechanism of B cell neoplasia, pp. 368-371, Editores Roche, Basel
21. Mushinski, J.F., Bauer, S.R., Potter, M., and Reddy, E.P. (1983): Proc. Natl. Acad. Sci. USA 80:1073-1077
22. Neuberger, M.S., and Calabi, F. (1983): Nature 305:240-243

23. Nikaido, T., Nakai, S., and Honjo, T. (1981): Nature (London) 292:845-848
24. Ohno, S., Babonits, M., Weiner, F., Spira, J., Klein, G., and Potter, M. (1979): Cell 18:1001-1007
25. Ohno, S., Migita, S., Weiner, F., Babonits, M., Klein, G., Mushinski, J.F., and Potter, M. (1984): J. Exp. Med. (in press)
26. Perry, R.P. (1983): Cell 33:647-649
27. Rabbitts, T.H., Hamlyn, P.H., and Baer, R. (1983): Nature (London) 306:760-765
28. Shen-Ong, G.L.C., Keath, E., Picolli, S.P., and Cole, M.D. (1982): Cell 31:443-452
29. Stanton, L.W., Watt, R., and Marcu, K.B. (1983): Nature 303:401-406
30. Stanton, L.W., Yang, J.Q., Eckhardt, L.A., Harris, L.J., Birshtein, B.K., and Marcu, K.B. (1984): Proc. Natl. Acad. Sci. USA 81:829-835
31. Taub, R., Kirsch, I., Morton, C., Lenoir, G., Swan, D., Tronick, S., Aaronson, S., and Leder, P. (1982): Proc. Natl. Acad. Sci. USA 79:7837-7841
32. Taub, R., Moulding, C., Battey, J., Murphy, W., Vasicek, T., Lenoir, G.M., and Leder, P. (1984): Cell 36:339-348
33. Watt, R., Nishikura, K., Sorrentino, J., ar-Rushdi, A., Croce, C., and Rovera, G. (1983): Nature (London) 303:725-728
34. Weiner, F., Ohno, S., Babonits, M., Sumegi, J., Wirschubsky, Z., Klein, G., Mushincki, J.F., and Potter, M. (1984): Proc. Natl. Acad. Sci. USA 81:1159-1163
35. Yang, J.Q., Mushinski, J.F., Stanton, L.W., Fahrlander, P.D., Tesser, P.C., and Marcu, K.B. (1984): In: Current Topics in Microbiology and Immunology, edited by M. Potter, F. Melchers, and M. Weigert. Springer Verlag, New York (in press).

Molecular Biology of Tumor Cells, edited by
B. Wahren et al. Raven Press, New York © 1985.

Disrupted Expression of the c-myc Oncogene in Burkitt's Lymphoma

*T. H. Rabbitts, *·†R. Baer, *A. Forster, and ‡P. H. Rabbitts

*MRC Laboratory of Molecular Biology, Cambridge CB2 2QH, United Kingdom; ‡Ludwig
Institute for Cancer Research, MRC Centre, Cambridge CB2 2QH, United Kingdom;
†Present address: Memorial Sloan Kettering Cancer Center, New York, New York 10021*

The human Burkitt's lymphoma (BL) is a tumour of B-cells characterized by the presence of specific chromo-some translocations always involving the long arm (q) of chromosome 8 at band position 8q24. It has recently been shown that the proto-oncogene c-myc (so-called be-cause of its homology to the avian myelocytomatosis viral transforming gene v-myc) is present at this posi-tion (7,11,16) and that activation of the c-myc onco-genic potential results from the chromosomal transloca-tion. The most predominant type of translocation in BL is the t8/14 which involves 14q32 at which is located the immunoglobulin heavy (H) chain locus. In this type of translocation the c-myc gene is included in the seg-ment of chromosome 8 which joins with the abnormal chromosome 14q+ (6,8) and results from a chromosomal breakage to the 5' side of the c-myc gene since the resulting 14q+ chromosome contains the c-myc and usually immunoglobulin heavy chain constant (C) region genes in opposite transcriptional orientations. The situation in the variant BL translocations /t2/8 which involves chromosome 2p and the kappa (k) light (L) chain locus or t8/22 which involves chromosome 22q and the lambda (λ) L chain locus7 is quite different since these do not involve any movement of c-myc from chromo-some 8 thereby demonstrating that the chromosomal break-point is on the 3' side of c-myc in these cases (5,6, 10).

The c-myc gene has three exons of which only the se-cond two encode for protein (3,9,18). In many cases of BL, there is no gross damage to this gene as a result

29

of translocation and, as discussed above, a remarkable
variability in the precise breakpoint with respect to
the c-myc gene exists. Any mechanism devised to account
for the activation of the c-myc gene must explain this
imprecise chromosomal disruption. In this paper we discuss some findings on the translocated c-myc gene in
BL and possible explanations for the activation of this
gene.

TRANSLOCATION POSITIONS IN VARIOUS BL CELL LINES

We have studied the positional effect of translocation in five different BL cell lines viz. Daudi (t8/14)
JI and LY91 (t2/8) LY67 and MAKU (t8/22). None of these
cell lines has an altered restriction site within the
proximity of the translocated c-myc gene (Figure 1).
When an exon 2 probe was used in Southern filter hybridisation experiments we could not detect any rearrangement of the c-myc gene either with EcoRl or
BamHI digested DNA (unpublished data). Furthermore,
flanking probes of the c-myc gene, as shown in Figure
1, also failed to detect rearrangement at the 5' end
of Daudi c-myc gene (t8/14) or the 3' of the c-myc gene
of JI, LY91, MAKU and LY67 (t2/8 or 8/22). This places
the chromosomal breakpoint at least 12 kb upstream of
c-myc in Daudi and at least 14 kb downstream of this
gene in the other cell lines. These rather large dis-
tances are not so frequently encountered in the analogous mouse myeloma translocations where a high proportion of breakpoints occur between exons 1 and 2 of
the c-myc gene (1,4,14,15).

A different cell line called Raji (t8/14) has been
studied and we have shown it to contain a translocated
c-myc gene associated with the $C_{\gamma 1}$ gene in chromosome
14 (9). This is unusual among BL translocated genes
which generally involve the $C\mu$ gene. However, as the
structure of the translocated gene shows (Figure 2),
the breakpoint of the translocation involves, not a
gene-line switch (S) sequence of γ_1 but an amalgamated
sequence consisting of $S\gamma_1$ and $S\mu$ with the break occurring in $S\mu$. This $S\mu/S\gamma$ feature is a characteristic of
an event which results from V_H segments switches from
$C\mu$ to $C\gamma$ in the class switch and its presence shows
that the c-myc gene did not directly join to an unrearranged $C\gamma_1$ gene in this cell.

The structures of the translocated c-myc gene in
Raji revealed several interesting features. The translocation point occurs about 2.5 kb upstream of the c-
myc gene and does not in itself interfere with the dual
promote (P1 and P2) system which we observed to be uti-
lized in BL cells (9). For example, BL cells CA46 and

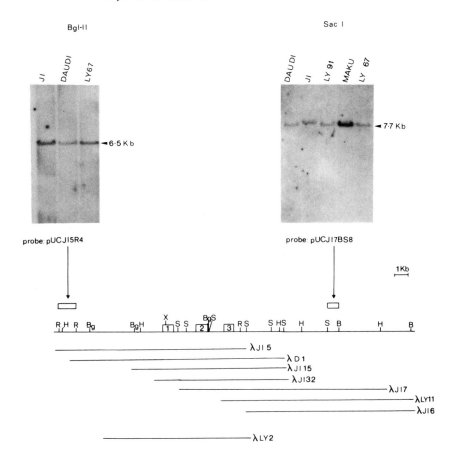

FIG. 1. Southern filter hybridisation of BL
DNA using c-myc gene flanking probes. A partial restriction map of the c-myc gene (derived from the overlapping clones shown below) is shown together with the location of
the flanking region probes used for the filter hybridisations. R = EcoRl; H = HindIII;
Bg = BglII; X = XhoI; S = SacI.

JD38 utilize the promoters Pl and P2 to about equal a-
mounts compared to the non-BL cell line HT29 which predominantly used P2 (9) whilst we also noted that Raji
c-myc mRNA comes predominantly from Pl. Severe sequence
alterations also exist in the transcribed region of the
Raji translocated c-myc gene (13) and one of them is a
deletion which removes the RNA splicing site at the 3'
end of exon 1 (which itself contains deletions). This
site is apparently replaced by a new site which for-
tuitously occurs in an almost analogous position resulting from the deletion. Since exon 1 is non-coding,
the occurrence of deletions has of course no effect on
protein reaching frames. The coding sequence of c-myc

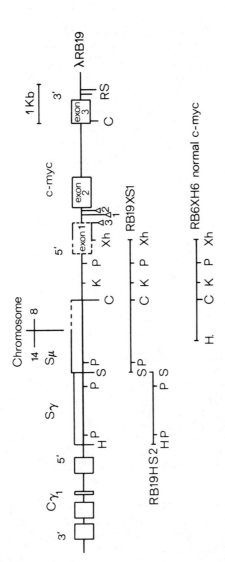

FIG. 2. Restriction map of the translocated c-myc gene from Raji (t8/14). The triangles indicated by 1, 2 and 3 are deletions within the intron between exons 1 and 2. H = HindIII; P = PstI; S = SacI; C = ClaI; K = KpnI; Xh = XhoI; R = EcoRI.

was, however, found to contain many nucleotide changes (25 in total, all in exon 2) which would generate 16 amino acid substitutions in the translocated c-myc gene product. There were no base substitutions at all in the third exon.

SEQUENCE CHANGES IN BL TRANSLOCATED C-MYC GENES

The critical observation that the normal c-myc allele is transcriptionally silent in cells containing translocated alleles (2,12) allows an indirect way of identifying translocated c-myc genes in cells where Southern blotting fails to show evidence of c-myc gene rearrangement. Our procedure was, therefore, based on cDNA cloning from BL mRNA which, in view of the above, will derive from the translocated allele. If such c-myc cDNA clones were to contain base substitutions, these would serve as markers for genomic clones derived from the relevant cell DNA. The results of an experiment like this are shown in Figure 3. An oligonucleotide primer was used to make cDNA which, when converted to double strands, was cloned into M13 phage. Direct sequencing of six clones isolated using LY67 mRNA showed them all to contain a T residue substitution altering codon 62 from ser→pro. An LY67 genomic clone was thus identified which contained this substitution and therefore represents the translocated allele from this cell. The proline substitution was the only coding region alteration in this gene. However, restriction site differences in and around exon 1 indicated that sequence alterations had occurred in this area. Indeed the sequence of exon 1 revealed 9 substitutions. Further, a cDNA clone made from Daudi mRNA (t8/14) showed 7.3% base difference in exon 1 compared to normal sequences (excluding a 35-base duplication). The common feature between the 3 BL cell lines appears to be sequence alteration, not in coding, but in non-coding exons. A similar survey of 4 other BL cell lines revealed other examples (17). These results, together with the finding that the normal c-myc allele is shut off in cells with translocated genes, suggest a model of c-myc gene trnscription in which the gene product, either directly or indirectly, controls its own transcription and possibly the transcription of other genes. Furthermore, that the effect of translocation is to disrupt this normal control pathway rather than to cause major quantitation differences in mRNA or protein levels. If this hypothesis is correct, then mutations in the myc protein (such as those evident in the Raji cell) might affect transcription causing inactivation of the normal c-myc allele.

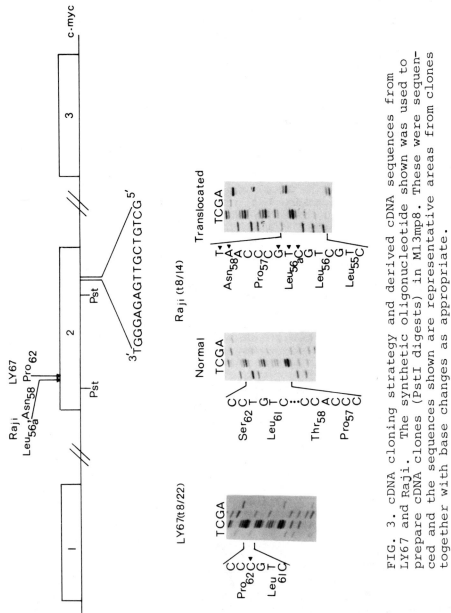

FIG. 3. cDNA cloning strategy and derived cDNA sequences from LY67 and Raji. The synthetic oligonucleotide shown was used to prepare cDNA clones (PstI digests) in M13mp8. These were sequenced and the sequences shown are representative areas from clones together with base changes as appropriate.

We have tested this in Raji cells using the cDNA cloning strategy shown in Figure 3. In this way we found two cDNA clones which represented transcription from both alleles, thereby demonstrating at least some activity from the normal allele. In order to quantitate the relative transcription levels we have used specific oligonucleotides in filter hybridisations of RNA from Raji and JI (t2/8) cells (Figure 4). Using a common 17-long oligonucleotide and a 17-long oligonucleotide specific for the translocated c-myc gene mRNA (Raji specific oligonucleotide) we were able to detect transcripts from both translocated and normal c-myc alleles in Raji cells. Furthermore, quantitation of the relative amounts of transcription in these cells show that about 35% of the c-myc mRNA is derived from the non-translocated c-myc gene. Therefore, it seems that in this cell line, unlike other BL cell lines, the normal c-myc gene is being transcribed at an appreciable level and that this transcription correlates with the presence of mutations in the protein product of the translocated c-myc allele.

CONCLUSION

The translocation of the c-myc gene in BL shows a remarkable variation in the breakpoint relative to this gene. Why does the gene always associate with the Ig locus to exert the detrimental effect on the gene? We have found no evidence for a quantitative change of c-myc transcriptional levels after translocation (9) nor do we find a quantitative alteration in protein levels when BL and EBV-transformed lymphoblastoid cell lines are compared (unpublished). Therefore, the oncogenic activation of the c-myc gene seems to be the result of changes in the mechanism by which the c-myc gene is normally controlled. The way in which translocation brings about this change is not yet established. It is apparently manifested by the alteration of the utilization of the P1/P2 promoters (9,17) and this may be mediated by loss of sequence recognition due to somatic mutation in the translocated c-myc gene. Such mutations do exist as shown above and the true significance can only be revealed by studies introducing the c-myc gene components into various host cell lines.

SUMMARY

Burkitt lymphoma cells show a marked variability of the chromosomal breakpoint with respect to the c-myc gene. Using an indirect procedure to identify the translocated c-myc gene we have found the occurrence of

A

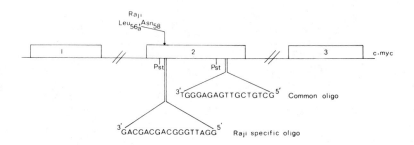

B.

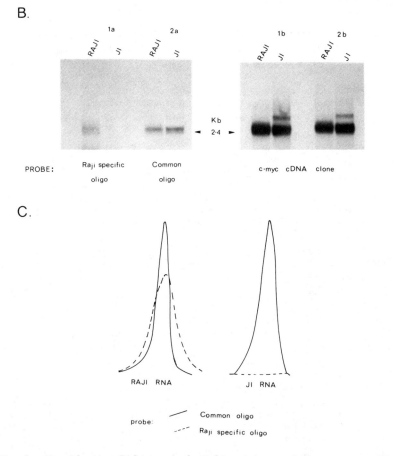

FIG. 4. Northern filter hybridisation with c-myc oligonucleotide probes. (A) Sequence and location of oligo-
nucleotides; (B) Autoradiographs of identical filters
containing Raji or JI RNA probed with either the common oligonucleotide or the Raji specific oligonucleotide and subsequently reprobed with a c-myc cDNA clone;
(C) Densitometer tracings from RNA lanes probed with
the c-myc oligonucleotides.

mutations in the first, non-coding exon from LY67 (t8/22) and Daudi (t2/8) as well as Raji (t8/14). Furthermore, Raji cells express c-myc mRNA from the untranslocated allele unlike other BL cells and this phenomenon correlates with alterations in the coding exons of the translocated allele. These results support the idea that the activation of the c-myc gene by translocation in BL results from changes in the control of this gene rather than quantitative alterations in mRNA or proteins.

ACKNOWLEDGEMENT

R. Baer is a recipient of a Lady Tata Memorial Research Fellowship.

REFERENCES

1. Adams, J.M., Gerondakis, S., Webb, E., Corcoran, L.M., and Cory, S. (1983): PNAS 80:1982-1986
2. Bernard, O., Cory, S., Gerondakis, S., Webb, E., and Adams, J.M. (1983): EMBO J 2:2375-2383
3. Colby, W.W., Chen, E.Y., Smith, D.H., and Levinson, A.D. (1983): Nature 301:722-725
4. Crews, S., Barth, R., Hood, L., Prehn, J., and Calame, K. (1982): Science 218:1319-1321
5. Croce, C.M., Thierfelder, W., Erikson, J., Nishikura, K., Finan, J., Lenoir, G.M., and Nowell, P.C. (1983): PNAS 80:6922-6926
6. Davis, M., Malcolm, S., and Rabbitts, T.H. (1984): Nature 308:286-288
7. Dalla-Favera, R., Bregni, M., Erikson, J., Patterson, D., Gallo, R.C., and Croce, C.M. (1982): PNAS 79:7824-7827
8. Erikson, J., Finan, J., Nowell, P.C., and Croce, C.M. (1982): PNAS 79:5611-5615
9. Hamlyn, P.H., and Rabbitts, T.H. (1983): Nature 304:135-139
10. Hollis, G.F., Mitchell, K.F., Battey, J., Potter, H., Taub, R., Lenoir, G.M., and Leder, P. (1984): Nature 307:752-755
11. Neel, B.G., Jhanwar, S.C., Chaganti, R.S.K., and Hayward, W.S. (1982): PNAS 79:7842-7846
12. Nishikura, K., AR-Rushdi, A., Erikson, J., Watt, R., Rovera, G., and Croce, C.M. (1983): PNAS 80:4822-4826
13. Rabbitts, T.H., Hamlyn, P.H., and Baer, R. (1983): Nature 306:760-765
14. Shen-Ong, G.L.C., Keath, E.J., Piccoli, S.P., and Cole, M.D. (1982): Cell 31:443-452

15. Stanton, L.W., Watt, R., and Marcu, K.B. (1983):
    Nature 303:401-406
16. Taub, R., Kirsch, I., Morton, C., Lenoir, G., Swan,
    D., Tronick, S., Aaronson, S., and Leder, P.
    (1982): PNAS 79:7837-7841
17. Taub, R., Moulding, C., Battey, J., Murphy, W.,
    Vasicek, T., Lenoir, G.M., and Leder, P. (1984):
    Cell 36:339-348
18. Watt, R., Stanton, L.W., Marcu, K.B., Gallo, R.C.,
    Croce, C.M., and Rovera, G. (1983): Nature 303:
    725-728.

Molecular Biology of Tumor Cells, edited by
B. Wahren et al. Raven Press, New York © 1985.

Interacting Oncogenes

Alan Schechter, David F. Stern, Lalitha Vaidyanathan,
Hartmut Land, Luis F. Parada, and Robert A. Weinberg

*Center for Cancer Research, Massachusetts Institute of Technology, and Whitehead Institute for
Biomedical Research, Cambridge, Massachusetts 02139*

Various experimental procedures have revealed a large group
of cellular oncogenes that appear to play important roles in
carcinogenesis. In all instances, these oncogenes have been
found to arise from normal cellular genes, termed proto-
oncogenes. The processes that cause the activation of these
proto-oncogenes appear to be, in all cases, somatic mutations
occurring in the target organs.

In our own laboratory, we have studied a series of
oncogenes of the ras gene family, which we detected by the
technique of gene transfer or "transfection." DNAs were
prepared from a series of tumor cell lines and shown to be able
to transform NIH3T3 cells when introduced into the latter by
transfection (1). Subsequent experiments in a number of
laboratories showed that these genes were, with rare exception,
members of the ras gene family (2, 3, 4). These genes had been
previously known from their association with the two rat
viruses, Harvey and Kirsten sarcoma virus (5). These viruses
have each acquired and activated a proto-oncogene from the rat
cellular genome. Each of these proto-oncogenes is homologous to
a sequence that can be activated in human cells during
spontaneous, nonviral carcinogenesis.

One area of our recent research concerned the effects of
these ras oncogenes on normal cells. Specifically, we were
interested in determining whether or not the ras gene could
fully transform normal cells to tumor cells. The normal cells
used in these experiments were rat embryo fibroblasts (REFs)
that had been explanted from embryos several days earlier. We
had isolated a ras oncogene (6) by molecular cloning and
attempted to introduce this into the REFs by transfection.

As we observed in our initial experiments, such an
introduced ras oncogene was not able to transform REFs.
Although these cells could exhibit anchorage independence and
an altered morphology, they showed limited ability to grow in
culture and were unable to form tumors in nude mice.
Consequently, we concluded that a ras oncogene, while perhaps
necessary for tumorigenesis, was hardly sufficient.

We reasoned that further changes in cellular phenotype were required in order to achieve the tumorigenic state. Such additional changes might well be supplied by other, cooperating oncogenes. As a consequence, we attempted to search for other oncogenes that might complement the activities of the ras oncogene.

One candidate for such a complementing oncogene was suggested by other work in which we had detected, by transfection, an N-ras oncogene in the human promyelocytic leukemia cell line HL-60. Others had found that these cells carry amplified copies of the cellular myc oncogene. This suggested a synergistic role between these two oncogenes (7, 8).

We constructed a series of myc oncogene clones and cotransfected each of these with the ras oncogene clone into REFs. We found that the resulting cells carrying two oncogenes were tumorigenic, while their singly transfected counterparts were not so. We concluded that each oncogene acts in a distinct fashion, and the two acting together are able to achieve tumorigenesis. This also suggested that the multiple steps which are known to be required for the conversion of normal cells into tumor cells may reflect the need for the sequential activation of a series of cellular proto-oncogenes (9).

This REF cotransfection test made it possible to address the functioning of a series of other oncogenes of cellular or viral origin. As we soon found out, the adenovirus Ela oncogene is able to replace myc in this cotransfection test. This is also true of the large T antigen of SV40 or polyoma. In contrast, the middle T oncogene of polyoma can work instead of ras in a cotransfection experiment.

Such results suggest the existence of at least two, distinctly acting groups of oncogenes. Of interest is the intracellular localization of their encoded proteins. Those of the ras group are cytoplasmic in their localization, while these of the myc group are to be found associated with the nuclear matrix. This may reflect the existence of two distinct targets within the cell, each of which must be acted upon, in order for full tumorigenicity to ensue.

****

The two classes of oncogenes of the ras and myc type may well reflect the existence of two distinct regulatory pathways that are responsible for controlling cellular proliferation. At the same time, a model involving two such pathways cannot explain the entirety of cellular growth control, as it ignores a vital element in growth regulation—the extracellular growth factors. Most cells would seem to require these factors in order to divide, and their interactions with the cell must trigger a series of cellular changes that ultimately affect the products encoded by the proto-oncogenes and oncogenes.

At the interface of the cell and the extracellular space lie receptors, whose function is to monitor the concentration of extracellular growth factors and to signal the cellular interior accordingly. A derangement of such receptors could in turn lead to deregulation of the cellular growth regulatory pathways. In fact, a recent report indicated that one cellular oncogene, the erbB, is an altered version of the cellular epidermal growth factor receptor (10). The suggested model is that such an altered receptor can stimulate cellular growth, even in the absence of its bound ligand.

Such findings rekindled interest in an oncogene and induced protein that we had studied in 1980 and 1981 (11, 12). This oncogene was detected upon transfection of DNA from a series of rat neuroblastomas. These neuroblastomas had been induced in rats by transplacental exposure to the carcinogen ethylnitrosourea (ENU). Such exposure, during the 15th day of gestation, creates tumors which appear 3-6 months postpartum.

These neuroblastoma oncogenes were found to be distinct from those of the ras group. Thus, Southern blotting analysis of the DNAs of transfected cells failed to reveal the presence of any novel, acquired ras sequences. While these neu oncogenes, as we called them, seemed not associated with the presence of a known oncogene, they affect the cell in one distinct and unique way, in that they induced synthesis of a novel antigen in transfected cells.

This antigen was detected by taking transfected cells and using them to seed tumors in young mice. Sera of the tumor-bearing mice were then used to immunoprecipitate the metabolically labeled lysates of transfected cells. All cells carrying a neu oncogene were found to express a protein of 185,000 daltons which could be precipitated by the anti-tumor serum. Sera of animals bearing other types of tumors, such as those induced by a ras oncogene, were unable to immunoprecipitate this antigen. Moreover, sera of the mice bearing the neu-induced tumor did not recognize specific determinants in the lysates of cells transformed by ras oncogenes.

All this indicated that the presence of the neu oncogene was tightly associated with the expression of a 185,000 dalton protein. Nevertheless, we had little direct proof that this protein was encoded by the oncogene, rather than simply being secondarily induced by the actions of the gene.

Characterization of the protein yielded several additional clues concerning its nature. The protein was a cell surface protein, in that mild trypsin treatment of intact cells destroyed the ability of the protein to be immunoprecipitated. This also suggested that its immunogenic domains were located in the extracellular portion of the protein. The protein was found to be phosphorylated. Moreover, synthesis in the presence of tunicamycin yielded a more rapidly migrating form (D.F. Stern, unpublished results). The latter result indicated that the protein was glycosylated and that the absence of carbohydrate groups did not impair its reactivity with antibody.

The protein induced by the neu oncogene bore many similarities with cell surface receptors. The aforementioned demonstration of homology of the EGFr gene and the <u>erbB</u> oncogene (10), caused us to renew our attempts at finding homology between the <u>neu</u> oncogene and the other known oncogenes. We did not need to survey a large array of oncogenes to detect homology. The <u>erbB</u> oncogene itself was found to be strongly homologous.

Thus, we must conclude that the <u>neu</u> oncogene is closely related to the gene encoding the EGFr. Moreover the protein present on the surface of <u>neu</u>-transfected cells must be related in some fashion to the EGFr. The p185 protein is thus, with high probability, encoded by the oncogene.

We have yet to undertake detailed structural analysis of the p185. But the implications of this homology are already apparent. A mutagen like ENU is able to alter a gene encoding a protein which behaves like a growth factor receptor. The resulting mutation appeared to yield an altered receptor protein, and this protein is able, in turn to act as a potent mediator of transformation. We hope over the next year to ascertain the nature of the protein and its activating lesion.

This finding of an apparently altered receptor protein compels us to attempt to relate its role and function to proteins known to be encoded by the other, similarly acting oncogenes. One way of conceptualizing these relationships stems from the previously mentioned importance of autonomy from growth factors.

This autonomy can be achieved in several ways that are suggested by the existing literature and the present results. A cancer cell may achieve autonomy from exogenous factors by manufacturing its own. The recently demonstrated homology between the <u>sis</u> oncogene and the cellular gene encoding PDGF (platelet-derived growth factor) is an example of this (14, 15). The implied "autocrine" mechanism allows the cell's growth to be stimulated by the very same growth factor that it has just secreted.

A second strategy for achieving autonomy may derive from alterations in the receptors that cells use to sense the presence of exogenous growth factors. Appropriate alterations of the receptors may cause them to emit growth regulatory signals constitutively, independent of ambient factor concentration. The erbB oncogene is one example of this (10). We propose that the presently described neu oncogene protein p185 represents yet another erbB encoded protein and is a drastically altered version of its normal cognate, the EGF receptor. We suspect, in contrast, that the neu-encoded protein is also structurally altered, but only minimally.

A third mechanism for achieving factor independence may arise from alterations in the intracellular signal pathway that is triggered by growth factor receptors. We suspect that oncogene proteins, like those specified by the ras genes, participate in the transduction of signals from cell surface receptors to critical intracellular targets. Use of biochemical and genetic tools should make it possible to demonstrate these interrelationships over the next several years.

Acknowledgement

The work described herein was supported by the American Business Cancer Foundation, by a grant from the Education Foundation of America, and by grants CA31649 and CA17537 from the U.S. National Cancer Institute. H.L. is a fellow of the Deutsche Forschungsgemeinschaft.

REFERENCES

1. Murray, M.J., Shilo, B.Z., Shih, C., and Weinberg, R.A. (1981): <u>Cell</u>, 25: 355.
2. Der, C.J. and Cooper, G.M. (1983): <u>Cell</u>, 32: 201.

3. Parada, L.F., Tabin, C.J., Shih, C., and Weinberg, R.A. (1983): <u>Nature</u>, 297: 474.

4. Shimizu, K. et al. (1983): <u>Proc. Natl. Acad. Sci. USA</u>, 80:383-387.

5. Ellis, R.W., Lowy, D.R., and Scolnick, E.M. (1982) In <u>Advanced Viral Oncology</u>, G. Klein (ed.), Raven Press, NY, pp. 107-126.

6. Shih, C. and Weinberg, R.A. (1982): <u>Cell</u> 29: 161.

7. Murray, M.J. et al. (1983): <u>Cell</u>, 33: 749-757.

8. Dalla Favera, R., Wong-Staal, F., and Gallo, R.C. (1982): <u>Nature</u>, 299: 61-63.

9. Land, H., Parada, L.F., and R.A. Weinberg (1983): <u>Nature</u>, 304: 596.

10. Downward, J. et al. (1984): <u>Nature</u>, 307: 521.

11. Shih, C., Padhy, L.C., Murray, M., and Weinberg, R.A. (1981): <u>Nature</u>, 290: 261.

12. Padhy, L.C., Shih, C., Cowing, D., Finkelstein, R., and Weinberg, R.A. (1982): <u>Cell</u>, 28:865.

13. Ullrich et al. (1984): <u>Nature</u>, 309: 418-430.

14. Doolittle, R.F. et al. (1983): <u>Science</u>, 221: 275-276.

15. Waterfield, M.D. et al. (1983): <u>Nature</u>, 304: 35-39.

Molecular Biology of Tumor Cells, edited by
B. Wahren et al. Raven Press, New York © 1985.

Pathogenetic and Clinical Significance of Chromosomal Aberrations in B-Cell Chronic Lymphocytic Leukemia

G. Gahrton, G. Juliusson, K.-H. Robèrt, *K. Friberg, and *L. Zech

*Division of Clinical Hematology and Oncology, Department of Medicine, Huddinge Hospital and Karolinska Institute, S-141 86 Huddinge, Sweden; *Institute of Medical Cell Genetics, Medical Nobel Institute, Karolinska Institute, S-104 01 Stockholm, Sweden*

ABSTRACT

Polyclonal B-cell mitogens such as Epstein-Barr virus (EBV), lipo-polysaccharide from E. coli (LPS) and 12-0-tetradecanylphorbol-13-acetate (TPA) stimulate B-cells in chronic lymphocytic leukemia to proliferation, which makes cytogenetic analysis of these cells possible. Of 55 patients studied by us, 43 yielded evaluable metaphases. 74% of these had clonal chromosomal aberrations and 53% of those with abnormal clones had an extra chromosome 12 either alone or together with other aberrations. A partial duplication (q13-q22) of chromosome 12 in one patient implicates a possible locus for the important genes on this segment. Structural aberrations were seen on chromosome 3,+del(3)(p13), in 2 patients with prolymphocytic leukemia; on chromosome 6 in 4 patients with different breakpoints in all; on chromosome 11 in 4 patients, 2 with deletion at q22; and on chromosome 12 in 3 patients. Oncogenes were assigned to all these involved chromosomes and breakpoints were in some of them close to the possible location of the oncogene. An extra chromosome 12 alone or together with other aberrations as well as the presence of several different aberrations were associated with aggressive disease.

INTRODUCTION

Chronic lymphocytic leukemia (CLL) is characterized by an increase in peripheral blood and bone marrow by monoclonal small lymphocytes with a low spontaneous mitotic index. In the great majority of cases, the lymphocytes are B-cells that carry monoclonal surface immunoglobulins (B-CLL). Only about 5% or less (5) of patients with CLL have monoclonal T-cell markers (T-CLL). In early studies only a small minority of patients with CLL were found to have chromosomal abnormalities with a random distribution among patients (28). Stimulation of the cells with commonly

45

used mitogens, such as phytohemagglutinin (PHA) generally resulted in the finding of a normal karyotype(20). In retrospect, this
was not amazing since the great majority of patients have B-CLL,
and the B-CLL leukemic cells cannot be stimulated to proliferate
with T-cell mitogens such as PHA.

In recent years a number of mitogens have been found to stimulate B-cells (21), and we could show that such B-cell activators
could stimulate the leukemic B-cells to proliferate in vitro (7,
25),which made cytogenetic typing of the B-cells possible (7). In
a series of studies we could then show that B-cell chronic lymphocytic leukemia is characterized by nonrandom chromosomal aberrations, the most common of which is an extra chromosome 12 (8,9,10,
11). Studies of this aberration as well as of other nonrandom
chromosomal abnormalities in B-CLL have contributed to the knowledge of pathogenetic mechanisms in this disease and to predic-
tion of outcome.

MITOGENIC STIMULATION OF B-CLL LYMPHOCYTES

A number of mitogens have been used for stimulation of the B-
cells in B-CLL (1,25,26). In our hands, the most successful stimulation for obtaining metaphases evaluable for chromosomal analysis have been Epstein-Barr virus (EBV) from the B95-8 cell line,
and lipopolysaccharide from E. coli (LPS). Lately we have also
used 12-0-tetradecanylphorbol-13-acetate TPA) with success. EBV
stimulation was performed by preincubating the cells with 1 ml of
the supernatant of the B95-8 cell line/10^7 cells for 1 h and
thereafter culture the cells for 4 days. LPS from E. coli was used
at a final concentration of 100 µg/ml and TPA was used to the
final concentration of 2×10^{-6}M. Both these mitogens were present
throughout the culture period for 4 days. Most other mitogens
that stimulate B-cells also have a considerable T-cell activating
capacity.

The Q-banding technique (6) was used by us for chromosome
identification.

CHROMOSOMAL ABNORMALITIES - TYPES AND FREQUENCY

We have now analysed 55 patients with B-CLL (previously reported
in 9 and 18). They were in different stages of the disease.
According to Rai (24), 10 patients were in stage 0, 20 in stage
I, 9 in stage II, 8 in stage III and 8 in stage IV. If classified
according to Binet (2), 27 patients were in stage A, 10 in stage
B and 18 in stage C. Cell-surface immunoglobulin phenotyping was
made in all cases. 7 were µκ, 22 µδκ, 6 γκ, 5 µλ, 12 µδλ, while 3
patients had too weak fluorescence to be properly typed. In 43 of
the 55 patients, a sufficient number of metaphases was found for
evaluation of chromosomal abnormalities. A clonal chromosomal
abnormality was defined according to the International System for
Human Cytogenetic Nomenclature (ISCN) (15), i.e.: (1) gain of a

specific chromosome in at least 2 cells; (2) loss of a specific chromosome in at least 3 cells; (3) identical structural aberration in at least 2 cells. If no clonal chromosomal aberrations were found in at least 12 evaluable metaphases, the karyotype was considered to be normal. As seen in Table 1, with this definition

TABLE 1. Chromosomal abnormalities in subgroups of B-CLL

Diagnoses	No. of patients		Clonal abnormalities	+12 or dup(12)
	Total patients	Total evaluable		
CLL-Kiel	22	17	12(71%)	6(35%)
Immunocytoma	29	22	16(73%)	10(45%)
Other	4	4	4(100%)	1(25%)
Total	55	43	32(74%)	17(40%)

74% of evaluable patients had clonal chromosomal abnormalities of which more than half were an extra chromosome 12. Of the 17 patients with an extra chromosome 12 (or in one patient part of chromosome 12, see below), 6 had this abnormality as the only aberration, while 11 had other abnormalities as well. One patient had a partial duplication of chromosome 12 (Fig. 1). Through

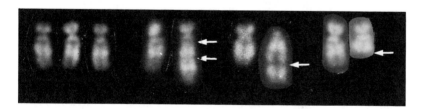

FIG. 1. Chromosomal abnormalities in chromosome 12 in B-CLL. +12, dup(12) (q13-q22), t(12;14)(q15;q22), +del(12)(q22).

a chromatid exchange the segment q13-q22 was duplicated on one chromosome 12, while the other was normal. One patient had +12 in two metaphases, but in three metaphases the extra chromosome 12 was deleted at 12q22. Fifteen patients had clonal chromosomal aberration (Fig. 2) that did not involve a duplication of chromo-

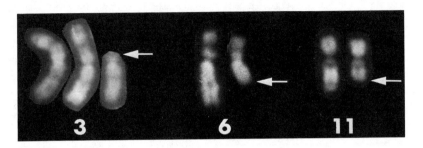

FIG. 2.   Chromosome abnormalities in B-CLL.+Del(3)(p13) in pro-lymphocytic leukemia (PLL), del(6)(q21) in CLL-Kiel, del(11)(q22) in immunocytoma (IC).

some 12. However, one of them had involvement of chromosome 12 in a translocation, t(12;14)(q15;q32) (Fig. 1). Thus, the breakpoint on 12 was close to the breakpoint found in the patient with the partial duplication. Six patients had a 14q+ marker chromosome, 4 patients had deletions of chromosome 6 with different break-points at p12, p21, q15, and q21. Four patients had deletions of chromosome 11, 2 of them with the same breakpoint at q22. The other two breakpoints were at q13 and q14. Two patients had a del(3) abnormality with the same breakpoint at p13. Seven pati-ents had a complex karyotype with 3 or more clonal aberrations, while 15 patients had only one single aberration. In 11 patients no apparent chromosomal aberration was found in at least 12 in-vestigated metaphases.

NORMAL AND ABNORMAL METAPHASES

In most patients with clonal chromosomal aberrations metaphases with abnormal and normal karyotypes coexisted. Only 4 patients had the same clonal chromosomal aberrations in all investigated metaphases (9-17 metaphases investigated), while in one patient only 5% of the metaphases had the clonal aberration. The median percentage of abnormal metaphases was 40%. This variation was found both in peripheral blood cells, bone marrow cells, lymph node cells, and spleen cells. In peripheral blood the frequency of abnormal metaphases was not directly correlated to the number of white blood cells (Table 2). Thus, patients with a high lymphocyte count could have a relatively low frequency of abnorm-al metaphases (patient 106) and those with a relatively low lymphocyte count could have a high frequency (patient 108). Thus, the nature of the normal metaphases is still unclear. They could

TABLE 2.   Frequency of abnormal metaphases   in two B-CLL patients
(see text)

Pat.	Lympho-cytes x10^9/l	E-RFC pos. cells x10^9/l (T-cells)	^{3}H-thymidine incorporation. Net count after mitogen stimulation		Abnormal meta-phases/ Total meta-phases	Karyotype
			EBV	LPS		
108	26.6	3.7	79.7	13.5	30/40 (75%)	46,XX/47,XX,del (14)(q24),+12
106	41.9	1.7	8.9	17.6	5/27 (19%)	46,XY/45(46),XY, del(11)(q22),+12, ±other markers

be normal T-cells, but this is less likely, since EBV and LPS are
known to be specific B-cell stimulators. They could be normal B-
cells. This would imply that normal B-cells are more easily
stimulated with the polyclonal B-cell stimulators. At present it
cannot be excluded that clonal chromosomal aberrations appear
during progression of the disease. Against this hypothesis speaks
our finding that two of the four patients with 100% abnormal
metaphases were only in stage I-II according to Rai, and A
according to Binet, while several patients with less than 30%
abnormal metaphases were in stage III and C, respectively. Thus,
the nature of the cells with normal metaphases in patients with
both normal and abnormal ones is still an open question.

RELATION TO ONCOGENES

Oncogenes have been mapped to all those chromosomes that are frequently involved in B-CLL (Fig. 3). Two oncogenes have been mapped to chromosome 12, the most frequently involved chromosome in
our study. KRAS 2 has been assigned to both the short arm at
p12.1 and the long arm, at q24.2 (16). Therefore, it is of particular interest that two of three breakpoints found on chromosome
12, i.e. in the patient with a partial duplication of the long
arm and in the patient with a deletion, were at 12q22. This is
close to one of the two possible locations of the KRAS 2. The
INT 1 oncogene has been assigned to the region 12pter-q14 (23),
thus including the second breakpoint at q13 in the patient with
the partial duplication of chromosome 12. In collaboration with
Dr. Roel Nusse (22), we investigated the possible expression of
the INT 1 gene, but none was found in patients with or without
the extra chromosome 12 or partially duplicated chromosome 12
abnormality. Chromosome 6 harbours 2 oncogenes, KRAS 1 at p23-q12
and MYB at q15-q24 (for review see 27). Thus, 2 of the breakpoints (q15 and q21) were found within the possible location of
KRAS 1. It is of interest that the aberration del(6)(q21) has in

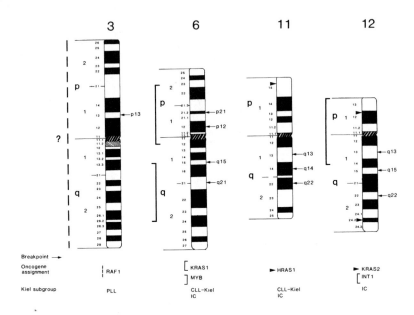

FIG. 3. Oncogene assignment and chromosomal breakpoints in leukemic cells in B-CLL. Chromosomes 3, 6, 11, and 12.

other studies been found in high frequency in large-cell lymphoma
(3). The HRAS 1 oncogene has been mapped to the short arm of
chromosome 11 (11p15.5-p15.1) (for review see 12). Although 4
patients were found with structural aberrations on 11, all the
breakpoints were on the long arm, 2 of them on q22. Chromosome
3 was found to be deleted at p13 in 2 of our patients. RAF 1 has
been mapped to this chromosome, but the exact location is not
known (4). Thus, although oncogenes are present on most chromosomes that are frequently engaged in CLL, the possible relationship between breakpoints in structural aberrations and the oncogene on the chromosome is unclear. However, the mere fact that
one, or in two cases, 2 oncogenes are present on those chromosomes which are most frequently involved in aberrations in B-CLL
may indicate an as yet unknown mechanism of importance for leukemogenesis. Our present aim is to investigate the expression of
the KRAS oncogenes and try to relate them to the specific abnormalities on the chromosomes involved.

RELATION TO SUBCLASS

Patients with CLL can be subclassified according to the Kiel
agreement (19). This classification is based on the cytological
and morphological picture and immunocytochemistry of specimens
from lymph nodes, spleen, bone marrow, and/or peripheral blood.
CLL in this setting (CLL-Kiel) is only a subgroup within the
low-grade malignant lymphocytic proliferative disorders with a
leukemic blood picture. Thus, according to this classification

(Table 1), our material contained 22 patients with CLL-Kiel, 29
with immunocytoma, 2 with prolymphocytic leukemia, one with
centrocytic lymphoma, while one patient could not be subclassified. The +12 abnormality as well as most other clonal chromosomal aberrations were seen within both main subgroups, CLL-Kiel
and immunocytoma, in about the same frequency. Although the
number of patients with other specific clonal aberrations was
small, no apparent difference in distribution of these aberrations between these two groups could be found. The +12 abnormality was also found in the patient with centrocytic lymphoma. The
only aberration that was more specifically assigned to one subtype was a+del(3)(p13) abnormality which was found in both patients with PLL. Thus, with the exception of this aberration,
chromosomal aberrations of specific type were not linked to any
of the B-CLL subgroups within the Kiel classification.

PROGNOSTIC IMPLICATION

Prognostic information was gained both by the type of chromosomal aberrations and from the number of different clonal aberrations in a single patient. Since the overall survival is long in
patients with B-CLL, the number of deaths in the material was
not large enough to make firm conclusions about differences in
survival. We have therefore chosen to investigate the time from
established disease to indication for treatment (therapy-free
survival). This time is an indication of the aggressiveness of
the disease since indications for treatment are fairly well established. In our hands(14), these indications are progressive disease with clear B-symtoms(fever above 38°, night sweats, or weight
loss >10% during 6 months), progressive disabling lymphadenopathy,
progressive anemia (hemoglobin level constantly >100 g/l) or
thrombocytopenia (platelet count decreasing below 100 x 10^9/1).
The +12 abnormality was associated with a significantly shorter
therapy-free survival than no abnormalities or other chromosomal
abnormalities or lack of evaluable metaphases (Fig. 4). Although

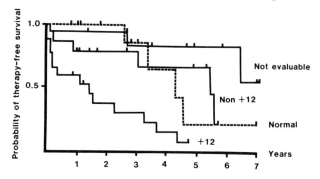

FIG. 4.   Therapy-free survival in patients with B-CLL. Not evaluated = patients with too few metaphases for evaluation (n=12);
normal = patients with a normal karyotype (n=11); non+12 = patients with other chromosomal abnormalities than +12 (n=15); +12 =
patients with +12 or dup(12) (n=17).

few patients could be compared, the +12 per se appeared to carry the same poor prognostic information as +12 together with other abnormalities. This finding has been challenged by others who found that the +12 per se did not hamper the survival more than if having a normal karyotype (13). Thus, this investigation indicated that it was the additional aberrations that were responsible for the poor prognosis in some patients with +12. However, in this study there were few patients and few deaths. Therefore, in our view it is too early to judge survival from this material. We found a significant difference in the therapy-free survival between patients with +12 as a single abnormality compared to patients with other single chromosomal abnormalities (17). The therapy-free survival of patients with such non+12 single abnormalities did not differ significantly from the therapy-free survival in patients with a normal karyotype.

The prognostic information of other types of chromosomal aberrations could not be clearly investigated in this study since each of them occur in too low frequency. However, if several different types of chromosomal aberrations appear in the same patient, this is a poor prognostic sign. In the present study, 3 or more clonal aberrations implies the most aggressive disease. Several of these patients have died and thus not only therapy-free survival but also survival was significantly shorter in this group than in patients who had none or only one single clonal aberration (18).

Thus, the conclusion is that an extra chromosome 12, alone or together with other chromosomal aberrations, is associated with a more aggressive disease. Also, several different clonal chromosomal aberrations in the same patient signifies a poor prognosis.

REFERENCES

1. Autio, K., Turunen, O., Pentillä, P., Erämaa, E., de la Chapelle, A., and Schröder, J. (1979); Cancer Genet. Cytogenet. 1:147-155.

2. Binet, J.L., Auquier, A., Dighiero, G., Chastang, C., Piquet, H., Goasguen, J., Vaugier, G., Potron, G., Colona, P., Oberling, F., Thomas, M., Tchernia, G., Jacquillat, C., Boivin, P., Lesty, C., Duault, M.T., Monconduit, M., Belabbes, S., and Gremy, F. (1981): Cancer 48:198-206.

3. Bloomfield, C.D. (1984): Second International Conference on Malignant Lymphoma, Lugano, Switzerland. June 13-16, 1984. Abstract No. 49, p. 43.

4. Bonner, T.I., Rapp, U.R., Nash, W.G., and O'Brien, S.J. (1984): Cytogenet. Cell Genet. 37:424.

5. Brouet,J.C., and Seligman, M. (1981): Pathology Research and Practice, 171:262-267.

6. Caspersson, T., Lomakka, G., and Zech, L. (1971): Hereditas 67:89-102.

7. Gahrton, G., Zech, L., Robèrt K.-H, and Bird, A.G, (1979): N. Engl. J. Med. 301:438-439.

8. Gahrton, G., Robèrt, K.-H., Friberg, K., Zech, L., and Bird. A.G. (1980): Lancet 1:146-147.
9. Gahrton, G., Robèrt. K.-H., Friberg, K., Zech, L., and Bird, A.G. (1980): Blood 56:640-647.
10. Gahrton, G., Robèrt, K.-H., and Zech, L. (1981): Blood 58: 859.
11. Gahrton, G., and Robèrt K.-H. (1982): Cancer Genet. Cytogenet. 6:171-181.
12. Gerald, P.S., and Grzeschik, K.H. (1984): Cytogenet. Cell. Genet. 37:103-126.
13. Han, T., Ozer, H., Sadamori, N., Emrich,L., Gomez, G.A., Henderson, E.S., Bloom, M.L., and Sandberg, A.A. (1984): N.Engl. J. Med. 310:288-292.
14. Ideström, K., Kimby, E., Björkholm, M., Mellstedt, H., Engstedt, L., Gahrton, G., Johansson, B., Killander, A., Robèrt, K.-H., Stalfelt, A.-M., Udén, A.-M., Wadman, B., and Wählby, S. (1982): Eur. J. Cancer Clin. Oncol. 18: 1117-1123.
15. ISCN (1978): Cytogenet. Cell Genet. 21:309-404.
16. Jhanwar, S.C., Neel, B.G., Hayward, W.S., and Chaganti, R.S.K. (1983): Proc. Natl. Acad. Sci. USA 80:4794-4797.
17. Juliusson, G., Robèrt, K-H., and Gahrton, G. (1984): N. Engl. J. Med., in press.
18. Juliusson, G., Robèrt, K.-H., Öst, Å., Friberg, K., Biberfeld, P., Nilsson, B., Zech, L., and Gahrton, G. (1984): Submitted for publication.
19. Lennert, K. (1978): Malignant lymphomas other than Hodgkin's disease. Handbuch der speziellen patologischen Anatomie und Histologie. 1. Band, Teil 3 B. Springer-Verlag, Berlin, Heidelberg, New York.
20. Mitelman, F., and Levan, G. (1977): Heredjtas 89:207-232.
21. Möller, G., editor (1975): Transplant Rev. 1-236.
22. Nusse, R.: Personal communication.
23. Nusse, R., v.´t Veer, L., Geurts van Kessel, A., van Agthoven, A., Bootsma, D., and Varmus, H. (1984): Cytogenet. Cell Genet. 37:556.
24. Rai, K.R., Sawitsky, A., Cronkite, E.P., Chanana, A.D., Levy, R.N., and Pasternack, B.S. (1975): Blood 46: 219-234.
25. Robèrt, K.-H., Möller, E., Gahrton, G., Eriksson. H., and Nilsson, B. (1978): Clin. exp. Immunol. 33:302-309.
26. Robèrt, K.-H. (1979): Immuol. Rev. 48:123-143.
27. Robson, E.B., and Lamm, L.U. (1984): Cytogenet. Cell. Genet. 37:47-70.
28. Sandberg, A.A. (1980): The chromosomes in human cancer and leukemia, pp. 349-353. Elsevier, New York.

Molecular Biology of Tumor Cells, edited by
B. Wahren et al. Raven Press, New York © 1985.

Molecular Mechanisms of Multistage Chemical Carcinogenesis

I. Bernard Weinstein, John Arcoleo, Michael Lambert,
Wendy Hsiao, Sebastiano Gattoni-Celli, Alan M. Jeffrey,
and Paul Kirschmeier

*Division of Environmental Sciences and Cancer Center/Institute of Cancer Research, Columbia
University, New York, New York 10032*

Recent studies demonstrating altered oncogenes in tumor
cells have raised new questions on the mechanism of action of
chemical carcinogens since these alterations can include not only
point mutations but also oncogene amplification, sequence
deletions and insertions, and chromosome translocations
(4,16,20,25,31,57,58,70). In addition, since many of these
changes were found in fully evolved malignant tumors it is not
yet clear at what stage in the multistage carcinogenic process
they occurred, and what role they play in the establishment
and/or maintenance of the tumor cell phenotype. In this paper we
will review recent findings on the mechanism of action of
chemical carcinogens and tumor promoters, emphasizing their
possible relevance to the activation of cellular oncogenes and to
altered states of gene transcription in tumor cells. We will
emphasize the concept that chemical and radiation carcinogenesis
involves changes in multiple cellular genes that evolve over a
prolonged period of time through a variety of molecular
mechanisms.

INITIATING CARCINOGENS, GENE AMPLIFICATION AND CHEMICAL-VIRAL SYNERGY

It is now well established that a variety of chemical
carcinogens act, at least in part, by yielding highly reactive
intermediates that bind covalently to cellular DNA (71). This,
and other findings, have led to the concept that they act by
producing mutations in somatic cells. We would caution, however,
that carcinogenesis probably involves much more complex changes
in DNA structure than simple point mutations at sites of
carcinogen-induced DNA damage. Supporting evidence includes:

the high apparent frequency of the initiation process, the long latent period in carcinogenesis, and the above mentioned evidence that cellular oncogenes in tumors can display various types of structural changes.

We have demonstrated that the carcinogen benzo(a)pyrene and its activated derivative benzo(a)pyrene 7,8 dihydrodiol 9,10-oxide (BPDE) induce a marked increase in the asynchronous replication of polyoma DNA in transformed rat cells containing integrated polyoma virus DNA (44,45). Furthermore, this effect does not require direct carcinogen damage to the polyoma DNA since we can induce viral DNA replication by fusing normal cells previously exposed to BPDE to the polyoma-transformed cells (44). In recent studies utilizing recombinant DNA constructs in which either the bacterial drug resistance gene gpt or the mammalian dihydrofolate reductase gene dhfr were linked to the polyoma DNA, we have found that when cells carrying these constructs were exposed to BPDE, then the latter genes also underwent asynchronous replication (45). These findings, and other evidence (44,45,47) suggest that carcinogen-induced damage to cellular DNA can induce the formation of a trans acting factor that can induce the asynchronous replication and amplification of specific genes. This phenomenon may be relevant to the finding of amplified oncogenes, amplified genes related to drug resistance, and other amplified DNA sequences in tumors.

We would also stress the fact that certain human tumors may result from synergistic interactions between DNA viruses and environmental chemicals (23,71,74). Possible examples include: an interaction between hepatitis B virus and aflatoxin in liver cancer causation, and papilloma virus and cigarette smoking in cervical cancer causation. Perhaps chemicals exert a synergistic effect by altering the replication and/or state of integration of viral DNAs. Certain tumor promoters can enhance the replication of EBV virus, and also enhance EBV-induced lymphocyte transformation. This, and other findings, have suggested a synergistic interaction between tumor promoters and EBV virus in the causation of nasopharyngeal cancer in Southern China (32,38). Other cases of chemical-viral synergy may play an important role in human cancer causation, acting either alone or in combination with direct effects of environmental chemicals on cellular genes (71,74).

TUMOR PROMOTERS

Inductive Effects and Activation of Protein Kinase C.
In contrast to initiating carcinogens and complete carcinogens, the potent tumor promoter 12-0-tetradecanoyl phorbol 13-acetate, and related compounds, do not produce direct damage to cellular DNA. There is now extensive evidence that their primary effects relate to changes in membrane structure and function (32,35,71) and that these effects may be mediated by the ability of these compounds to bind to and enhance the activity of the phospholipid dependent enzyme protein kinase C (PKC) (for review see 7,12,55,72).

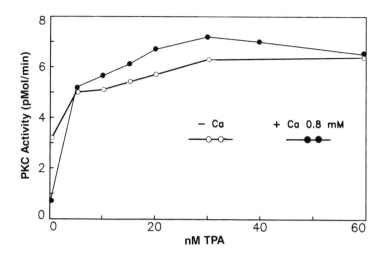

FIG. 1. Effect of TPA on PKC activity in the presence and
absence of Ca^{2+}. Assays were done with a partially purified
preparation of bovine brain PKC. The 0.2 ml assay system
contained: 2.5 nmoles ^{32}P-ATP (2x10^6 cpm), 24 μg PKC extract, 2.0
μg brain phosphatidylserine (Sigma), 40 μg histone (Sigma IIIS),
25mM PIPES buffer (pH 6.5), 10 mM MgCl$_2$, 200 μM EGTA, 200 μM
EDTA, 1mM 2-mercaptoethanol, and either 0 or 0.8mM CaCl$_2$. The
reaction was incubated at 30°C for 10 min., terminated by
spotting a 75 μl aliquot onto 6.25 cm^2 pieces of PC81 paper
(Whatman) and the papers were washed in 1 liter of water. The
radioactivity on the paper was counted in a scintillation counter
in 6 ml of Hydroflour (National Diagnostics). For additional
details see text and ref. 1.

We have recently studied the effects of various types of
tumor promoters on the activity of PKC *in vitro* (1). The enzyme
was partially purified from bovine brain and displayed a high
dependence on added phospholipid and Ca^{2+}. Other details of the
assay are described in *Figure 1*. A striking finding is that
maximum stimulation (>10 fold) of PKC activity by TPA occurs in
the presence of phospholipid, but in the absence of added Ca^{2+}
(Fig. 1). In effect, nM concentrations of TPA substitute for mM
concentrations of added Ca^{2+}, and the two agents are not
synergistic. Biologically active analogs of TPA such as phorbol
dibutyrate (PDBu), 12-0-hexadecanoyl-16-hydroxyphorbol-13-acetate
(HHPA) (38), and mezerein were also effective activators of PKC,
as were the chemically unrelated tumor promoters teleocidin and
aplysiatoxin (67), when tested at nM concentrations in the
absence of added Ca^{2+} (Table 1). On the other hand, the
biologically inactive compounds phorbol and 4α-phorbol-12, 13-
didecanoate (4αPDD) did not affect PKC activity in the absence of
Ca^{2+} (Table 1). These and additional results are consistent with
our previously proposed stereochemical model (see *Figure 2* and

Table 1

Effects of Various Tumor Promoters on PKC Activity
In the Absence and Presence of Added Ca^{2+}

	$-Ca^{2+}$	$+Ca^{2+}$
Experiment 1		
Control	0.65	3.60
TPA	4.29	3.60
Teleocidin	4.45	4.20
PDBu	2.49	3.55
Phorbol	0.83	3.25
4-α-PDD	0.68	3.75
Experiment 2		
Control	0.5	19.0
Aplysiatoxin	12.2	21.9
Debromoaplysiatoxin	14.4	22.2
Lyngbyatoxin A	12.0	20.9
Anhydrodebromoaplysiatoxin	2.1	20.5
Experiment 3		
Control	0.8	1.56
TPA	2.17	2.18
Mezerein	2.33	2.33
HHPA	2.19	2.11
HHPA 13,20-diacetate	0.72	1.63
HHPA 1,2-dihydro, 20-deoxy	0.63	1.29

Values are expressed as pMol/min of ^{32}P incorporated into histone. All compounds were tested at 100 nM in the absence and presence of added Ca^{2+} (0.8mM), but always in the presence of added phospholipid. For additional details see Figure 1 and ref. 1
PKC: protein kinase C
TPA: tetradecanoyl phorbol acetate
PDBu   phorbol dibutyrate
PPD: phorbol didecanoate
HHPA: hexadecanoyl-hydroxyphorbol acetate

ref. 36,73) in which the structurally similar hydrophilic domains of certain diterpenes, teleocidin and aplysiatoxin interact specifically with a protein receptor (in this case PKC apoenzyme), while their less specific hydrophobic domains interact with phospholipid, thus forming an enzymatically active ternary complex. In intact cells these tumor promoters might

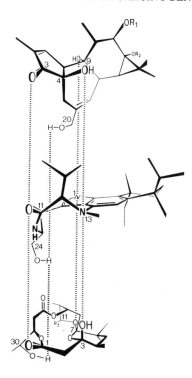

FIG. 2. Perspective drawings of TPA (top), dihydroteleocidin B (middle) and aplysiatoxin (bottom). The dotted lines connect heteroatoms whose spatial positions might correspond with one another, and represent residues that could interact with protein kinase C (PKC) apoenzyme. The hydrophobic R_1 residue on TPA (myristate), the hydrophobic ring system on the right side of dihydroteleocidin B and the phenolic side chain of aplysiatoxin might interact with the phospholipid cofactor for PKC. The stereochemistries of dihydroteleocidin B and aplysiatoxin were chosen arbitrarily to maximize their similarity to TPA. Further studies are required to establish their actual stereochemistries. For additional details see 73.

bind first to lipid domains in cell membranes thus inducing changes in lipid structure which enhance binding to and activation of PKC. This sequence could explain the finding that when intact cells are exposed to TPA there appears to be a migration of the cytosolic apoenzyme to the membrane fraction (42). The ability of tumor promoters to substitute for added Ca^{2+} in the activation of PKC may also be of significance in terms of their action in intact cells. There is previous evidence that TPA lowers the Ca^{2+} requirement for the growth of certain cell types in cell culture (71).

Several findings suggest that there may be heterogeneity (or subclasses) of receptors for phorbol esters and related tumor

promoters. Scatchard analyses of [^{3}H]-PDBu-receptor binding to
intact cells are consistent with at least two classes of binding
sites (35). Although the compound mezerein is quite potent with
respect to certain biologic effects including activation of PKC
(1), it competes less well than TPA in inhibiting [^{3}H]-PDBu-
receptor binding, and also is much weaker than TPA as a complete
tumor promoter on mouse skin (19,32). Therefore, some cell types
may have a subset of receptors that discriminate between TPA and
mezerein. Differential effects of aplysiatoxin and
debromoaplysiatoxin (36,67) are also consistent with receptor
heterogeneity. In a study with C3H 10T1/2 cells we found that
the dose response curves for TPA, PDBu and teleocidin inhibition
of the binding of [^{3}H]-PDBu to high affinity receptors were quite
different than those obtained when the same compounds were tested
for their ability to alter membrane lipid fluidity in the same
cells, as measured with fluorescence polarization probes (69).
Receptor heterogeneity could contribute to the tisssue
specificity and pleiotropic effects of these compounds. The
basis for this heterogeneity is not known but it could involve
the following mechanisms: 1) heterogeneity of PKCs; 2) variations
in lipid domains associated with PKC; and 3) interactions of
tumor promoters with other lipid-modulated enzymes, in addition
to protein kinase C.

Certain hormones and growth factors induce the turnover of
polyphosphatidyl inositol, which can generate transient increases
in diacylglycerol and inositol triphosphate (55). The former
compound could activate PKC and the latter could act as a second
messenger to cause the release of intracellular Ca^{2+} (11,55).
Thus, a number of factors, including alterations in dietary
lipids (71,74), might indirectly mimic the action of the phorbol
ester tumor promoters and thus play a role in multistage
carcinogenesis. Recent studies indicating that pp60^{sarc} (66) and
p68^{v-ros} (51) can phosphorylate phosphatidyl inositol, and other
lipids, suggest that these oncogene products could also produce
effects similar to those of the tumor promoters. Although the
idea that diacylglycerol is an endogenous analog of certain tumor
promoters is an attractive one, we should stress that TPA and
related compounds are about 10^4 times more potent than DAG in
activating PKC (12,55) and also in competing for high affinity
binding (7). Perhaps this is because diacylglycerol lacks the
hydrophilic residues so characteristic of the potent tumor
promoters (see Fig. 2). Furthermore, the chemical structures of
compounds, like mezerein, teleocidin and aplysiatoxin do not
display any resemblence to diacylglycerol, and yet these
compounds are potent activators of PKC (1). It would seem
worthwhile, therefore, to search for more complex amphiphilic
cellular lipids as possible endogenous analogs of these tumor
promoters.

A fundamental area for future research is the identification
of specific cellular proteins phosphorylated by PKC, particularly
those that are critical to the process of tumor promotion. A
related question is whether or not the multiple effects of tumor

promoters represent a simple linear cascade of events. The circuitry may be quite complex. For example tumor promoters induce phospholipid turnover (53) which may be associated with the release of diacylglycerol, itself an activator of PKC (55); and alterations in ion flux (i.e., Ca^{2+}) (71) could also further modulate protein kinase and phospholipic activities. Recent studies indicate that treatment of cells with TPA can alter the state of phosphorylation of epidermal growth factor (EGF) receptors (14,39) and also the receptors for insulin and somatomedin C (40). These effects are presumably mediated via activation of PKC and could explain the fact that TPA treatment leads to an indirect inhibition of EGF-receptor (48) and insulin-receptor binding (40). Other recently identified potential targets for phosphorylation by PKC, that may be relevant to tumor promotion, include the ribosomal S6 protein (49), the cytoskeletal protein vinculin (76) and a retinoid binding protein (17). Furthermore, even though PKC does not phosphorylate tyrosine residues, the exposure of cells to TPA can also enhance the phosphorylation of tyrosine residues on a 43K protein, the same protein which is a target for the action of pp60 sarc (5,27). It appears, therefore, that in addition to its effect on PKC TPA can enhance, either directly or indirectly, the activity of a cellular tyrosine-specific protein kinase.

<u>Irreversible Effects and Synergy with Oncogenes.</u>
Although our research group has stressed the membrane and cytoplasmic effects of tumor promoters, other investigators have provided evidence that the phorbol ester tumor promoters can also produce chromosomal aberrations and DNA damage, perhaps via activated forms of oxygen (for review see 21,32). These effects, however, are most prominent in inflammatory cells and may reflect the specialized responses (i.e., oxidative burst) of these cells to various activators. Furthermore, certain effects of TPA can be seen in the absence of detectable DNA damage (26). We would also stress that since the process of tumor promotion on mouse skin is often reversible (3), it seems unlikely that the early events during tumor promotion involve DNA damage and chromosomal aberrations. It is possible, of course, that with prolonged exposure to TPA chromosomal changes might occur and contribute to the process of tumor progression, particularly since chromosomal anomalies are more prominent during the late rather than the early stages of carcinogenesis.

A related question is whether tumor promoters act entirely via inductive or hormone-like effects, thus mediating clonal expansion of previously mutated cells, or whether they can themselves produce stable and heritable changes in cell phenotype. Although most of the pleiotropic effects produced by tumor promoters in cell culture are dependent upon the continuous presence of the promoter (71), there are a few examples in which the action of tumor promoters is associated with irreversible effects. These include: 1) the enhancement of cell transformation induced by certain oncogenic viruses, including adenovirus, Epstein-Barr virus, SV40 virus and polyoma virus (23,32); 2) the enhancement of anchorage independent growth of either adenovirus transformed rat fibroblasts (24) or of certain murine epidermal cell lines (15); and 3) enhancement of the outgrowth of cell variants displaying amplified genes for dihydrofolate reductase (2) or metallothionein (30). In addition, the papillomas and carcinomas induced by initiation and promotion on mouse skin can become autonomous with respect to the promoter (3).

We have carried out a series of experiments to see if tumor promoters might interact synergistically with oncogenes to enhance stable cell transformation (74 and Hsiao, W., Gattoni-Celli, S. and Weinstein, I.B., unpublished studies). We have found that when C3H 10T1/2 cells are transfected with the cloned human bladder cancer c-ras^H oncogene growth of the cells in the presence of TPA or teleocidin, but not phorbol, enhances the number of transformed foci obtained at least tenfold (Table 2). In addition, in the presence of the tumor promoter the foci appear earlier and they are larger. Parallel transfection studies with the drug resistance gene gpt indicate that TPA does not enhance, and even tends to inhibit, the number of gpt$^+$ colonies obtained (Table 2). Thus the enhancement of foci obtained with the transfected oncogene does not appear to be a generalized effect of tumor promoters on the transfection process per se. Time course studies with teleocidin support this conclusion. Thus, it is possible that tumor promoters can act synergistically with cellular oncogenes during multistage carcinogenesis. We presume that they do so by activating the expression of other cellular genes and are currently attempting to identify these genes.

Recent studies indicate that DNA damaging agents are more effective than tumor promoters in enhancing the progression of papillomas to carcinomas on mouse skin (33). This suggests that the evolution of a fully malignant tumor during multistage carcinogenesis may involve more than one cycle of damage to DNA, rather than a simple linear sequence of DNA damage induced by the initiator and subsequent non-genomic effects induced by the promoter. It also seems likely that tumor progression involves rather extensive genomic changes including gene amplification (58) and gross chromosomal abnormalities. This is, however, a highly speculative area since even less is known about the mechanism of tumor progression than about the earlier stages of initiation and promotion. In future studies it will be important to focus on this question because at a clinical level the major therapeutic challenges presented by tumors are related to invasion and metastasis, aspects of the tumor phenotype that probably result from the process of tumor progression.

CELLULAR GENES INVOLVED IN MULTISTAGE CARCINOGENESIS

The complexity of multistage carcinogenesis predicts that the evolution and maintenance of malignant cancer cells involves

Table 2

Transfection Frequencies Obtained with pT24 and psSV2-gpt

Plasmid DNAs in C3H 10T1/2 Cells in the Absence and

Presence of TPA

	gpt$^+$ colonies	T24 transformed foci
minus TPA	313	6
+100 ng/ml TPA	82	92

Cells transfected with pSV2-gpt DNA were scored for gpt$^+$
colonies as previously described (52); cells transfected
with the T24 plasmid containing the mutated human bladder
cancer c-ras^H oncogene (28), were scored for
morphologically transformed foci. Where indicated, TPA (100
ng/ml) was present throughout the transfection and
subsequent growth stages. Values represent colonies or
foci per plate. Similar results were obtained with
teleocidin but phorbol was inactive. The presence of
integrated human c-ras^H oncogene in the transformed cells
was confirmed by Southern blot analysis (Hsiao, W-L. W.,
Gattoni-Celli, S., and Weinstein, I.B., manuscript submitted
for publication).

changes in multiple types of cellular genes (71,73). Indeed, as
emphasized at the beginning of this paper there is accumulating
evidence that tumor cells display a wide variety of alterations
in the state of integration and/or expression of several cellular
oncogenes, as well as alterations in the expression of cellular
sequences analogous to the LTR sequences of retroviruses (41).
DNA transfection studies also indicate that the conversion of
normal cells to tumor cells requires the action of at least two
oncogenes (46,54,59). Furthermore, since only about 20% of human
tumors examined yield DNA which is active in the NIH 3T3
transformation assay (16,70) it is possible that in the majority
of human tumors the tumor phenotype is a complex function of
multigene interactions, both positive and negative (for
supporting evidence see 13,64,65).

We discovered that murine cells transformed by chemical
carcinogens or radiation express constitutively a series of poly
A$^+$ RNAs that contain murine leukemia virus LTR-like sequences
(41). Carcinogen-transformed murine cells also express RNAs
homologous to endogenous VL30 (34), and intracisternal (IAP) (43)
sequences, both of which are moderately repetitive retrovirus-
like sequences present in the mouse genome. These findings have
led us to suggest that carcinogenesis involves a disturbance in
mechanisms controlling the function of multiple classes of
cellular DNA enhancer sequences. Table 3 summarizes evidence

that tumor cells display rather widespread disturbances in the
control of gene expression and differentiation. In terms of
targets for the action of chemical carcinogenesis it is worth
noting that, although there are about 18 known cellular
oncogenes, the normal mouse genome contains over 1200 copies of
various types of LTR-sequences per haploid genome. The
structural resemblence of LTRs to known transposable elements
(6,63,68), their ability to enhance the transcription of a
variety of genes (6,68), and the phenomena of viral LTR-
promoter-insertion (31,56) and of insertion-mutation by
endogenous intracisternal A-particle sequences (25,43,57,62),
indicate the capacity of LTRs to act as mobile elements. Thus
these elements, and other transcriptional enhancer sequences yet
to be identified, constitute a major repertoire for potential
aberrations in the control of gene expression during the course
of chemical carcinogenesis. The switch on in transcription of
retrovirus-like sequences may, in part, be related to alterations
in the state of methylation of cytidine residues in DNA, which
are often associated with carcinogen action and tumor formation
(9,37,50,77). Furthermore, since endogenous retrovirus-like
sequences can also code for reverse transcriptase, once their
expression is switched on the RNA transcripts might undergo
reverse transcription and the resulting DNA copies might then be
reinserted into foreign sites in the genome, thus producing
insertion mutations and further abnormalities in gene expression.
There is evidence that analogous mechanisms might be involved in
gene transposition by the copia element of Drosophila (60,63).
Thus an epigenetic event (i.e. activation of transcription of
endogenous retrovirus-like elements) could lead to a stable
genetic event. We are currently examining whether this
postulated mechanism plays a role in tumor promotion or
progression.

Table 3

Types of Genes Expressed Aberrantly in Carcinogen and

Radiation Transformed Cells

1. MLV-like LTR sequences (41)
2. MLV ENV genes (8,22,41)
3. VL30 sequences (18)
4. A particle sequences (43)
5. Multigene "TS DNA" Family (29)
6. "Set 1" repetitive element, Qa/Tla MHC antigen (10)
7. Fetal genes and inappropriate differentiation genes
    (71)

MLV: mouse leukemia virus
LTR: long terminal repeat
ENV: envelope
MHC: major histocompatibility

Finally, we would stress that although we have speculated about several qualitatively different mechanisms to explain the actions of carcinogens and tumor promoters, these mechanisms need not be mutually exclusive because of the complexity of the process of multistage carcinogenesis and the pervasive phenomenon of tumor heterogeneity.

SUMMARY

The evolution of a fully malignant tumor is a multistep process resulting from the action of multiple factors, both environmental and endogenous, and involves alterations in the function of multiple cellular genes. Chemical carcinogens that initiate this process appear to do so by damaging cellular DNA. In addition to producing simple point mutations, this damage appears to induce the synthesis of a <u>trans</u> acting factor that can induce asynchronous DNA replication. This response may result in gene amplification and/or gene rearrangement. This phenomenon may also play a role in synergistic interactions between chemicals and viruses in the causation of certain cancers. The primary target of the tumor promoters 12-0-tetradecanoyl phorbol 13-acetate (TPA), teleocidin, and aplysiatoxin appears to be cell membranes. All three of these agents act, at last in part by, enhancing the activity of the phospholipid-dependent enzyme protein kinase C. We have proposed a stereochemical model to explain the interaction of these amphiphilic compounds with the PKC system. We have found that TPA and teleocidin markedly enhance the transformation of C3H 10T1/2 mouse fibroblasts when these cells are transfected with the cloned H-ras human bladder cancer oncogene. Thus tumor promoters can act synergistically with an activated oncogene to enhance cell transformation. Furthermore, carcinogen-transformed rodent cells display aberrations in the expression of various endogenous retrovirus-related sequences. Activation of some of these sequences may lead to insertion mutations and further aberrations in gene expression. These findings are discussed in terms of a multistep model that involves progessive changes in cellular oncogenes and aberrrations in the function of DNA transcription enhancer sequences.

Acknowledgement

This research was supported by DHS, NCI Grants CA 021111 and CA 26056, funding from the National Foundation for Cancer Research, and funds from the Dupont Company and the Alma Toorock Memorial for Cancer Research. We thank Dr. Y. Ito for providing the HHPA compounds, Dr. R. E. Moore for the aplysiatoxin and Dr. H. Fujiki for the teleocidin. We are grateful to G. Vande Woude for providing c-mos probes. We thank John Mack for the art work shown in Figure 2 and Evelyn Emeric for assistance in preparing this manuscript.

REFERENCES

1. Arcoleo, J. and Weinstein, I. B. (1984):
    Proc. Amer. Assoc. Cancer Res., 25:142 (Abstract).

2. Barsoum, J. and Varshavsky, A. (1983):
    Proc. Natl. Acad. Sci. USA, 80:5330-5334.

3. Berenblum, I. (1982): In: Cancer: A Comprehensive Treatise,
    Vol. 1 (2nd Edition), edited by F. F. Becker. Plenum
    Publishing Corp.

4. Bishop, J. M. (1983): Cell, 32:1018-1020.

5. Bishop, R., Martinez, R., Nakamura, K. D. and Weber, M. J.
    (1983): Biochem. Biophys. Res. Commun. 115:536-543.

6. Blair, D. G., Oskarsson, M., Wood, T. G., McClements, W. L.,
    Fischinger, P. J. and Vande Woude, G. F. (1981): Science,
    212:941-943.

7. Blumberg, P.M., Jaken, S., Konig, B., Sharkey, N. E., Leach,
    K. L., Jeng, A. Y. and Yeh, E. (1984): Biochem. Pharm.,
    33:933-940.

8. Boccara, M., Souyri, M., Magarian, C., Stavnezer, E. and
    Fleissner, E. (1983): J. of Virology, 48:102-109.

9. Boehm, T. L. J. and Drahovsky, D. (1983):
    J. Natl. Cancer Inst. 71: 429-434.

10. Brickell, M., Latchman, S., Murphy, W. and Rigby, W. J.
    (1983): Nature, 306:756-760.

11. Burgess, G. M., Godfrey, P.P., McKinney, J. S., Berridge, M.
    J., Irvine, R. F. and Putney, J.W. (1984): Nature, 309:63-
    66.

12. Castagna, M., Takai, U., Kaibuchi, K., Sano, K., Kikkawa, U.
    and Nishizuka, Y. (1982): J. Biol. Chem., 257:7847-7851.

13. Cavenee, W. K., Dryja, T. P., Phillips, R. A., Benedict, W.
    F., Bodbout, R., Gallie, B. L., Murphree, A. L., Strong, L.
    C. and White, R. L. (1983): Nature, 305:779-784.

14. Cochet, C., Gill, G. N., Meisenhelder, J., Cooper, J. A. and
    Hunter, T. (1984): J. Biol. Chem., 259:2553-2558.

15. Colburn, N. H., Former, B. F., Nelson, K. A. and Yuspa, S. H.
    (1979): Nature, 281:589-591.

16. Cooper, G. M. (1982): Science, 218:801-806.

17. Cope, F. O., Staller, J. M., Mahsem, R. A. and Boutwell, R. K. (1984): Biochem. Biophys. Res. Commun., 120:593-601.

18. Courtney, M. G., Schmidt, L. J. and Getz, M. J. (1982): Cancer Res., 42:569-576.

19. Delclos, K. B., Nagle, D. S. and Blumberg, P. M. (1980): Cell, 19:1025-1032.

20. Duesberg, P. H. (1983): Nature, 304:219-225.

21. Emerit, I., Levy, A. and Cerutti, P. (1983): Mutation Res., 110:327-335.

22. Fischinger, P. J., Thiel, H. J., Lieberman, M., Kaplan, H. S., Dunlop, N. M. and Robey, W. G. (1982): Cancer Res. 42:4650-4657.

23. Fisher, P. B. and Weinstein, I. B. (1980: In: Molecular and Cellular Aspects of Carcinogens Screening Tests, edited by R. Montesano, L. Bartsch, and L. Tomatis, pp. 113-131. IARC Scientific Publ., No. 27, Lyon France.

24. Fisher, P. B., Bozzone, J. H. and Weinstein, I. B. (1979): Cell, 18:695-705.

25. Gattoni-Celli, S., Hsiao, W-L, and Weinstein, I. B. (1983): Nature, 306:795.

26. Gensler, H. L. and Bowden, G. T. (1983): Carcinogenesis, 4:1507-1511.

27. Gilmore, T. and Martin, G. S. (1983): Nature, 306:487-490.

28. Goldfarb, M., Shimizu, K., Perucho, M. and Wigler, M. (1982): Nature, 296:404-409.

29. Hanania, N., Shaool, D., Harel, J., Wiels, J. and Trusz, T. (1983): EMBO J. 2:1621-1624.

30. Hayashi, K., Fujiki, H. and Sugimura, T. (1983): In: Cellular Interactions by Environmental Tumor Promoters, edited by H. Fujiki et al., Japan Sci. Soc. Press, Tokyo, in press.

31. Hayward, W. S., Neel, B. G. and Astrin, S. M. (1981): Nature 290:475-480.

32. Hecker, E., Fusenig, N. E., Kunz, W., Marks, F. and Thielmann, H. W. (Editors) (1982):

Carcinogenesis: A Comprehensive Survey, Vol. 7, Raven Press, NY.

33. Hennings, H., Shores, R., Wenk, M. L., Spangler, E. F., Tarone, R. and Yuspa, S. (1983): Nature 304:67-69.

34. Hodgson, C. P., Elder, P. K., Ono, T., Foster, D. N. and Gertz, M. J. (1983): Cellular Biology, 3:2221-2234.

35. Horowitz, A., Greenebaum, E. and Weinstein, I. B. (1981): Proc. Natl. Acad. Sci. USA 78:2315-2319.

36. Horowitz, A., Fujiki, H., Weinstein, I. B., Jeffrey, A., Okin, E., Moore, R. E. and Sugimura, T. (1983): Cancer Res. 43:1529-1535.

37. Hsiao, W., Gattoni-Celli, S., Kirschemeir, P. and Weinstein, I. B. (1984): Molecular and Cellular Biol., 4:634-641.

38. Ito, Y., Yanase, S., Tokuda, H., Kishishita, M., Ohigashi, H., Hirota, M. and Koshimizu, K. (1983): Cancer Letts., 18:87-95.

39. Iwashita, S. and Fox, C. F. (1984): Jl. Biol. Chem. 259:2559-2567.

40. Jacobs, S., Sayyoun, N. E., Saltiel, A. R. and Cuatracasas, P. (1983): Proc. Natl. Acad. Sci. USA, 80:6211-6213.

41. Kirschmeier, P., Gattoni-Celli, S., Dina, D. and Weinstein, I. B. (1982): Proc. Natl. Acad. Sci. USA, 79:273-277.

42. Kraft, A. A. and Anderson, W. B. (1983): Nature, 301:621-623.

43. Kuff, E. L., Feenstra, A., Lueders, K., Smith, L., Harvey, R., Hozumi, N. and Shulman, M. (1983): Proc. Natl. Acad. Sci. USA 80: 1992-1996.

44. Lambert, M. E., Gattoni-Celli, S., Kirschmeier, P and Weinstein, I. B. (1983): Carcinogenesis 4:587-594.

45. Lambert, M., Pelligrini, S., Gattoni-Celli, S. and Weinstein, I.B. (1984): "Cold Spring Harbor Meeting on DNA Tumor Viruses", Cold Spring Harbor, N.Y., in press (Abstract).

46. Land, H., Parada, L. F. and Weinberg, R. A. (1983): Nature, 304: 596-602.

47. Lavi, S. and Etkin, S. (1981): Carcinogenesis 2:417-423.

48. Lee, L. S. and Weinstein, I. B. (1980): Carcinogenesis, 1:669-679.

49. Le Peuch, C. J., Ballester, R., and Rosen, O. M. (1983): Proc. Natl. Acad. Sci. USA, 80:6858-6862.

50. Lu, L. J. W., Randerath, E. and Randerath, K. (1983): Cancer Letts., 19:231-239.

51. Macara, I. G., Marinetti, G. V. and Balduzzi, P. C. (1984): Proc. Natl. Acad. Sci. USA, in press.

52. Mulligan, R. C. and Berg, P. (1981): Proc. Natl. Acad. Sci. USA, 78:2072-2076.

53. Mufson, R. A., Okin, E. and Weinstein, I. B. (1981): Carcinogenesis 2:1095-1102.

54. Newbold, R. F. and Overell, R. W. (1983): Nature, 304:648-651.

55. Nishizuka, Y. (1984): Nature, 304:648-651.

56. Payne, G. S., Bishop, J. M. and Varmus, H. E. (1982): Nature, 295:209-214.

57. Rechavi, G., Givol, D., Canaani, E. (1982): Nature, 300:607-611.

58. Robertson, M. (1984): Nature, 300:149-152.

59. Ruley, H. E. (1983): Nature, 304:602-606.

60. Ryo, H., Shiba, T., Fukunaga, A., Kondo, S. and Gateff, E. (1984): Gann, 75:22-28.

61. Sharkey, N. A., Leah, K. L., and Blumberg, P. M. (1984): Proc. Natl. Acad. Sci. USA, 81:607-610.

62. Shen-ong, G. L. C. and Cole, M. D. (1984): J. of Virology, 49:171-177.

63. Shiba, T. and Saigo, K. (1983): Nature, 302:119-124.

64. Solomon, E. (1983): Nature, 309:111-112.

65. Stanbridge, E. J., Der, C. J., Doerson, C. J., Nishimi, Y., Peehl, D. M., Weissman, E. and Wilkinson, J. E. (1982): Science, 215:252-259.

66. Sugimoto, Y., Whitman, M., Cantley, I.C. and Erikson, R. I. (1984): Proc. Natl. Acad. Sci. USA, 81:2117-2121.

67. Sugimura, T. (1982): Gann, 73:499-507.

68. Temin, H. M. (1982): Cell, 28:3-5.

69. Tran, P. L., Castagna, M., Sala, M., Vassent, G., Horowitz, A. D., Schachter, D. and Weinstein, I. B. (1983): European J. of Biochem., 130:155-160.

70. Weinberg, R. A. (1983): Scientific American, 249:126-142.

71. Weinstein, I. B. (1981): J. of Supramol. Structure and Cellular Biochem., 17:99-120.

72. Weinstein, I. B. (1983): Nature, 302:750.

73. Weinstein, I. B., Gattoni-Celli, S., Kirschmeier, P., Hsiao, W., Horowitz, A. and Jeffrey, A. (1984): Federation Proc., 43:2287-2294.

74. Weinstein, I. B., Arcoleo, J., Backer, J., Jeffrey, A. M., Hsiao, W., Gattoni-Celli, S., and Kirschmeier, P. (1984): In: Cellular Interactions of Environmental Tumor Promoters, edited by H. Fujiki et al. Japan Sci. Soc. Press, Tokyo, in press.

75. Weiss, R., Teich, N., Varmus, H. and Coffin, J. (Editors) (1982): Molecular Biology of Tumor Viruses, Second Edition, RNA Tumor Viruses, Cold Spring Harbor Laboratory, Cold Spring Harbor, NY.

76. Werth, D. K. Niedel, J. E. and Pastan, I. (1983): J. Biol. Chem., 258:11423-11426.

77. Wilson, V. L. and Jones, P. A. (1983): Cell, 32:329-346.

Molecular Biology of Tumor Cells, edited by
B. Wahren et al. Raven Press, New York © 1985.

Subversion of Growth Factor Signal Transduction by Oncogenes

M.D. Waterfield

*Protein Chemistry Laboratory, Imperial Cancer Research Fund,
London WC2A 3PX, United Kingdom*

ABSTRACT

Growth factors interact with specific cell surface
receptors to induce a complex cascade of biochemical
events which can result in stimulation of DNA synthesis
and proliferation of target cells. Studies of the
structure and function of platelet derived growth factor (PDGF) and of the receptor for epidermal growth
factor (EGF) have revealed two different but related
mechanisms for subversion of the control of cell proliferation by oncogenes. The sis oncogene encodes a
growth factor related to PDGF and thus could stimulate
proliferation by an autocrine mechanism while the erb-B
oncogene encodes a defective EGF receptor which could
be delivering a continuous proliferation signal in
transformed cells. Other oncogenes may encode proteins
which interact at other steps in the growth factor induced mitogenic cascade.

INTRODUCTION

The control of cell proliferation involves a number
of interacting regulatory pathways inside the cell
which can be influenced by a variety of extracellular
signals through signal transduction at the cell surface
A productive approach to deciphering the regulation of
cell proliferation in normal and neoplastic cells has
been to identify extracellular signal molecules and to
study the process of signal transduction from the membrane into the cell. It has become clear that a struc-

turally diverse set of polypeptide growth factors are involved in extracellular signalling. Either alone or through synergistic interactions these factors can induce DNA synthesis and proliferation of certain target cells. In this review the factors which are involved in maturation and differentiation of immune effector functions will not be discussed. The search for the factors required by cells in culture, where serum is added to support proliferation, led to the discovery of certain growth factors (e.g. PDGF) while others were initially characterised using biological assays which employed whole animals (e.g. EGF) or various in vitro systems. Perhaps the best characterised growth factor is EGF which was originally detected in extracts of male mouse submaxillary gland during a search for nerve growth factor (for reviews see 9,10). PDGF was identified as the major mitogen in serum for connective tissue cells (see 12,13,50). A whole series of fundamental observations have been made with EGF and PDGF which have suggested general mechanisms for growth factor action.

EGF and other growth factors such as PDGF and Insulin like growth factor (IGF-I), interact with specific cell surface receptors present necessarily on the surface of target cells (for recent reviews see 23). An important concept which is stressed by Rozengurt (39) is that synergistic responses between growth factors are often observed and perhaps required to induce a response in particular target cells.

A number of events which occur rapidly after interaction of different growth factors with their specific receptors have been documented and these can be divided into 4 categories.

1. Rapid changes in ion fluxes that lead to an alkalinisation of intracellular pH through extrusion of H+ probably mediated by a Na+/H+ antiport system (28,32, 38). Changes in Ca^{2+} movements have also been observed which possibly result from mobilisation from internal compartments (27,28). Such changes in ion concentrations could have far reaching effects on several biochemical pathways (see below).

2. Changes in phosphorylation of the receptors themselves and of a variety of other proteins occur. In the case of EGF, PDGF, Insulin and IGF-I, autophosphorylation of tyrosine residues has been documented. As yet however the functional significance of this protein kinase activity is unclear. The most important part of this observation is perhaps to suggest a link between these receptors and the transforming proteins of the src family, many of which share an ability to phosphorylate tyrosine residues and a region of matching amino acid sequence (reviewed in 4). That a close rela-

tionship between these proteins exist has been further supported by observations on the structure of the EGF receptor which show that the oncogene erb-B encodes a truncated avian EGF receptor (see later). It is clerly possible that other members of the src family encode other membrane associated signal molecules.

3. <u>Membrane phospholipid breakdown</u>, which can result in the formation of prostaglandins that can produce a variety of diverse effects including increased cAMP levels (39) or the degradation of inositol lipids to form phosphoinositides and diacyl glycerol. It was originally suggested by Mitchell (31) that changes in calcium gating and inositol lipid breakdown accompany signal transduction associated with a variety of receptors and in an as yet unknown fashion growth factors may mediate some of their effects through these pathways. Diacylglycerol which together with phosphoserine and Ca^{2+} will activate protein kinase C - an enzyme which has well documented functions in the platelet, (reviewed by Nishizuka, 33), is known to be the receptor for phorbol esters (35) and may mediate various important phosphorylations relevant to signal transductions (e.g. receptor phosphorylation (11,22) or to metabolic regulation (S6 ribosomal protein phosphorylation). A further link which stresses the relevance of inositol lipids is provided by the observation that the oncogenes src and ros may encode proteins involved in inositol lipid metabolism (30,44).

4. <u>Changes in the aggregation state of receptors</u> which may be both the signal for internalisation and degradation of the receptor ligand complex (40) and part of the process of transduction of the mitogenic signal across the membrane. This process may be mimicked by some monoclonal antibodies (41) suggesting that inter receptor interactions are involved in signal transduction.

The diverse biochemical studies briefly outlined above gives some idea of the directions which are being explored in understanding the relationship between growth factor signal transduction and the control of proliferation. To elucidate how these events may be perturbed in transformed cells or in neoplasia a multi-faceted approach has been taken which has paid off in unexpected ways as is well illustrated by the structural studies of the growth factor PDGF and the receptor for EGF which I will review here. As a result of the interaction of the fields of study including virology, cell biology, biochemistry and computer studies we have been able to show how growth factor signal transduction may be subverted by two different retroviruses which have acquired cellular sequences which encode PDGF or a truncated EGF receptor.

AUTOCRINE GROWTH REGULATION INVOLVING PDGF

The concept that a target cell having receptors for a particular growth factor may respond to synthesis of that growth factor by the cell itself and thus overcome the need for an extracellular signal came from the studies of Temin and Todaro and their colleagues.

The suggestion that certain tumour derived cell lines and other transformed cells might produce growth factors similar to PDGF stems from two lines of investigation. It was shown that the major mitogen for cells of connective tissue origin was PDGF through fractionation studies of mitogens in serum, and since it had been known for some time that transformed cells needed less serum for optimum proliferation than normal cells, it was suggested that these cells may elaborate their own growth factors. In the case of cells of connective tissue origin the factor could be a PDGF like molecule (see reviews 13,50).

As part of a study to characterise the PDGF like factor produced by an SV40 transformed cell line (PDGF produced by SV40-BHK28 cells) (5,8,14,43) we set out, in collaboration with the laboratories of Deuel and of the Swedish group of Heldin, Wasteson and Westermark, to study the structure of human PDGF. As a result of this study (47) and through subsequent analysis of PDGF (24) we have established a partial amino acid sequence of 2 polypeptide chains purified from PDGF - a summary of the data is shown in Fig. 1. Through the use of protein and nucleic acid sequence data banks (15) and the National Biomedical Research Foundation, April, 1983) we were able to find that the sequence of PDGF closely matched that of the transforming protein of the simian sarcoma virus (SSV) putative transforming protein p28 sis whose amino acid sequence had previously been predicted from sequence analysis of the viral genome. A similar observation was reported almost simultaneously by Doolittle et al., (16) who analysed the structural data of Antoniades & Hunkapiller (1). Subsequently the partial nucleotide sequences of the human gene for PDGF has been reported by Josephs et al., (25) and Johansson et al., (24) confirming the data obtained by protein sequencing of PDGF. SSV transformed cells produce a mitogen functionally (13) and antigenically (37) related to PDGF. Particularly interesting was the observation that certain human tumour cell lines were expressing mRNA transcripts of the PDGF gene (18) which correlates with the observation that similar cell lines produce PDGF like mitogens (3,20,34,49).

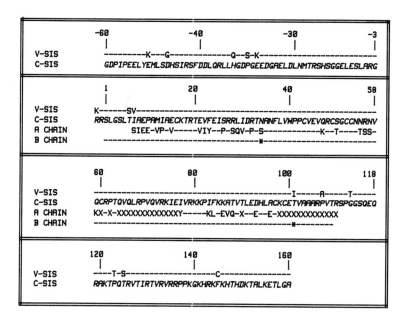

FIG. 1. The deduced sequences of the products of the c-sis v-sis genes are compared with the amino acid sequences of PDGF A and B chains.

These results suggested that expression of the PDGF gene in either SSV transformed cells or in various tumour cell lines could be important and that aberrant autocrine secretion of PDGF could influence the proliferation of target cells having receptors.

A number of important concepts came out of this work whose implications have yet to be fully evaluated. It has been shown that SSV transformed cells and certain tumour derived cells produce mitogens like PDGF but we do not know if they exert their effect only by signal transduction through the receptor, implying a need for secretion. What is clear, if external receptor interactions are needed, is that only a subset of cells with expressed receptors could respond to autocrine synthesis of PDGF. The preliminary survey of Eva et al., (18) suggests that the majority of human cell lines expressing mRNA transcripts of the c-sis gene are those that normally have receptors i.e., connective tissue and glial cell lines. However, as shown by Eva et al., (18) certain lymphocytes transformed by human tumour leukemia virus (HTLV), which are not usually considered to have PDGF receptors, do express c-sis transcripts. It remains to be seen what the role of PDGF in these cells is.

The normal function of PDGF is thought to be in tissue repair processes through action as a chemoattractant for cells and as a mitogen (see 6). It is conceptually interesting that PDGF is thought to be produced by the megakaryocyte - a cell which becomes multinucleate and disrupts to form platelets thus ensuring that the cell producing PDGF is destroyed. It is also perhaps relevant that PDGF is delivered to damage sites where it is released in blood clots by a non-viable subcellular vehicle - the platelet. This suggests a mechanism has been developed to ensure that PDGF is not produced at a wound site by a viable cell. It is perhaps important to ensure that such a potent mitogen is only made under very carefully controlled conditions. Perhaps synthesis at the wrong place and wrong time could have disastrous consequences such as neoplasia.

SUBVERSION OF GROWTH FACTOR RECEPTOR SIGNAL TRANSDUCTION

A key step in signal transduction by a growth factor is clearly its interaction with a specific cell surface receptor. To help unravel the nature of the transduction process we set up a program to determine the structure and function of the epidermal growth factor receptor. This receptor was studied because, due to the pioneering work of Cohen and his colleagues, it is the best characterised of any of the growth factor receptors. An additional reason for studying this receptor is that it is expressed at high levels on the placenta and on the A431 vulval carcinoma cell line. To carry out detailed studies of receptor biosynthesis, expression and purification, the monoclonal antibody Rl has been employed (46). This antibody was raised using A431 cells as an immunogen, and several lines of evidence suggest that Rl recognises an external conformation dependent polypeptide determinant on the receptor which is distinct from the EGF binding site (19,29,46). This monoclonal has been used to develop a radioimmunoassay which employs radioiodinated EGF and Staphylococcus aureus protein A to measure amounts of receptor after solubilization in neutral detergents (19).

Biosynthesis of the EGF receptor

The biosynthesis of the receptor was studied in A431 cells using radiolabelled precursors and metabolic inhibitors and with monoclonal antibody Rl to immunoprecipitate precursor polypeptides (22). At early labelling times two receptor related polypeptides were detected of apparent molecular weights (MWs) of 95.000 and 160.000. Pulse chase studies showed that the 95.000 MW polypeptide was almost certainly not a pre-

cursor of the 160.000 MW polypeptide which itself could
be chased into the mature receptor protein of MW
175.000. Using tunamycin and endoglycosidase it was
shown that the first detectable polypeptides which
lacked N-linked sugar side chains were of MWs 138.000
and 68.000 and, since preliminary evidence suggests
there are no o-linked oligosaccharides on the receptor,
we suggested that two receptor related polypeptides of
about 1250 and 650 amino acids (aa) are synthesised in
A431 cells. Evidence was obtained that the 650 aa polypeptide is glycosylated and secreted into the medium.
Subsequently we have been able to show that this polypeptide corresponds to the external domain of the receptor synthesised from an mRNA of 2.8 kb which is distinct to those of 6.8 and 10.5 kb which encode the intact receptor (45). This observation has been confirmed by other groups (26,48).

Purification of the EGF receptor

The receptor in A431 cells and placenta was solubi-
lised from total cell detergent lysates or from membrane preparations and purified by immunoaffinity (17),
lectin affinity or EGF affinity chromatography (7). The
RIA was used to monitor receptor degradation and recovery during purification. In the case of A431 cells the
recovery of receptor from membranes made by the method
of Thom et al., was very low, while for placenta a 50
fold purification and 30% yield was achieved using syn-
cytotrophoblastic vesicles prepared by the method of
Smith et al., (42). In both cases the receptor maintained its EGF stimulated protein kinase activity and
was not proteolytically degraded. To recover sufficient
quantities of receptor from A431 cells a total cell lysate solubilized in neutral detergent was used and the
RIA was employed again to monitor receptor yields and
overcome problems caused by proteolysis. It was found
that by working fast, using affinity resins in the
batch mode, including EDTA to remove Ca++ (thus inhibiting the calcium activated protease) and by maintaining
initial pHs at values of 8.5 the receptor could be recovered in sufficient amounts for structural analysis.
The need for alkaline pHs is presumed to be to inhibit
acid proteases released from lysozomal compartments
within the cell that are perhaps involved in normal degradation of internalised receptor. An outline of the
purification, including examples of SDS polyacrylamide
gel analysis of the receptor at different stages of purification is shown in Fig. 2.

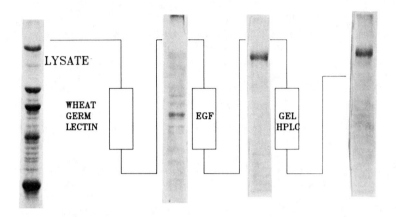

FIG. 2. Purification of the placental EGF receptor.

A431 and placental receptor are similar in structure

To show that receptor purified by immuno and ligand affinity chromatography from A431 and placental cells have similar structures we carried out high performance liquid chromatographic (HPLC) analysis of tryptic peptides using reverse phase columns. The majority of the peptides, from the different receptor preparations were indeed similar in their elution characteristics (see 17). Slight differences between peptide maps of A431 and placenta receptors may relate to A431 specific oligosaccharide determinants which are added to the receptor polypeptide (35). These results showed that monoclonal R1 and immobilised ligand purified very similar polypeptides.

Structural analysis of the EGF receptor

To determine the amino acid sequence of regions of the EGF receptor the affinity purified protein was fully reduced and alkylated, fractionated by gel permeation HPLC in 6 M guanidine solutions, cleaved into peptides with trypsin or cyanogen bromide and the mixtures of peptides fractionated by reverse phase HPLC. Twenty different peptides were purified and their partial or complete amino acid sequences determined (17,45). The amino acid sequence of one cyanogen bromide peptide was used to construct an oligonucleotide probe and to screen cDNA banks constructed from mRNA isolated from A431 cells (45).

The complete amino acid sequence of the EGF receptor and of the truncated external domain (MW 115.000, see above) was deduced from nucleotide sequence analysis of

```
EGF R   GTAGAALLAL LAALCPASRA LEEKKVCQGT SNKLTQLGTF EDHFLSLQRM FNNCEVVLGN LEITYVQRNY DLSFLKTIQE VAGYVLIALN TVERIPLENL
EGF R   QIIRGNMYYE NSYALAVLSN YDANKTGLKE LPMRNLQEIL HGAVRFSNNP ALCNVESIQW RDIVSSDFLS NMSMDFQNHL GSCQKCDPSC PNGSCWGAGE
EGF R   ENCQKLTKII CAQQCSGRCR GKSPSDCCHN QCAAGCTGPR ESDCLVCRKF RDEATCKDTC PPLMLYNPTT YQMDVNPEGK YSFGATCVKK CPRNYVVTDH
EGF R   GSCVRACGAD SYEMEEDGVR KCKKCEGPCR KVCNGIGIGE FKDSLSINAT NIKHFKNCTS ISGDLHILPV AFRGDSFTHT PPLAPQELDI LKTVKEITGF
EGF R   LLIQAWPENR TDLHAFENLE IIRGRTKQHG QFSLAVVSLN ITSLGLRSLK EISDGDVIIS GNKNLCYANT INWKKLFGTS GQKTKIISNR GENSCKATGQ
EGF R   VCHALCSPEG CWGPEPRDCV SCRNVSRGRE CVDKCNLLEG EPREFVENSE CIQCHPECLP QAMNITCTGR GPDNCIQCAH YIDGPHCVKT CPAGVMGENN
Erb-B                                                                                      MKCAH FIDGPHCVKA CPAGVLGEND

EGF R   TLVWKYADAG HVCHLCHPNC TYGCTGPGLE GCPTNGPKIP SIATGMVGAL LLLLVVALGI GLFMRRRHIV RKRTLRRLLQ ERELVEPLTP SGEAPNQALL
Erb-B   TLVRKYADAN AVCQLCHPNC TRGCKGPGLE GCP-NGSKTP SIAAGVVGGL LCLVVVGLGI GLYLRRRHIV RKRTLRRLLQ ERELVEPLTP SGEAPNQAHL

EGF R   RILKETEFKK IKVLGSGAFG TVYKGLWIPE GEKVKIPVAI KELREATSPK ANKEILDEAY VMASVDNPHV CRLLGICLTS TVQLITQLMP FGCLLDYVRE
Erb-B   RILKETEFKK VKVLGSGAFG TIYKGLWIPE GEKVKIPVAI KELREATSPK ANKEILDEAY VMASVDNPHV CRLLGICLTS TVQLITQLMP YGCLLDYIRE

EGF R   HKDNIGSQYL LNWCVQIAKG MNYLEDRRLV HRDLAARNVL VKTPQHVKIT DFGLAKLLGA EEKEYHAEGG KVPIKWMALE SILHRIYTHQ SDVWSYGVTV
Erb-B   HKDNIGSQYL LNWCVQIAKG MNYLEERRLV HRDLAARNVL VKTPQHVKIT DFGLAKLLGA DEKEYHAEGG KVPIKWMALE SILHRIYTHQ SDVWSYGVTV

EGF R   WELMTFGSKP YDGIPASEIS SILEKGERLP QPPICTIDVY MIMVKCWMID ADSRPKFREL IIEFSKMARD PQRYLVIQGD ERMHLPSPTD SNFYRALMDE
Erb-B   WELMTFGSKP YDGIPASEIS SVLEKGERLP QPPICTIDVY MIMVKCWMID ADSRPKFREL IAEFSKMARD PPRYLVIQGD ERMHLPSPTD SKFYRTLMEE

EGF R   EDMDDVVDAD EYLIPQQGFF SSPSTSRTPL LSSLSATSNN STVACIDRNG LQSCPIKEDS FLQRYSSDPT GALTEDSIDD TFLPVPEYIN QSVPKRPAGS
Erb-B   EDMEDIVDAD EYLVPHQGFF NSPSTSRTPL LSSLSATSNN SATNCIDRNG QGH-PVREDS FVQRYSSDPT GNFLEESIDD GFLPAPEYVN QLMPKKPSTA

EGF R   V-QNVPYHNQ PLNPAPS-R- DPHYQDPHST AVGNPEYLNT VQPTCVNSTF DSPAHWAQKG SHQISLDNPD YQQDFFPKEA KPNGIFKGST AENAEYLRVA
Erb-B   MVQNQIYNFI SLTAISKLPM DSRYQNSHST AVDNPEYLNT NQSPLAKTVF ESSPYWIQSG NHQINLDNPD YQQDFLPTSC S

EGF R   PQSSEFIGA
```

FIG. 3. The amino acid sequence of the EGF receptor and the erb-B transforming protein showing matching aa residues:
●-carbohydrate attachment sites,
_____-transmembrane sequence (putative).

a variety of cDNA clones. The deduced sequence is shown
in Fig. 3 together with the location of the peptides
sequenced.

The amino acid sequence of the EGF receptor

The EGF receptor precursor contains a signal sequence which would allow transmembrane orientation of the
polypeptide during biosynthesis. The mature receptor
can be divided into two domains by the assignment of a
transmembrane hydrophobic sequence located near the linear centre of the polypeptide chain. This is the only
obvious stretch of sequence capable of assimung an $\propto$
helical structure similar to that thought to be transmembrane in other proteins. The receptor appears to
have an external EGF binding domain of 641 aas and a
cytoplasmic domain of 542 aas. The external domain contains stretches of sequences extremely rich in cyste-
ines which are somewhat related in sequence perhaps reflecting the evolutionary origin of the protein. The
internal domain contains features perhaps related to an
ATP binding site similar to that deduced in studies of
bovine cyclic AMP dependent protein kinase (2) and is
presumably the domain which has tyrosine specific protein kinase activity.

Relationship between the EGF receptor and the v-erb-B transforming protein

Using the rapid search technique of Wilbur & Lipman
(51) and an oncogene data base set up at ICRF we found
(17) that six receptor petides we had sequenced showed
a 90% identity to sequences of the v-erb-B transforming
protein established by Yamamoto et al., (52). Our subsequent analysis of other peptides and of the predicted
amino acid sequence from nucleotide sequence analysis
of cDNA clones confirms and extends the original observation (45). The complete sequences are presented in
Fig. 3. The data suggest that avian erythroblastosis
virus has acquired cellular sequences for the gene
which encodes the avian EGF receptor. Since in the
chicken and in man (26,45) there appears to be a single
gene encoding this receptor, this suggestion is almost
certainly correct.

A comparison of the two sequences (Fig. 3) shows
that the erb-B protein may be a truncated version of
the avian receptor which lacks the majority of the external EGF binding domain but maintains the transmembrane region thus allowing association of the protein
with internal and plasma membranes as observed by
Hayman et al., (21) and Privalsky et al., (36). A model
illustrating the differences between the EGF receptor

and the erb-B transforming protein is shown in Fig. 4.
No information is yet available on the avian receptor
polypeptide or its amino acid sequence so that we cannot ascertain the meaning of differences in amino acid
sequence between the erb-B transforming protein and its
normal equivalent in the human:

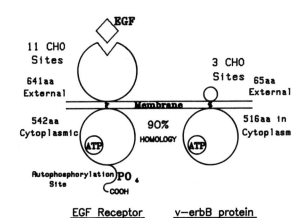

Fig. 4. A model of the putative structures of the EGF receptor and
the v-erb-B transforming protein.

Certain hypothetical concepts can however be formu-
lated. Since the erb-B transforming protein lacks the
EGF binding domain it may be unable to interpret the on
and off signals normally generated by EGF binding. Thus
if signal transduction or removal of a positive signal
by downregulation involves aggregation (40) and subsequent internalisation which are functions of the external domain, then any signal which the truncated receptor may be providing could be continuously generated.
Since the erythroblastoid cells transformed by AEV in
vivo are not thought to normally express EGF receptors,
it is possible that AEV introduces a transformation
signal through expression of a truncated receptor which
provides a signal that can be interpreted by the
normal biochemical pathways in these cells that is
used to transduce receptor signals. This signal is presumably common to other receptors which at different
stages in differentiation are expressed and their signal interpreted by this cell lineage to promote proliferation and or differentiation.
The only known intrinsic receptor function associated with the EGF receptor is an EGF stimulated tyrosine
specific protein kinase. This activity has not been de-

tected in the erb-B protein perhaps for technical reasons but perhaps also because it has been lost or modified in the acquisition of avian receptor (and other?)
sequences. Since the EGF receptor and transforming proteins of the src family, including of course erb-B,
share a region of matching sequence and because other
growth factor receptors share the ability to phorphory-
late tyrosine residues it is possible that the oncogenes which encode these proteins are derived from cellular sequences which encode other proteins involved in
transduction of growth factor signals.

CONCLUSION

Two distinct but related mechanisms described here
show that subversion of normal growth factor signals
may be used by retroviral oncogenes to cause some of
the manifestations of neoplasia. The concepts illustrated by these studies are illustrated in Fig. 5. Recently Kelly et al., (1983) have shown that PDGF may induce
transcription of the myc gene suggesting that other oncogenes subvert normal pathways involved in growth factor stimulated proliferation.

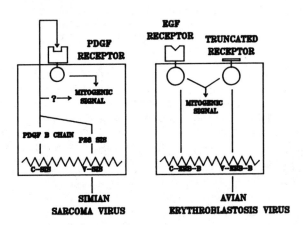

FIG. 5. A cartoon to show the alterna-
        tive methods of subversion of
        signal transduction by the
        oncogenes sis and erb-B.

ACKNOWLEDGEMENTS

The studies described here are the result of a series of productive and friendly collaborations. I am
indebted to my colleagues in the Protein Chemistry Laboratory (P. Stroobant, E. Mayes, W. Gullick, P. Parker,

P. Stockwell, P. Bennett, R. Philp, S. Young, N. Totty, G. Scrace, J. Downward, J. Marsden) who together with our collaborators at Uppsala(A. Johnsson, C. Heldin, A. Wasteson and B. Westermark), at the Weizmann Institute (T. Libermann, Y. Yarden and J. Schlessinger), at St. Louis (T. Deuel and J. Huang) and at Genentech (A. Ullrich, P. Seeburg, L. Coussens, J. Hayflick, T. Dull, A. Gray, L. Tam) have made the work reviewed here possible.

REFERENCES

1. Antoniades, H.N., and Hunkapiller, M.W. (1983): Science 220:963
2. Barker, W.C., and Dayhoff, M. (1982): Proc. Nat. Acad. Sci. 79:2836
3. Betsholtz, C., Heldin, C-H., Nister, M., Ek, B., Wasteson, A., and Westermark, B. (1983): Biochem. Biophys. Res. Comm. 117:176
4. Bishop, J.M. (1983): Rev. Biochem. 52:301
5. Bourne, H., and Rozengurt, E. (1976): Proc. Nat. Acad. Sci. 73:4555
6. Bowen-Pope, D.F., and Ross, R. (1983): Clin. Endocrinol. Metab. 13:191
7. Bubrow, S.A., Cohen, S., and Staros, J.V. (1982): J. Biol. Chem. 258:7824.
8. Burk, R.R. (1973): Proc. Nat. Acad. Sci. 70:369
9. Carpenter, G. (1981): Handbook of Experimental Pharmacology 57:89
10. Carpenter, G., and Cohen, S. (1984): Trends in Biochem. Sci. 169
11. Cochet, C., Gill, G.N., Meisenhelder, J., Cooper, J.A., and Hunter, T. (1984): J. Biol. Chem. 259:2553
12. Deuel, T.F., Huang, J.S., Huang, S.S., Stroobant, P., and Waterfield, M.D. (1983): Science 221, 1348
13. Deuel, T.F., and Huang, J.S. (1983): Prog. Hematol. 13 (In press)
14. Dicker, P., Pohjanpelto, P., Pettican, P., and Rozengurt, E. (1981): Exp. Cell Res. 135:221
15. Doolittle, R.F. (1981): Science 214:149
16. Doolittle, R.F., Hunkapiller, M.W., Hood, L., Devare, S.G., Robbins, K.C., Aaronson, S.A., and Antoniades, H.N. (1983): Science 221:275
17. Downward, J., Yarden, Y., Mayes, E., Scrace, G., Totty, N., Stockwell, P., Ullrich, A., Schlessinger, J., and Waterfield, M.D. (1984): Nature 521

18. Eva, A., Robbins, K.C., Anderson, P.R., Srinilasan, A., Tronick, S.R., Reddy, E.P., Ellmore, N.W., Galen, A.T., Lautenberger, S.A., Papas, T.S., Weston, E.H., Wong-Staal, F., Gallow, R.C., and Aaronson, S.A. (1982): Nature 295:116

19. Gullick, W.J., Downward, J.H., Marsden, J.J., and Waterfield, M.D. (1984): Analyt. Biochem. (In press)

20. Heldin, C-H., Westermark, B., and Wasteson, A. (1980): J. Cell Physiol. 105:235

21. Hayman, M.J., Ramsay, G.M., Savin, K., Kitchener, G., Graf, T., and Beug, H. (1983): Cell 32:579

22. Iwashita, S., and Fox, C.F. (1984): J. Biol. Chem. 259:2559

23. James, R., and Bradshaw, R.A. (1984): Ann. Rev. Biochem. (In press)

24. Johnsson, A., Heldin, C-H., Wasteson, A., Westermark, B., Deuel, T.F., Huang, J.S., Seeburg, P.H., Gray, A., Ullrich, A., Scrace, G., Stroobant, P., and Waterfield, M.D. (1984): EMBO J. 3:921

25. Josephs, S.F., Guo, C., Ratner, L., and Wong-Staal, F. (1984): Science 223:487

26. Lin, C.R., Chen, W.S., Kruiger, W., Stolarsky, L.S., Weber, W., Evans, R.M., Verma, I.M., Gill, G.N., and Rosenfeld, M.G. (1984): Science 224: 843

27. Lopez-Rivas, A., and Rozengurt, E. (1983): Biochem. Biophys. Res. Comm. 114:240

28. Lopez-Rivas, A., and Rozengurt, E. (1984): Am. J. Physiol. (In press)

29. Mayes, E.L.V., and Waterfield, M.D. (1984): EMBO J. 3:531

30. Macara, I.G., Marientti, G.U., and Balduzzi, P.C. (1984): Proc. Nat. Acad. Sci. (In press)

31. Mitchell, R.H. (1983): Biochim. Biophys. Acta 415: 81

32. Mollenaar, W.H., Tslen, R.Y., Van der Saag, P.T., and De Laat, S.W. (1983): Nature 304:645

33. Nishizuka, Y. (1984): Trends in Biochem Sci. 163

34. Nister, M., Heldin, C-H., Wasteson, A., and Westermark, B. (1984): Proc. Nat. Acad. Sci. 81: 926

35. Parker, P.J., Young, S., Gullick, W.J., Mayes, E.L.V., Bennett, P., and Waterfield, M.D. (1984): J. Biol. Chem. (In press)

36. Privalsky, M.L., Sealy, L., Bishop, J.M., McGrath, J.P., and Levinson, A.D. (1983): Cell 32:1257

37. Robbins, K.C., Antoniades, H.N., Devare, S.G., Hunkapiller, M.W., and Aaronson, S.A. (1983): Nature 305:605

38. Rothenberg, P., Glaser, L., Schlessinger, P.,
    Cassel, D. (1983): J. Biol. Chem. 258:4883
39. Rozengurt, E. (1983): Molecul. Biol. Med. 1:169
40. Schlessinger, J. (1978): Proc. Nat. Acad. Sci. 75:
    1659
41. Schreiber, A.B., Lax, I., Yarden, Y., Eschar, Z.,
    and Schlessinger, J. (1981): Proc. Nat. Acad.
    Sci. 78:7535
42. Smith, C.H., Nelson, D.M., King, B.F., Donahue,
    T.M., Ruzycki, S.M., and Kelly, L.K. (1977): Am.
    J. Obstet. Gynecol. 128:190
43. Stroobant, P., Whittle, N., Waterfield, M.D., and
    Rozengurt, E. (1984): Nature (In press)
44. Sugimoto, Y., Whitman, M., Cantley, L.C., and
    Erikson, R.L. (1984): Proc. Nat. Acad. Sci. 81:
    2117
45. Ullrich, A., Coussens, L., Hayflick, J.S., Dull,
    T.J., Gray, A., Tam, L.J., Yarden, Y., Liverman,
    T.A., Schlessinger, J., Downward, J., Mayes,
    E.L.V., Whittle, N., Waterfield, M.D., and
    Seeburg, P.H. (1984): Nature (In press)
46. Waterfield, M.D., Mayes, E.L.V., Stroobant, P.,
    Bennett, P.L.P., Young, S., Goodfellow, P.,
    Banting, G.S., and Ozanne, B. (1982): J. Cell
    Biochem. 20:149
47. Waterfield, M.D., Scrace, G.T., Whittle, N.,
    Stroobant, P., Johnson, A., Wasteson, A.,
    Westermark, B., Helding, C-H., Huang, J.S., and
    Deuel, T.F. (1983): Nature 304:35
48. Weber, W., Gill, G.N., and Spiess, J. (1984):
    Science 224:294
49. Westermark, B., and Wasteson, A. (1975). Adv. Me-
    tabol. Disorders 8:85
50. Westermark, B., Heldin, C-H., Ek, B., Johnsson, A.,
    Mellström, K., and Wasteson, A. (1983): In:
    Guroff, G. (ed.) Growth & Maturation Factors,
    Wiley & Sons, vol. 1, pp. 73
51. Wilbur, W.J., and Lipmann, D.J. (1983): Proc. Nat.
    Acad. Sci. 80:726
52. Yamamoto, T., Nishida, T., Miyajima, N., Kawai, S.,
    Ooi, T., and Toyoshima, K. (1983): Cell 35:71

Molecular Biology of Tumor Cells, edited by
B. Wahren et al. Raven Press, New York © 1985.

Platelet-Derived Growth Factor: Comments on the Structural and Functional Relationship with the Transforming Protein of Simian Sarcoma Virus

Bengt Westermark, *Ann Johnsson, Christer Betsholtz, *Åke Wasteson, and *Carl-Henrik Heldin

*Department of Pathology, and *Department of Medical and Physiological Chemistry, University of Uppsala, S-751 85 Uppsala, Sweden*

Studies on the interaction of pure polypeptide growth factors with their target cells has led to a growing understanding of the molecular biology of mitogenesis. In particular, epidermal growth factor (EGF) and platelet derived growth factor (PDGF) have been instrumental in these studies (for reviews, see 3, 22, 26). These factors bind to specific, high affinity, cell surface receptors and thereby initiate a program of cellular responses which precede the onset of DNA replication. Both the EGF (2) and the PDGF (14) receptors appear to be integral membrane proteins with an intracellular, catalytic domain displaying tyrosylkinase activity.

Recent studies suggest that normal mitogenesis has several features in common with neoplastic transformation. Several lines of evidence imply that transformation may involve an undue expression of any of the regulatory components along the normal mitogenic pathway: the growth factor itself, the growth factor receptor or the intracellular signal system which controls events in the prereplicative phase of the cell cycle (reviewed in ref. 15). The findings of an amino acid homology between the v-sis gene product (p28[sis]) and PDGF B chain (8, 9, 17, 24) on one hand and that between the erbB gene product and the EGF receptor (10) on the other hand are particularly impressive. These observations show that the corresponding retroviruses (simian sarcoma virus, SSV, and avian erythroblastosis virus, AEV) have obtained transforming capacity by aquiring cellular gene sequences encoding a growth factor and a growth factor receptor, respectively.

In the present communication we will focus on PDGF, its structure, function and relationship with the transforming gene product of simian sarcoma virus.

THE SUBUNIT COMPOSITION OF PDGF

Purification protocols for human PDGF have been worked out by several laboratories (reviewed in ref. 26). SDS gel electrophoresis of pure PDGF under non-reducing conditions reveals a broad band in the M_r 30,000 region (12). Biologically active material can be recovered from this entire region. This result suggests that PDGF undergoes a limited proteolysis when stored in the platelet or during the course of preparation. PDGF consists of two disulfide bonded polypeptide chains which we have designated A and B (16). The subunit composition of the molecule has not been worked out in detail. We have proposed that PDGF is a heterodimer (A-B) but the possibility that the factor occurs as a mixture of A-A and B-B homodimers has not been ruled out. It should be mentioned that an intact dimer structure is required for the biological activity of PDGF; all mitogenic activity is abolished by reduction and alkylation.

After reduction and alkylation, the subunit polypeptide chains can be separated on HPLC (16). SDS gel electrophoresis of separated B chains reveals a distinct band migrating as an M 16,000 component whereas separated A chains give rise to multiple species in the M_r 12,000 - 17,000 range. Hence, the heterogeneity of the intact PDGF molecule appears to be due to a partial degradation of the A chain.

AMINO ACID SEQUENCE OF PDGF

A 109 amino acid residue stretch of the B chain has been sequenced; this probably constititutes the entire B chain (17). This sequence shows a 97% homology with the predicted sequence of $p28^{sis}$, the putative transforming protein of simian sarcoma virus (8). Sequence data has also provided evidence for a structural homology within the PDGF molecule; the 54 amino terminal residues of the A chain sequenced so far are about 60% homologous to the B chain (17). These data imply that the gene sequences encoding PDGF A and B chain have evolved through duplication of an ancestral gene and, moreover, that SSV has aquired PDGF B chain gene sequences.

STRUCTURAL AND FUNCTIONAL RELATIONSHIP BETWEEN $p28^{sis}$ AND PDGF

The normal human c-<u>sis</u> gene, which has been located to chromosome 22 (5, 23), includes six regions of homology with v-<u>sis</u> (6,18), the nucleotide sequences of which have been determined (17,19). A schematic representation of the structural relationship between the predicted v-<u>sis</u> and c-<u>sis</u> gene products is given in Fig. 1. The open reading frame of c-<u>sis</u> predicts an amino acid sequence which is virtually

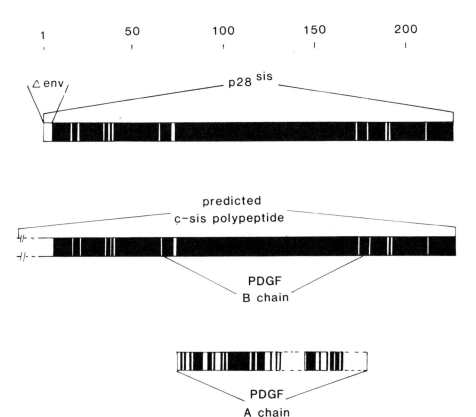

FIG. 1. Schematic representation of the structural
relationship between p28 [sis] (8), the predicted c-sis
polypeptide (17, 19) and the subunit chains of PDGF (17). The
sequences of p28[sis] and the c-sis polypeptide are deduced from
the respective genomic nucleotide sequences. Their carboxy
termini are defined by the presence of termination codons at
the corresponding positions. The amino terminus of p28[sis] is
defined by a candidate initiator codon, derived from the viral
env gene (8). An initiator codon in c-sis has not been located;
possibly, the predicted c-sis polypeptide constitutes the
carboxy terminus of a putative PDGF precursor protein. p28 [sis]
is apparently a precursor polypeptide which is processed by
dimer formation and proteolytic cleavage to form a p24 [sis]
species. In view of the extensive homology between v-sis and
c-sis, the processed parts of p28 [sis] may have counterparts in
the putative PDGF precursor; p24 [sis] would then be virtually
identical to a PDGF B-B homodimer.
Filled areas, sequence identity; Open areas, non-identity;
dashed lines, relation unknown.

identical to that of p28^{sis}. The B chain sequence covers a 109
amino acid residue stretch within this polypeptide and is
flanked by amino and carboxy terminal sequences. In addition,
p28^{sis} contains a short amino terminal sequence, derived from
the viral env-gene.The open reading frames of v-sis and c-sis,
respectively, terminate at the same position (8, 17, 19). A
candidate initiator codon has been identified in the env
sequence of the viral gene (8); the location of the initiator
codon in the cellular gene has not yet been determined. The
predicted c-sis polypeptide probably represents the carboxy
terminus of a putative PDGF precursor molecule. It is not known
whether the A chain is contained within the amino terminus of
this putative precursor.

The metabolic processing of p28^{sis} in SSV transformed cells
has been elucidated by Robbins et al. (21). These investigators
found that p28^{sis}, which is a single polypeptide chain, rapidly
forms a 56 kDa dimer, which is proteolytically cleaved to a
p24^{sis} species. This molecule can be expected to be structurally
very similar to a putative PDGF B-B homodimer. Because of the
homology between the two PDGF chains, such a B-B homodimer might
also be expected to have a similar functional activity as
authentic PDGF, and stimulate SSV transformed cells in an
autocrine fashion. Some experimental support for this view has
been obtained; SSV transformed cells contain in their cytoplasm
a growth factor which is antigenically related to PDGF (7).
Moreover, in our laboratory we have found that SSV transformed
marmoset cells secrete a growth factor which has all functional
properties of PDGF (Johnsson et al., in preparation).

Although addition of PDGF to Balb/c 3T3 cells (26) and human
glial cells (20) induces certain phenotypic changes resembling
those of transformed cells, it appears that PDGF alone, at any
concentration, will not induce a fully transformed phenotype.
What is then the difference in cellular action of exogenously
added PDGF and endogenously synthesized p28^{sis} and its
derivatives? In the following, two main alternatives will be
discussed: 1) p28^{sis} and its derivatives have other functional
properties in addition to those of authentic PDGF which make
them transforming rather than only growth promoting factors. 2)
co-expression of a mitogen and the corresponding receptor in the
same cell leads to an uncontrolled mitogenic signal.

Ad 1). It appears unlikely that the amino terminal env
portion of p28^{sis} (c.f. Fig 1) is of any functional
significance for transformation. Likewise, it is unlikely that
the other amino acid substitutions of p28^{sis} are essential for
the transforming properties of the viral gene product. This view
is based on experiments by Clarke et al. (4) who constructed a

plasmid with a 2.7 kb c-sis cDNA insert, derived from the 4.2 kb
c-sis transcript from human T-cells, transformed by human T cell
leukemia virus (HTLV). Since this plasmid, which was also
equipped with an SV40 promoter, was able to transform NIH 3T3
cells in gene transfer experiments, one might draw the
conclusion that c-sis sequences have transforming potential.
At present one should not neglect the possibility that
the amino and carboxy terminal peptides that are apparently
cleaved off during the maturation of p28^{SIS} are biologically
active and may operate in the transformation process; these
sequences are also contained within the 2.7 kb cDNA fragment
referred to above (4). Finally, there is the possibility that a
B-B homodimer (p24^{SIS}) has other functional properties than
authentic PDGF, that appears to be an A-B heterodimer, making
the viral product transforming rather than only growth
promoting.

Ad 2). PDGF mediated stimulation of cell replication is
initiated by the binding of PDGF to its cell surface receptor,
followed by a rapid internalization and degradation in the
lysosomes. It is conceivable that co-expression of a PDGF
agonist and PDGF receptor in the same cell leads to a growth
factor-receptor interaction at an aberrant subcellular site,
such as in an intracellular compartment. The activated receptor
may then elude growth regulatory mechanisms, associated with the
cell membrane, and thus cause an aberrant growth stimulus.

EXPRESSION OF THE c-sis GENE IN HUMAN TUMOR CELLS

An involvement of the c-sis gene in human malignancy is
suggested by the finding of sis related transcripts in certain
cell lines and the concomitant production of a PDGF like factor.
We reported several years ago than the human osteosarcoma cell
line U-2 OS releases a growth factor which was termed
osteosarcoma-derived growth factor (13, 25). As we made progress
in the purification of this factor parallel to our work on PDGF,
we became aware of a striking resemblance between the tumor
cell-derived factor and PDGF. We have now obtained data which
strongly suggest that U-2 OS cells express the c-sis gene and
release PDGF to the culture medium. This factor, after metabolic
labeling and immunoprecipitation with PDGF antibodies, migrates
as a 31 kDa species on SDS gel electrophoreses under
non-reducing conditions (1). After reduction, this protein is
converted to faster migrating species of M_r 17,000 and 16,500.
Thus, the molecule manufactured by osteosarcoma cells is
composed of two disulfide bonded polypeptide chains as is PDGF.
However, its is not known whether the two peptides that appear
after reduction are in fact identical to the two subunit chains
of PDGF.

Using a ^{32}P-labeled c-<u>sis</u> probe (kindly provided by Dr. Dalla-Favera), we have recently identified c-<u>sis</u> transcripts on Northern blots of polyA$^+$ RNA isolated from U-2 OS cells and other sarcoma and glioma cell lines (Betsholtz et al., unpublished). These results confirm those published by Eva et al. (11) who reported on the expression of <u>sis</u> transcripts in a number of such cell lines. It is conceivable that an undue expression of the c-sis gene and synthesis of PDGF leads to an autocrine stimulation of growth of these tumor cells. Indeed, gliomas and sarcomas are derived from PDGF responsive tissues.

Expression of c-<u>sis</u> is not a constant feature of gliomas and sarcomas (ref. 11 and Betsholtz el al., unpublished), although it occurs at a rather high frequency, especially in sarcoma cell lines. We have proposed that any of the regulatory components in the chain of events linked to normal growth factor action may have oncogenic properties if inappropriately expressed or activated (15). Thus, an undue expression of c-<u>sis</u> and PDGF production may represent only one of several mechanisms of constitutive mitogenesis in glioma and sarcoma cells.

Acknowledgement

Our own work was supported by grants from the Swedish Medical Research Council (4486) and the Swedish Cancer Society (689, 786, 1794).

REFERENCES

1.   Betsholtz, C., Heldin, C.-H., Nistér, M., Ek, B., Wasteson, Å. and Westermark, B. (1983): <u>Biochem. Biophys. Res. Commun</u>. 117:176-182

2.   Buhrow, S.A., Cohen, S. and Staros, J.V. (1982): <u>J. Biol. Chem</u>. 257:4019-4022

3.   Carpenter, G. and Cohen, S. (1979): <u>Ann. Rev. Biochem</u>. 48:193-216

4.   Clarke, M.F., Westin, E., Schmidt, D., Josephs, S.F., Ratner, L., Wong-Staal, F., Gallo, R.C. and Reitz, M.S., Jr. (1984): <u>Nature</u> 308:464-467

5.   Dalla-Favera, R., Gallo, R.C., Giallongo, A. and Croce, C.M. (1982): <u>Science</u> 218:686-688

6.   Dalla-Favera, R., Gelman, E.P., Gallo, R.C. and
     Wong-Staal, F. (1981): <u>Nature</u> 292:31-35.

7.   Deuel, T.F., Huang, J.S., Stroobant, P. and Waterfield,
     M. (1983): <u>Science</u> 221:1348-1350

8.   Devare, S.G., Reddy, E.P., Law, J.D., Robbins, K.C. and
     Aaronson, S.A. (1983): <u>Proc.Acad. Sci. USA</u> 80:731-735

9.   Doolittle, R.F., Hunkapiller, M.W., Hood, L.E., Devare,
     S.G., Robbins, K.C., Aaronson, S.A. and Antoniades, H.N.
     (1983): <u>Science</u> 221:275-277

10. Downward, J., Yarden, Y., Mayes, E., Scrace, G., Totty,
     N., Stockwell, P., Ullrich, A., Schlessinger, J. and
     Waterfield, M.D. (1984): <u>Nature</u> 307:521-527

11. Eva, A,. Robbins. K.C., Andersen, P.R., Srinivasan, A.,
     Tronick, S.R., Reddy, E.P., Ellmore, N.W., Galen, A.T.,
     Lautenberger, J.A., Papas, T.S., Westin, E.H.,
     Wong-Staal, F., Gallo, R.C. and Aaronson, S.A. (1982):
     <u>Nature</u> 295:116-119

12. Heldin, C.-H., Westermark, B. and Wasteson, Å. (1979):
     <u>Proc. Natl. Acad. Sci. USA</u> 76:3722-3726

13. Heldin, C.-H., Westermark, B. and Wasteson, Å. (1980):
     <u>J. Cell. Physiol.</u> 105:235-246

14. Heldin, C.-H., Ek, B. and Rönnstrand, L. (1983): <u>J.
     Biol. Chem.</u> 258:10054-10061

15. Heldin, C.-H. and Westermark, B. (1984): <u>Cell</u> 77:9-20

16. Johnsson, A., Heldin, C.-H., Westermark, B. and
     Wasteson, Å. (1982): <u>Biochem. Biophys. Res. Comm.</u>
     104:66-74

17. Johnsson, A., Heldin, C.-H., Wasteson, Å., Westermark,
     B., Deuel, T.F., Huang, J.S., Seeburg, P.H., Gray, A.,
     Ullrich, A., Scrace, G., Stroobant, P. and Waterfield,
     M. (1984): <u>EMBO J.</u> 3:921-928

18. Josephs, S.F., Dalla-Favera, R., Gelmann, E.P., Gallo,
     R.C. and Wong-Staal, F. (1983): <u>Science</u> 219:503-505

19. Josephs, S.F., Guo, C., Ratner, L. and Wong-Staal, F.
     (1984); <u>Science</u> 223:487-491

20.   Mellström, K., Höglund, A.-S., Nistèr, M., Heldin, C.-H., Westermark, B. and Lindberg, U. (1983): *J. Muscl. Res. & Cell Motility* 4:589-609

21.   Robbins, K.C., Antoniades, H.N., Devare, S.G., Hunkapiller, M.W. and Aaronson, S.A. (1983): *Nature* 305:605-608

22.   Stiles, C.D. (1983): *Cell* 33:653-655

23.   Swan, D.C.. McBride, O.W., Robbins, K.C., Keithley, D.A., Reddy, E.P. and Aaronson, S.A. (1982): *Proc. Natl. Acad. Sci. USA* 79:4691-4695

24.   Waterfield, M.D., Scrace, G., Whittle, N., Stroobant, P., Johnsson, A., Wasteson, Å., Westermark, B., Heldin, C.-H., Huang, J.S. and Deuel, T.F. (1983): *Nature* 304:35-39

25.   Westermark, B. and Wasteson, Å. (1975): *Adv. Metab. Disord.* 8:85-100

26.   Westermark, B., Heldin, C.-H., Ek, B., Johnsson, A., Mellström, K., Nistèr, M. and Wasteson, Å. (1983): In: Growth and Maturation Factors, edited by G. Guroff, pp. 73-115. John Wiley and Sons, New York

Molecular Biology of Tumor Cells, edited by
B. Wahren et al. Raven Press, New York © 1985.

Phosphorylation-Dephosphorylation Events in Cells Transformed by Rous Sarcoma Virus

R. L. Erikson, John Blenis, Jordan G. Spivack, and Y. Sugimoto

*Department of Cellular and Developmental Biology, Harvard University,
Cambridge, Massachusetts 02138*

The work that I describe in this talk was initiated at the
University of Colorado, where I had many valuable discussions
with James Maller, and continued at Harvard for the past year.
Retrovirus transforming genes and their products have now been
extensively characterized. To date oncogene products fall into
two large classes. One subsumes many distinct products that are
found in the cytoplasm and/or on the plasma membrane. Many of
these have been found to be protein kinases specific for tyrosine
residues. Despite the increasing knowledge about these enzymes
the biochemical events leading to malignancy remain largely
unknown. In this paper I will describe experiments aimed at
characterizations of transformed cells with a focus on
phosphorylation events as well as additional studies on the Rous
sarcoma virus transforming product $pp60^{v-src}$. Although a great
deal of attention has been focused on tyrosine phosphorylation in
the past few years there are also a number of quantitative
changes in the levels of serine residues phosphorylated in
certain proteins. One such protein is S6, a protein found in the
40S ribosomal subunit.

Interest in S6 phosphorylation was initially stimulated by
observations demonstrating a temporal correlation between
phosphorylation of this protein and the initiation of protein
synthesis when quiescent cells are treated with serum or several
mitogens (8,12). In contrast to normal cells, serum-starvation
of many oncogenically transformed cells does not lead to a
decrease in S6 phosphorylation. In serum-starved Rous sarcoma
virus (RSV)-transformed chicken embryo fibroblasts (CEF),
expression of the src gene is responsible for S6 phosphorylation
(3,6). Although $pp60^{v-src}$ is a tyrosine-specific protein kinase
(5,10), S6 is phosphorylated on serine in biosynthetically
labeled cells (3,6) Moreover, the ability of $pp60^{v-src}$ to alter

_____

This lecture was also presented at the Sigrid Juselius
Symposium: Gene Expression During Normal and Malignant
Differentiation, May 20-24, 1984 in Helsinki, Finland.

S6 phosphorylation has also been demonstrated in <u>Xenopus laevis</u> oocytes after microinjection of purified enzyme (15).   Based on these results it has been proposed that pp60[v-src] directly or indirectly interacts with a pathway operative in normal cells which regulates the state of S6 phosphorylation.

The tumor promoter, 12-0-tetradecanoyl phorbol 13-acetate (TPA), when added to normal cells induces the expression of many properties common to oncogenic transformation and to cells treated with growth factors (4,9,19).   In CEF for example, TPA, serum growth factors and functional pp60[v-src] are mitogenic, stimulate glucose uptake, induce uridine and thymidine utilization and modulate the expression of plasminogen activator (4,9,19).

Nishizuka and coworkers (11) have described a novel enzyme denoted C-kinase that requires Ca^{2+} and phospholipid but, at physiological concentrations of Ca^{2+}, depends on diacylglycerol for its activation. Recently it has been suggested that the tumor-promoting phorbol esters activate C-kinase by substituting for diacylglycerol, thus this enzyme may play a role in the proliferative and tumor-promoting effects of these agents.

Little is known about the regulation of the enzymes involved in diacylglycerol synthesis and degradation, however, it seems clear that most diacylglycerol is produced by hydrolysis of phosphatidylinositol (PtdIns) by a phosphodiesterase and is removed by rephosphorylation to phosphatidic acid (for review, see Berridge, 1). Regulation of the hydrolysis of PtdIns may involve a kinase that phosphorylates PtdIns in the inositol head group to form phosphatidylinositol 4-phosphate (PtdIns4P) and phosphatidylinositol 4,5-bisphosphate (PtdIns4,5P$_2$). Because PtdIns4,5P$_2$ seems to be the best substrate for the phosphodiesterase, a plasma membrane kinase may be an important component in the regulation of PtdIns turnover and diacylglycerol production.

In view of the capacity of pp60[v-src] to phosphorylate glycerol and of the observation that PtdIns turnover is stimulated in RSV-transformed cells (7), we investigated the relevant lipids as pp60[v-src] substrates, in order to determine if it could stimulate PtdIns turnover directly.

MATERIALS AND METHODS

All of the details concerning the experiments described here have recently been published by us in Sugimoto <u>et al</u>. (16) and Blenis <u>et al</u> (3).

RESULTS

TPA Stimulation of S6 Phosphorylation.

The effect of TPA on S6 phosphorylation was evaluated in normal chicken embryo fibroblasts (CEF) and in a murine cell line,

C127. Both cell types are quiescent when confluent and serum-starved. The S6 phosphoprotein in ^{32}P-labeled ribosomes isolated from these cells was analyzed by SDS-polyacrylamide gel electrophoresis and autoradiography and is shown in Fig. 1. Phosphorylation of S6 in serum-starved CEF (Fig. 1A, lane 1), serum-starved CEF incubated with 100 ng/ml phorbol, which is inactive as a tumor promoter (Fig. 1A, lane 4), serum-starved C127 murine cells (Fig. 1B, lane 1), and serum-starved C127 cells treated with 100 ng/ml phorbol (Fig. 1B, lane 4) was greatly reduced in comparison to that observed in CEF incubated in the presence of 5% (v/v) bovine calf serum and 100 ng/ml TPA (Fig. 1A, lanes 2 and 3, respectively) and in C127 murine cells treated with 5% serum or 100 ng/ml TPA (Fig. 1B, lanes 2 and 3, respectively). Figure 1C shows analysis of S6 phosphorylation in serum-starved CEF infected with a temperature-sensitive mutant of Rous sarcoma virus 72-4 (ts-CEF), at the nonpermissive temperature (Fig. 1C, lane 1) and transferred to the permissive temperature for 2h (Fig 1C, lane 2). This result demonstrates that stimulation of S6 phosphorylation is observed in TPA- or serum-stimulated cells, and in serum-starved oncogenically-transformed cells under the experimental conditions described in the legend to Fig. 1. Similar results were obtained when cells were prelabeled from 6-18 h before stimulation.

In vitro, TPA interacts with and activates the Ca^{2+}- and phospholipid-dependent protein kinase, protein kinase C (17). This apparently occurs in a manner similar to that observed with diacylglycerol, the endogenous protein kinase C activator, to which TPA has structural similarity (13). We therefore analyzed the effect of an exogenously added diacylglycerol 1-oleoyl-2-acetylglycerol (OAG) on S6 phosphorylation. Figure 2 shows the results obtained when serum-starved ts-CEF were prelabeled at 41° (nonpermissive temperature) and were untreated (lane 1), transferred to 35° (permissive temperature) (lane 2); treated with 100 ng/ml TPA (lane 3), 250 µg/ml OAG (lane 4) and 500 µg/ml OAG (lane 5) at 41°. As shown, OAG does stimulate phosphorylation of S6 in serum-starved cells, however, the degree of S6 phosphorylation obtained with these high concentrations of OAG (approximately 2-fold stimulation) did not reach the level obtained with TPA (approximately 4-fold stimulation in this experiment). This may be due to the poor solubility of diacylglycerol and/or its inability to enter the cell.

Comparison of S6 Phosphorylation Stimulated by TPA, Serum and RSV Transformation

Phosphorylation of S6 was characterized and compared by: 1) analysis of phosphoamino acids, 2) two-dimensional ribosomal gel electrophoresis, 3) limited proteolysis with S. aureus V8 protease, and 4) two-dimensional thin layer electrophoresis of chymotryptic phosphopeptides.

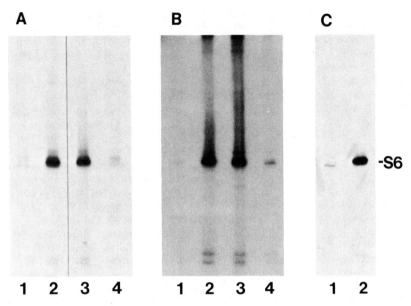

Fig. 1 Analysis of S6 phosphorylation stimulated by serum, TPA
and activated pp60^{v-src}. Confluent CEF, C127 murine cells and
CEF infected with a temperature-sensitive mutant of RSV, 72-4,
were serum-starved at 41°for 24 h, ^{32}P-labeled (1 mCi/plate) and
treated with serum, TPA, phorbol or active pp60^{v-src} for 2 h.
Ribosomes were isolated as described (6). Equal amounts of
ribosomal protein were analyzed by 12% polyacrylamide SDS-gel
electrophoresis. Phosphorylated proteins were visualized by
autoradiography. (A) S6 phosphorylation in serum-starved,
uninfected CEF which were untreated (lane 1), 5% serum-stimulated
(lane 2), incubated with 100 ng/ml TPA in 0.1% DMSO (lane 3) and
100 ng/ml phorbol in 0.1% DMSO (lane 4). (B) S6 phosphorylation
in C127 murine cells treated as in (A). (C) S6 phosphorylation
in serum-starved CEF infected with a temperature-sensitive mutant
of RSV, 72-4, and labeled for 2 h at the nonpermissive
temperature (lane 1) or during a 2 h shift to the permissive
temperature (lane 2).

Phosphoamino acids obtained by acid hydrolysis of ^{32}P-labeled
S6 from serum-stimulated, TPA-stimulated and serum-starved
RSV-transformed CEF were identical (data not shown). Greater
than 95% of the phosphoamino acids was phosphoserine and less
than 5% was phosphothreonine. No phosphotyrosine was detected.
    S6 can exist in multiple phosphorylated forms which can be
resolved in the two dimensional acrylamide/urea gel system (11).
Using this system up to five moles of phosphate per mole of S6
have been detected in biosynthetically-labeled cells (18). We
therefore examined the extent of S6 phosphorylation induced by

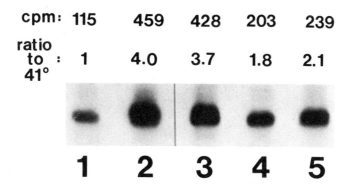

Fig. 2 Phosphorylation of S6 by incubation with diacylglycerol.
Confluent CEF infected with a temperature-sensitive mutant of RSV
(ts-CEF) were serum-starved at 41° for 24 h, prelabeled with 1.2
mCi ^{32}P for 6.5 h, treated as described below for 2.5 h, followed
by isolation of ribosomes, SDS-gel electrophoresis,
autoradiography and determination of radioactivity associated
with S6 for quantitation. Equal amounts of ribosomal protein
were analyzed. Lane 1, ts-CEF at 41°; lane 2, ts-CEF transferred
to 35° for 2.5 h; lane 3, ts-CEF at 41° treated with 100 ng/ml
TPA in 0.1% DMSO for 2.5 h; lane 4, ts-CEF at 41° incubated with
250 ng/ml 1-oleoyl-2-acetylglycerol (OAG) in 0.1% DMSO for 2.5 h;
lane 5, ts-CEF at 41° incubated with 500 ng/ml OAG in 0.2% DMSO
for 2.5 h. OAG was sonicated for 3 x 3 min in 1 ml medium before
addition of suspension to prelabeled cells.

the stimuli described here. As shown in Figure 3,
serum-stimulation (panel B), TPA-stimulation (panel D), and
RSV-transformation (panel E) all produced the highly
phosphorylated species of S6 (4-5 moles phosphate, d + e),
whereas in serum-starved (panel A) or phorbol-treated (panel C)
cells, S6 phosphorylated with 1-2 moles of phosphate was the
predominant form detected after a much longer exposure. Thus by
this analysis, the same degree of S6 phosphorylation was induced
by the stimuli under investigation.
    To determine if the sites of phosphorylation are identical,
S6-phosphopeptides generated by complete digestion with
chymotrypsin and separation by two-dimensional thin layer
electrophoresis were analyzed. Limited proteolysis patterns of
^{32}P-labeled S6 from TPA-, serum- and RSV-stimulated cells were
identical to each other and to results previously observed in
many serum-starved virally-transformed cells (data not shown,
12). Analysis of chymotryptic S6-phosphopeptides is shown in
figure 4. This analysis demonstrates that identical chymotryptic
S6-phosphopeptides were phosphorylated in serum-stimulated CEF
(Fig. 4A), TPA-stimulated CEF (Fig. 4B) and CEF infected with a
temperature-sensitive mutant of RSV and cultured at the
permissive temperature for 2 h (Fig. 4C). Figure 4D represents a
mix of S6 phosphopeptides from figures 4A, B, and C. In
addition, separation of chymotryptic S6 phosphopeptides by high

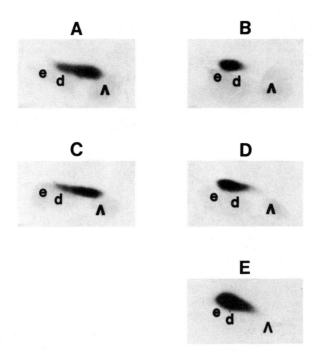

Fig. 3 Analysis of S6 phosphorylation by two-dimensional
ribosomal gel electrophoresis. Confluent CEF and ts-CEF were
serum-starved for 24 h, labeled with 2 mCi ^{32}P for 2 h in
phosphate-free medium and treated as described below.
Radiolabeled ribosomal proteins were analyzed by two-dimensional
ribosomal gel electrophoresis as described (11) using ribosomes
from unfertilized <u>Xenopus laevis</u> eggs as carrier and marker for
S6. d and e represent the positions of S6 phosphorylated with 4
and 5 moles phosphate per mole S6. Λ represents the position of
unphosphorylated S6. Panel A, untreated CEF. Panel B, CEF
treated with 5% serum. Panel C, CEF treated with 100 ng/ml
phorbol in 0.1% DMSO. Panel D, CEF treated with 100 ng/ml TPA in
0.1% DMSO. Panel E, ts-CEF transferred to the permissive
temperature for 2 h. Panels A and C required 4-10 times longer
exposure to film than panels B, D, and E to obtain an
autoradiogram of approximately equal exposure.

pressure liquid chromatography has yielded identical elution
profiles for the samples described above (data not shown). Thus,
these experiments suggest that the same sites are phosphorylated
in S6 from CEF stimulated by TPA, serum and RSV transformation.
However, quantitative differences in the degree of
phosphorylation of some peptides were observed and are under
study.
    To further support the notion that the same sites were being
phosphorylated in S6 upon stimulation of CEF with TPA, serum or
transformation, the effects of a combination of the stimulatory
factors were investigated. These studies again suggest that the
same amino acids are phosphorylated in CEF by the three stimuli

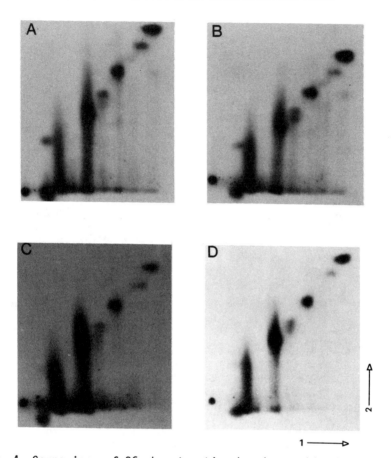

Fig. 4 Comparison of S6 chymotryptic phosphopeptides by
two-dimensional thin-layer electrophoresis. Radiolabeled S6 was
excised and eluted from an SDS-polyacrylamide gel, digested with
chymotrypsin, and the chymotryptic phosphopeptides analyzed as
described in Materials and Methods. The directions of
electrophoresis are indicated in the figure. Panel A, S6
chymotryptic phosphopeptides from 5% serum-stimulated CEF. Panel
B, S6 chymotryptic phosphopeptides from 100 ng/ml TPA-stimulated
CEF. Panel C, S6 chymotryptic phosphopeptides from serum-starved
CEF infected with the temperature-sensitive mutant of RSV, 72-4,
and transferred to the permissive temperature for 2 h. Panel D,
an equal mix (cpm) of the above samples.

investigated as any combination of two factors increased S6
phosphorylation only slightly over TPA-, serum-, or
pp60^{v-src}-induced S6 phosphorylation alone. This small increase
was not deemed significant when compared to the large increase
observed with one stimulating factor alone.

Phosphorylation of Lipids

When purified pp60^{v-src} was incubated with [γ-^{32}P]ATP in the
presence of PtdIns, phosphorylated compounds were produced as

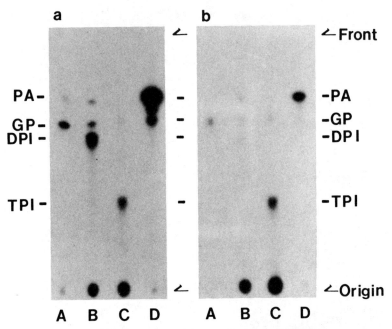

Fig. 5 Thin layer chromotographic analysis of lipids radiolabeled with $[\gamma-^{32}P]$ATP. pp60^{v-src} (a) or the catalytic subunit of cAMP-dependent protein kinase (b) in 10 mM potassium phosphate, pH 7.1, 1 mM EDTA was preincubated with lipid substrate for 15 min at 4°. The reaction was then started by addition of $[\gamma-^{32}P]$ATP and MgCl$_2$ to a final concentration of 20 µM and 20 mM, respectively. After incubation for 30 min at 30°, the reaction was terminated and lipid was extracted as described in the text. A tracks, no substrate; B tracks, PtdIns (200 µg/ml); C tracks, PtdIns4P (200 µg/ml); D tracks, 1,2-dioleoylglycerol (200 µM). PA, phosphatidic acid; GP, glycerolphosphate; DPI, PtdIns4P; TPI, PtdIns4,5P$_2$.

shown in Figure 5. The major phosphorylated product migrated with PtdIns4P upon thin layer chromatography. In addition, a slight amount of radioactivity, <10% of the major product, migrated with PtdIns4,5P$_2$. When PtdIns4P was used as a substrate, the major phosphorylated product migrated with PtdIns4,5P$_2$. This activity of pp60^{v-src} was about 50% of its PtdIns phosphorylating activity. We note in lanes B and C that a highly phosphorylated product(s) remains at the origin, but it has not been characterized. Furthermore, 1,2-dioleoylglycerol and 1,3-dioleoylglycerol were both phosphorylated by pp60^{v-src} to yield products that migrated with phosphatidic acid. 1,2-Dioleoylglycerol, a natural substrate for phosphatidic acid production, was phosphorylated at 3 times the rate of 1,3-dioleoylglycerol. Although 1,3-dioleoylglycerol is likely to be contaminated with 1,2-dioleoylglycerol, this amount of phosphorylation suggests that 1,3-dioleoylglycerol is also a substrate of pp60^{v-src}. We have not succeeded in separating β-phosphatidic acid from α-phosphatidic acid by thin layer chromatography. The phosphorylated products were further characterized by two-dimensional thin layer chromatography supporting the identification (data not shown). Thus, pp60^{v-src} is capable of phosphorylating a variety of diacylated glycerol substrates.

When the purified catalytic subunit of cAMP-dependent protein kinase was similarly tested at a concentration that had α-casein-phosphorylating activity comparable to that of pp60^{v-src}, the phosphorylation of PtdIns and diacylglycerols occurred at 1-3% of the level seen with pp60^{v-src}. On the other hand, PtdIns4P was phosphorylated by the catalytic subunit to 20% of the level obtained with pp60^{v-src}. Thus pp60^{v-src} shows relative specificity for phosphorylation of hydroxyl groups on PtdIns and on diacylglycerols.

Inhibition of the Phosphorylation of PtdIns and 1,2-Dioleoylglycerol

Evidence that the lipid kinase activities described above are indeed due to pp60^{v-src} and not to an impurity in the preparation is provided by inhibition experiments with antibodies raised against pp60^{v-src}. Preincubation of pp60^{v-src} with TBR-IgG specifically decreased the α-casein phosphorylation to 16% of that with normal IgG as control. Similarly the phosphorylation of PtdIns and 1,2-dioleoylglycerol was decreased to 19% and 9% of the control, respectively. TBR-IgG did not inhibit the casein kinase activity of the catalytic subunit of cAMP-dependent protein kinase, indicating that the inhibition by TBR-IgG is not due to a nonspecific kinase inhibitor in the IgG preparation (data not shown).

Quercetin, an inhibitor of pp60^{v-src} similarly inhibited the phosphorylation of PtdIns, 1,2-dioleoylglycerol and α-casein with Ki values of approximately 10 μM. In addition, all three kinase activities were inactivated in parallel when pp60^{v-src} was preincubated at 41°. These data support the contention that the phosphorylation of PtdIns and of 1,2-dioleoylglycerol is due to pp60^{v-src} itself.

DISCUSSION

In this report we show that tumor promoters, serum growth factors or the RSV-transforming protein pp60^{v-src} stimulate the phosphorylation of the 40S ribosomal protein S6 in a similar manner. The results suggest the same serine-specific enzymes are regulated by these diverse stimuli or alternatively, if more than one pathway is involved, they yield the same result.

The stimuli used in this study have in common several biochemical properties which may be linked to their ability to stimulate cell proliferation. The RSV src gene product, pp60^{v-src}, has tyrosine kinase activity as well as the ability to phosphorylate phosphatidylinositol in vitro which then could be metabolized to diacylglycerol and inositol triphosphate, apparent second messengers which may initiate a signal cascade (1). The potential for pp60^{v-src} to directly or indirectly function in this manner in vivo is supported by the observation that phosphatidylinositol turnover is stimulated in RSV-transformed cells (7). Several growth factor receptors also have associated tyrosine kinase activity and interaction with the polypeptide growth factors not only activates the kinase activity but also results in altered phosphoinositide metabolism (14). Furthermore, because of the apparent structural similarity between diacylglycerol and TPA the tumor promoter may replace the putative second messenger in activating kinases involved in growth regulation. In view of these findings, it is clear that identification of the modifications or alterations responsible for elevated S6 phosphorylation may answer several key questions concerning growth control in both normal and cancerous cells.

Acknowledgement: This research was supported by NIH grant CA34943 and an award from the American Business Cancer Research Foundation. J. Blenis was supported by a Damon Runyon-Walter Winchell postdoctoral fellowship, J.G. Spivack is a NRSA postdoctoral fellow (CA07168-01) and R.L. Erickson is an American Cancer Society Professor of Cellular and Developmental Biology.

REFERENCES

1. Berridge, M. J. (1984). Inositol trisphosphate and diacylglycerol as second messengers. Biochem. J. 220, 345-360.

2. Blenis, J. and Erikson, R. L. (1984). Phosphorylation of the ribosomal protein S6 is elevated in cells transformed by a variety of tumor viruses, J. Virol. 50, 966-969.

3. Blenis, J., Spivack, J.G. and Erikson, R.L. (1984). Phorbol ester, serum and the Rous sarcoma virus transforming gene product induce similar phosphorylations of the ribosomal protein S6, Proc. Natl. Acad. Sci. USA, in press.

4. Blumberg, P. M. (1981). In vitro studies on the mode of action of the phorbol esters, potent tumor promoters, CRC Critical Rev. Toxicol. 8, 153-234.

5. Collett, M. S., Purchio, A. F. and Erikson, R. L. (1980). Avian sarcoma virus-transforming protein, pp60^{src} shows protein kinase activity specific for tyrosine, Nature (London) 285, 167-169.

6. Decker, S. (1981). Phosphorylation of ribosomal protein S6 in avian sarcoma virus-transformed chicken embryo fibroblasts, Proc. Natl. Acad. Sci. USA 78, 4112-4115.

7. Diringer, H. and Friis, R.R. (1977). Changes in phosphatidylinositol metabolism correlated to growth state of normal and Rous sarcoma virus-transformed Japanese quail cells, Cancer Res. 37, 2979-2984.

8. Haselbacher G. K., Humbel R. E. and Thomas, G. (1979). Insulin-like growth factor: insulin or serum increase phosphorylation of ribosomal protein S6 during transition of stationary chick embryo fibroblasts into early G_1 phase of the cell cycle, FEBS Lett. 100, 185-190.

9. Heldin, C.-H. and Westermark, B. (1984). Growth factors: mechanism of action and relation to oncogenes, Cell 37, 9-20.

10. Hunter, T. and Sefton, B. M. (1980). Transforming gene product of Rous sarcoma virus phosphorylates tyrosine, Proc. Natl. Acad. Sci. USA 77, 1311-1315.

11. Kaltschmidt, E. and Wittman, H. G. (1970). Ribosomal proteins: VII: Two-dimensional polyacrylamide gel electrophoresis for fingerprinting of ribosomal proteins, Anal. Biochem. 36, 401-412.

12. Lastick, S. M. and McConkey, E. H. (1980). Control of ribosomal protein phosphorylation in HeLa cells, Biochem. Biophys. Res. Commun. 95, 917-923.

13. Nishizuka, Y. (1984). The role of protein kinase C in cell surface signal transduction and tumour promotion. Nature (London) 308, 693-698.

14. Sawyer, S.T. and Cohen, S. (1981) Enhancement of calcium uptake and phosphatidylinositol turnover by epidermal growth factor in A-431 cells, Biochemistry 20, 6280-6286.

15. Spivack, J. G., Erikson, R. L. and Maller, J. L. (1984). Microinjection of purified pp60[v-src] into Xenopus oocytes increases the phosphorylation of ribosomal protein S6, Mol. Cell. Biol., in press.

16. Sugimoto, Y., Whitman, M., Cantley, L. C. and Erikson, R.L. (1984) Evidence that the Rous sarcoma virus transforming gene product phosphorylates phosphatidylinositol and diacylglycerol, Proc. Natl. Acad. Sci. USA, 2117-2121.

17. Takai, Y., Kishimoto, A., Iwasa, Y., Kawahara, Y., Mori, T.
     and Nishizuka, Y. (1979). Calcium-dependent activation of
     a multifunctional protein kinase by membrane phospholipids,
     J. Biol. Chem. <u>254</u>, 3692-3695.

18. Thomas, G., Siegmann, M. and Gordon, J. (1979). Multiple
     phosphorylation of ribosomal protein S6 during transition
     of quiescent 3T3 cells into early G_1, and cellular
     compartmentalization of the phosphate donor, Proc. Natl.
     Acad. Sci. USA <u>76</u>, 3952-3956.

19. Weinstein, B., Wigler, M., Fisher, P. B., Siskin, E. and
     Pietropaolo, C. (1978). Cell culture studies on the
     biologic effects of tumor promoters. In "Carcinogenesis"
     (Eds. T. J. Slaga, A. Sivak, and R. K. Boutwell) Vol. 2,
     pp. 313-333. Raven Press, NY.

Molecular Biology of Tumor Cells, edited by
B. Wahren et al. Raven Press, New York © 1985.

Retroviral *onc* Gene Proteins: Intracellular Localization and Studies on Transformation Mechanisms

L. R. Rohrschneider, V. M. Rothwell, L. M. Najita, C. H. Ooi, and R. L. Manger

Fred Hutchinson Cancer Research Center, Seattle, Washington 98104

Acute retroviruses are a group of RNA-containing viruses that have acquired an oncogenic potential through the acquisition of a normal cellular gene. More than 20 such viruses have now been isolated and their transforming genes characterized and corresponding proteins identified (20,26). Very rapid progress has been made in the past few years on the analysis of the various viral genes and gene products, and the major challenge ahead now turns from trying to understand the virology to attempting to unravel the cell biology of transformation. The major question becomes: In what manner, shape, and form do the transforming proteins of these viruses interact with the normal cell to initiate and maintain the transformed state?

Our approach to that question has employed mainly the Rous sarcoma virus (RSV) system but we have studied other viral systems as well. We have been concerned with the intracellular locations of various transforming proteins and how these locations might be involved in the induction of particular transformation parameters. In this paper we will introduce the transforming protein of RSV and describe its intracellular target sites. Other transforming proteins will then be described and categorized based on their common intracellular localizations. Finally, we will return to the RSV system and describe experiments on the functional analysis of the RSV transforming protein (pp60^{src}) with a particular target site, the cellular adhesion plaques.

METABOLISM OF pp60^{src}

Rous sarcoma virus (RSV) has been one of the first and foremost retroviruses in the study of the mechanism of transformation and the synthesis and metabolism of its transforming protein have been extensively studied (for review see ref. 18). The transforming gene of RSV is termed v-src and the protein product, pp60^{src}, is synthesized on free cytoplasmic polyribosomes. Shortly after synthesis, pp60^{src} transiently associates with two host cell phosphoproteins of 50 kDa and 90 kDa before final deposition on the cytoplasmic face of the plasma membrane (5,6). The transit time between synthesis and association with the membrane is relatively rapid, about 15 min., and includes phosphorylation at ser #17 by a cAMP-dependent protein kinase, and myristilation near the amino terminal end of pp60^{src} (6,29). The latter modification is believed to be important for membrane association although it is not entirely clear whether pp60^{src} is directly affiliated with the lipid bilayer, or rather, bound to cytoskeletal elements subjacent to the plasma membrane. pp60^{src} ultimately becomes phosphorylated on tyrosine #416 concomitant with its acquisition of tyrosine kinase activity. This step is presumably due to autophosphorylation.

LOCALIZATION OF pp60^{src} AND RELATED ONC PROTEINS

The cytoplasmic face of the plasma membrane is the principal cellular location of pp60^{src}. Perhaps as much as 80% of pp60^{src} may be found in the plasma membrane depending on cell type studied and method of analysis. The src protein is uniformly distributed throughout the cytoplasmic face of the membrane, and most interestingly, also concentrated at very specialized regions of the membrane that govern substratum attachment, cell shape, and possibly intercellular communication (19,24,25,33). These specialized regions are the focal adhesion plaques and the cell-cell junctions (25). The former structures serve as focal points for microfilament bundle organization within the cell and fibronectin attachment on the outside of the cell (18,26). It is interesting that adhesion plaques are connected with several properties of a cell that becomes altered upon RSV-induced transformation and therefore the location of pp60^{src} at these sites suggests that this interaction could be responsible for at least some properties of the transformed cell.

The transforming protein of RSV is not the only onc protein that has been found in the substratum adhesion areas of the infected cell. Rather, the RSV pp60^{src} is but the prototype of a group of viruses that encode related onc proteins and express those proteins at related subcellular sites. The results in Fig. 1a demonstrate the adhesion plaque localization of pp60^{src} in RSV transformed cells. The transforming proteins of both Abelson MuLV (A-MuLV) and Esh sarcoma virus (ESV) are related to the src protein at both the nucleotide and protein sequence levels (16,23) and the results in Figs. 1b and 1c demonstrate that, like pp60^{src}, the transforming proteins of these viruses are also situated in focal adhesion areas of cells infected with the respective virus (12,27). In addition, Yamaguchi 73 (Y73) virus has acquired the same oncogene as Esh and its transforming protein also has been detected in adhesion plaques (12). These data indicate that a class of onc proteins exists that shares a common intracellular target site and may induce at least some transformation parameters by a common mechanism through the cellular adhesion plaques.

All the onc proteins that localize in substratum adhesion areas contain an associated tyrosine-specific kinase activity. This localization, however, does not appear to be a property of tyrosine kinases per se because not all onc proteins with this activity are found at these sites. For example, Fujinami sarcoma virus (FuSV) and other related viruses that carry the fps (or fes) oncogene show a high degree of homology to the src protein, contain a tyrosine-specific kinase activity but are not detectable in cellular adhesion areas (26) (Fig. 1d). Instead, these proteins are cytoplasmic and exhibit a salt dependent association with the plasma membrane (11). This again argues that some special features of the src-class of proteins determine their localization and transformation mechanisms.

OTHER CLASSES OF ONC PROTEINS BASED ON INTRACELLULAR LOCALIZATION

Still other onc proteins are found at cellular sites that clearly distinguish them from the previously mentioned proteins. The fms protein is encoded in the genome of the McDonough strain of

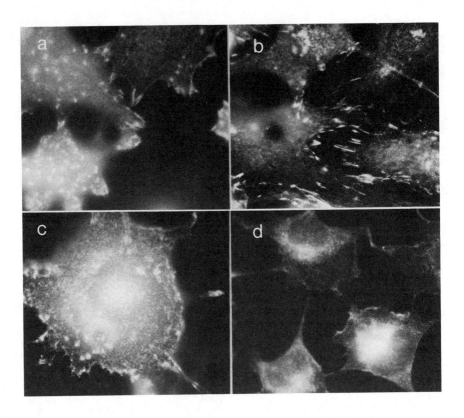

Fig. 1.   Localization of retroviral onc proteins by
indirect   immunofluorescence.   a.)   pp60^{src} in
RSV-transformed   chicken   embryo   cells   (CEC)   b.)
P80$^{gag-yes}$ in Esh sarcoma virus transformed CEC.   c.)
P120$^{gag-abl}$ in   A-MuLV   transformed   normal   rat   kidney
(NRK) cells.   d.) P85$^{gag-fes}$ in ST-FeSV transformed
NRK cells.   All but the P85$^{gag-fes}$ can be detected in
substratum adhesion structures.

feline sarcoma virus (Sm-FeSV) and is expressed as a
set   of   three   glycoproteins   termed   gp180$^{gag-fms}$,
gp140^{fms},   gp120^{fms} (3,13).   Antibodies   to   these
transforming   proteins   stain   the   surface   of   SM-FeSV
transformed   cells   indicating   that   at   least   one   of
these proteins is expressed on the cell surface (21)
(Fig. 2a).   Both cell surface iodination studies as
well as galactose oxidase followed by tritiated NaBH$_4$
reduction were used to specifically label and identify
the gp140^{fms} as the cell surface expressed species
(21).   Further results indicate that gp140^{fms} may be
found in clathrin-coated endocytotic pits and vesicles

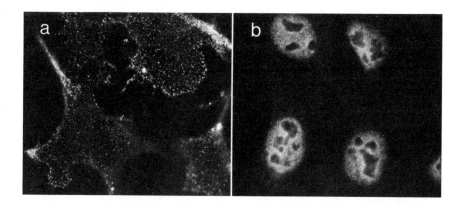

Fig. 2. Localization of other retroviral onc proteins by indirect immunofluorescence. a.) The transforming protein of SM-FeSV (gp140^{fms}) is found on the external surface of transformed mink cells. b.) Nuclear localization of the myc-containing transforming proteins of OK10 virus.

(21). This suggests that gp140^{fms} could represent another modified growth factor receptor as first described for the erb-B protein of avian erythroblastosis virus.

In addition to the plasma membrane localization, the nucleus also serves as a target for several other onc proteins derived from both mammalian and avian species. The first of these nuclear onc proteins to be described was the myc protein of myelocytomatosis virus (MC29) (1,7), and an example of this localization is shown in Fig. 2b. The other transforming proteins found primarily in the nucleus are listed in Table 1, and described in ref. 26.

Results from several sources are presented in Table 1 and it is clear that the various transforming proteins can be categorized according to their intracellular target site. This classification also implies functional differences in transforming mechanisms that may aid in our understanding of pathways that control normal cell growth. One class of proteins, typified by pp60^{src}, is found on the cytoplasmic face of the plasma membrane but with the unique additional attribute of localizing in cellular

TABLE 1.   Retroviral transforming protein
classification based on intracellular localization.
onc-gene proteins are listed in categories determined
by common intracellular locations.   Other proteins
from onc genes such as raf, fgr, ros, rel, ski, and
ets may also fit in these or additional categories
when their target sites are determined. ros has been
included in the fps group because the nucleotide
sequence data suggest a closer relation to these
proteins (L.H. Wang, personal communication).   For
additional details see ref. 26.

src (RSV)	$pp60^{src}$	membrane-adhesion plaque
yes (Y73)	$P90^{gag-yes}$	" "
abl (A-MuLV)	$P120^{gag-abl}$	" "
fps (PRCII)	$P110^{gag-fps}$	cytoplasm-membrane
fps (FuSV)	$P140^{gag-fps}$	" "
fes (ST-FeSV)	$P85^{gag-fes}$	" "
?ros (UR2)	$P68^{gag-ros}$	" "
fms (SM-FeSV)	$gp140^{fms}$	cell-surface
erbB (AEV)	$gp74^{erbB}$	"
fos (FBJ-virus)	$pp55^{fos}$	nuclear
myc (MC29)	$P110^{gag-myc}$	"
(CMII)	$P90^{gag-myc}$	"
(MH2)	$p60^{myc}$	"
(OK10)	$P200^{gag-myc}$	"
myb (AMV)	$p48^{myb}$	"
Ha-ras (HaMSV)	$pp21^{ras}$	membrane
Ki-ras (KiMSV)	$pp21^{ras}$	"
sis (SSV)	$gp28^{sis}$	growth factor analogue
mos (Mo-MSV)	$pp37^{mos}$	cytoplasmic

adhesion structures. A related class of proteins (prototype P140$^{gag-fps}$ of FuSV) share the plasma membrane localization but these proteins show no special affinity for adhesion plaques or related structures. The previous two classes of proteins are situated on the cytoplasmic side of the membrane. A third class of onc proteins (prototype gp75^{erb-B} of AEV) can be detected on the external surface of the cell and represent modified growth factor receptors (4,9). The nuclear proteins (prototype P110$^{gag-myc}$ of MC29) comprise another group in this classification and one could also argue for a separate class for all the ras proteins with their potential relationship to G proteins that activate adenylate cyclase (2). The remainder of the proteins fall into individual classes, the most notable of which is gp28^{sis} because of its homology with the growth hormone PDGF (8,32).

These groups suggest that distinct transformation mechanisms exist but this is perhaps more a function of our current state of understanding than a reflection of reality. Whereas distinct target sites now exist, future results will, no doubt, reveal underlying molecular associations and connections between and among these various sites. Transformation can most likely result from lesions at numerous points along inter-related molecular pathways.

pp60^{src} AND ADHESION PLAQUES

As described above, the adhesion plaque location of pp60^{src} was one of the most intriguing target sites for the RSV transforming protein. These small specialized regions of the membrane were associated with several changes commonly found in RSV transformed cells. To determine whether any properties of a transformed cell could be attributed to the interaction of pp60^{src} with adhesion plaques, several mutants of RSV were studied for pp60^{src} localization and resultant transformed phenotype (28).

Initially, one mutant (CU12) was found that did not express pp60^{src} in adhesion plaques even though cells infected with the mutant virus expressed high levels of tyrosine kinase activity, grew in soft agar and formed tumors in animals. The phenotype of CU12-infected cells, however, was different. These cells were fusiform in morphology (see Fig. 3) and fibronectin was present in the extracellular matrix. Other mutants of RSV that also induced the fusiform transformed morphology were checked and again all failed to show localization of pp60^{src} in adhesion plaques, and all expressed extracellular matrix fibronectin at near normal levels (in preparation). These results suggested that the binding of pp60^{src} to adhesion plaques might be related in some way to the expression of fibronectin and the fusiform morphology. Although other explanations also are possible, this notion seemed particularly plausible because of the direct connection reported between cellular adhesion areas and fibronectin, and the fact that fibronectin alone is sufficient to induce the fusiform morphology in RSV transformed cells (14,34) and may also regulate gene expression in some cells (30).

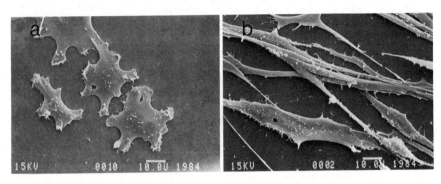

Fig. 3.   Scanning electron micrographs of RSV transformed CEC.   a.) CEC transformed with wild-type B77 strain of RSV.   b.) CEC transformed with CU12, a fusiform mutant of RSV.

WILD-TYPE vs. FUSIFORM TRANSFORMED MORPHOLOGY

In experiments originally designed to measure the conversion of fusiform transformed cells to the wild-type morphology upon superinfection with a wild-type virus, it was discovered that the fusiform morphology was, in fact, dominant to the wild-type transformed morphology in the system employed. If chicken embryo cells (CEC) were initially transformed with the fusiform mutant CU12 and, when completely transformed, superinfected with the wild-type virus B77, no change in cellular morphology could be detected (see Fig. 4).   If, however, CEC were initially transformed with the wild-type B77 virus and then superinfected with the fusiform CU12 virus, conversion to the fusiform morphology began within three days and was complete after one-to-two passages when 80-90% of the cells had converted to the fusiform morphology.

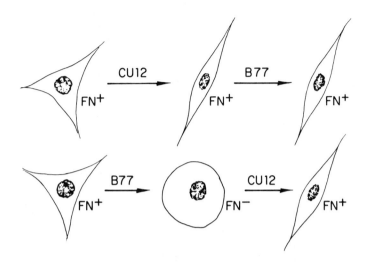

Fig. 4. Superinfection experiments to test the dominance of the wild-type vs. the fusiform transformed morphology. Normal CEC on the left are transformed with either CU12 or B77 virus then superinfected with the other virus. The morphology of the transformed cells is shown. FN refers to the expression of fibronectin in the extracellular matrix, other details are described in the text.

The time course for the conversion to the fusiform morphology following superinfection was similar to that observed following infection with CU12 alone. This suggested that the effect could not be due to mutation or recombination but instead represented a dominance of the fusiform morphology over the wild-type transformed morphology.

Another interesting and pertinent observation concerning the conversion to the fusiform morphology is that fibronectin (FN) expression also is coordinately regulated in the conversion to the fusiform morphology. Cells transformed with RSV virus exhibit a greatly reduced expression of fibronectin in the extracellular matrix and have reduced levels of fibronectin mRNA (10). Upon superinfection with CU12 and coordinately with conversion to the fusiform morphology, the cells re-express fibronectin in the matrix at elevated levels. Further analyses indicate that neither fibronectin mRNA levels nor fibronectin

translation rates are affected suggesting that the
re-expression is controlled at a post-translational
stage.   This finding is consistent with the previous
results on all other fusiform transformed cells and
again argues for the involvement of fibronectin in
determining the fusiform transformed morphology.

The dominance of the fusiform morphology is
probably not universal but confined to particular
combinations of viruses or experimental conditions.
CU12 is also dominant to certain clones of
Schmidt-Ruppin (subgroup D) strain of RSV as well as
Prague C, however, other clones of wild-type virus are
not converted to the fusiform morphology upon
superinfection with CU12.   This argues that the CU12
pp60^{src} is trans-dominant for morphological conversion
to the fusiform cell shape but that other undefined
factors are also at play in this process.   This view
is consistent with results presented more than 20
years ago by Temin (31).

POSSIBLE MECHANISMS FOR THE CONTROL OF
THE TRANSFORMED MORPHOLOGY

The finding that the fusiform transformed
morphology can act in a trans-dominant fashion is
surprising and we have considered several possible
mechanisms to account for this behavior.   The basic
premise in these mechanisms is that the wild-type and
fusiform pp60^{src} proteins must directly compete
against each other.   There seems no alternative
explanation especially considering that one protein is
derived from the other and their functions must be
related.

The first possibility that we considered was that
the fusiform src protein is able to block the
transport of the wild-type src protein to a particular
target site (Fig. 5) thus preventing complete
transformation and resulting in the fusiform
morphology.   This mechanism is possible, however, our
preliminary results suggest that the transport of
wild-type pp60^{src} to the adhesion plaque sites is not
blocked by the fusiform pp60^{src}.   Transport to other
sites may still be blocked but this is not obvious, at
least from immunofluorescence results.

Another possible mechanism could involve direct
competition for binding specific cellular targets.   If

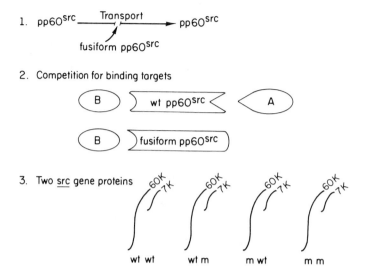

Fig. 5. Possible mechanisms to explain the transdominance of the CU12 fusiform morphology over the B77 wild-type transformed morphology. Further details are given in the text.

we assume that pp60^{src} normally has two separate sites for binding two different cellular proteins, then the fusiform mutation could be envisioned as a destruction of one of those binding sites (Fig. 5, mech. #2). If the host protein "A" were situated in the adhesion plaques (for example) and the host protein "B" were cytoplasmic, then the wild-type pp60^{src} could still bind to the adhesion plaque sites but the fusiform pp60^{src} would effectively compete for binding the "B" host protein and block the function of wild-type pp60^{src}. This could also explain the fact that the fusiform pp60^{src} does not localize in adhesion plaques.

Results from both genetic and biochemical studies on various fusiform mutants of RSV serves as the basis for yet another possible mechanism to explain the fusiform morphology and its trans-dominance over the wild-type transformed morphology. Work by Mardon and Varmus (22) has suggested that the src-gene may synthesize a second gene protein of 7 kDa from a reading frame different than that used to synthesize pp60^{src}. The interesting point concerning this protein is that a fusiform mutant is generated by deletion of the region that codes for the 7 kDa protein (15,17). This suggests that the 7 kDa src protein might exist and that it might be involved in regulating fibronectin expression and the transformed cell morphology.

The third mechanism presented in Fig. 5, therefore, proposes that the 60 kDa and 7 kDa src protein operate together to induce the total transformed phenotype. Perhaps then, mutations in the 60 kDa src protein or deletion of the 7 kDa src protein would produce the fusiform morphology. The trans-dominance of the fusiform over the wild-type morphology could then occur through phenotypic mixing of mutant (m) and wild-type (wt) 60 kDa and 7 kDa protein resulting in impaired src-gene function.

SUMMARY

The mechanism of transformation by retroviruses has been studied by examining the intracellular localization of the transforming proteins from these viruses. Distinct classes of transforming proteins can be defined based on their intracellular localization at specific target sites. One such class includes the src-gene product of RSV, the abl-gene product of A-MuLV, and the yes-gene protein of Y73 and Esh viruses. This class is distinguished by its unique localization in cellular adhesion plaques along with adherence to the cytoplasmic face of the plasma membrane. Analysis of src gene mutants of RSV suggested that the interaction of pp60^{src} with adhesion plaques was associated with the expression of extracellular fibronectin and morphological transformation and possible mechanisms were considered to explain the fusiform morphology and its trans-dominance over the wild-type transformed morphology.

Acknowledgement

This work was supported by Public Health Service grants CA 20551 and CA 28151 from the National Cancer Institute. R.L.M. was supported by a postdoctoral fellowship from an N.I.H. training grant.

REFERENCES

1. Abrams, H.D., Rohrschneider, L.R. and Eisenman, R.N. (1982): Cell, 29: 427-439.

2. Alberts, B., Bray, D., Lewis, J., Roff, M., Roberts, K. and Watson, J.D. (1983): Molecular Biology of the Cell, Chs. 6 and 13. Garland Publishing, New York.

3. Anderson, S.J., Furth, M., Wolff, L., Ruscetti, S.K. and Sherr, C.J. (1982): J. Virol., 44: 696-702.

4. Beug, H. and Hayman, M.J. (1984): Cell, 36: 963-972.

5. Brugge, J.S., Yonemoto, W. and Darrow, D. (1983): Mol. Cell. Biol., 3: 9-19.

6. Courtneidge, S.A. and Bishop, M.J. (1982): Proc. Natl. Acad. Sci. USA, 79: 7117-7121.

7. Donner, P., Greiser-Wilke, I. and Moelling, K. (1982): Nature (London), 296: 262-266.

8. Doolittle, R.F., Hunkapiller, M.W., Hood, L.E., Devare, S.G., Robbins, K.C., Aaronson, S.A. and Antoniades, H.N. (1983): Science, 221: 275-277.

9. Downward, J., Yarden, Y., Mayes, E., Scrace, G., Totty, N., Stockwell, P., Ullrich, A., Schlessinger, I. and Waterfield, M.D. (1984): Nature (London), 307: 521-527.

10. Fagen, J.B., Sobel, M.E., Yamada, K.M., deCrombrugghe, B. and Pastan, I. (1981): J. Biol. Chem., 256: 520-525.

11. Feldman, R.A., Wang, E. and Hanafusa, H. (1983): J. Virol. 45: 782-791.

12. Gentry, L.E. and Rohrschneider, L.R. (1984): J. Virol., 51:in press.

13. Hampe, A., Gobet, M., Sherr, C.J. and Galibert, F. (1984): Proc. Natl. Acad. Sci. USA, 81: 85-89.

14. Hsieh, P. and Chen, L.B. (1983): J. Cell. Biol. 96: 1208-1217.

15. Iwashita, S., Kitamura, N. and Yoshida, M. (1983): Virology, 125: 419-431.

16. Kitamura, N., Kitamura, A., Toyoshima, K., Hirayama, Y. and Yoshida, M. (1982): Nature (London), 297: 205-208.

17. Kitamura, H. and Yoshida, M. (1983): J. Virol., 46: 985-992.

18. Krueger, J.G., Garber, E.A. and Goldberg, A.R. (1983): In: Current Topics in Mircobiology and Immunology, Vol. 107, pp. 52-124. Springer Verlag.

19. Krueger, J.G., Wang, E. and Goldberg, A.R. (1980): Virology, 101: 25-40.

20. Land, H., Parada, L.R. and Weinberg, R.A. (1983): Nature (London), 222: 771-778.

21. Manger, R.L., Nichols, E., Hakomori, S. and Rohrschneider, L.R. (1984): manuscript in preparation.

22. Mardon, G. and Varmus, H.E. (1983): Cell, 32: 871-879.

23. Reddy, E.P., Smith, M.J. and Srinivasan, A. (1983): Proc. Natl. Acad. Sci. USA, 80: 3623-3627.

24. Rohrschneider, L.R. (1979): Cell, 16: 11-24.

25. Rohrschneider, L.R. (1980): Proc. Natl. Acad. Sci. USA, 77: 3514-3518.

26. Rohrschneider, L.R. and Gentry, L.E. (1984): In: Advances in Viral Oncology, Vol. 4, edited by G. Klein, pp. 269-306. Raven Press.

27. Rohrschneider, L.R. and Najita, L.M. (1984): J. Virol., 51:in press.

28. Rohrschneider, L.R. and Rosok, M.J. (1983): Mol. Cell. Biol., 3: 731-746.

29. Sefton, B.M., Trowbridge, I.S., Cooper, J.A. and Scolnick, E.M. (1982): Cell, 31: 465-474.

30. Spiegelman, B.M. and Ginty, G.A. (1983): Cell, 35: 657-666.

31. Temin, H.M. (1961): Virology, 13: 158-163.

32. Waterfield, M.D., Scrace, G.T., Whittle, N., Stroobant, P., Johnsson, A., Wasteson, A., Westermark, B., Helden, C.-H., Huang, J.S. and Deuel, T.F. (1983): Nature (London), 304: 35-39.

33. Willingham, M.C., Jay, G. and Pastan, I. (1979): Cell, 18, 125-134.

34. Yamada, K.M., Yamada, S.S. and Pastan, I. (1976): Proc. Natl. Acad. Sci. USA, 73: 1217-1221.

Molecular Biology of Tumor Cells, edited by
B. Wahren et al. Raven Press, New York © 1985.

Human Tumor Antigens

Hilary Koprowski and Meenhard Herlyn

The Wistar Institute of Anatomy and Biology, Philadelphia, Pennsylvania 19104

ANTIGENS OF MELANOMA

Human tumors present an advantage for the study of the process of carcinogenesis in vivo particularly when it is possible to observe development of cancer from the precursor cell through benign tumors, precancerous lesions and malignant neoplasms. The best example of this tumor progression (4) is the study of pigmented lesions of the skin from normal melanocytes, through benign lesions referred to as nevi, to precancerous lesions exemplified by dysplastic nevus, and finally, to two types of malignant neoplasm: radial growth phase melanoma with low competence for metastasis, and vertical growth phase melanoma which gives rise to metastasis in the vast majority of cases (7).

The purpose of studying tumors of pigmented lesions was to characterize, if possible, each stage of the malignant process and to use this information as the basis for investigations about the transformation process within this closed system of human carcinogenesis. In our initial efforts at characterization, we investigated the antigenic makeup of cells representing various stages of the neoplastic process by immunological means. In those studies, Balb/c mice were immunized with either live cells, or cell extracts, or culture medium from cells of tumors obtained either from donors or maintained in tissue culture for various lengths of time. Following immunization, spleen cells of mice were processed and fused with cells of non-secreting variants of P3 x 63 Ag8 mouse myeloma (21) to produce hybridomas secreting monoclonal antibodies (MAb). Table 1 shows the repertoire of MAbs generated after immunization of mice with melanoma cells (15).

Several conclusions can be drawn from the examination of the variety of antigens recognized by MAbs binding to the surface of either normal cells (melanocytes) or cells obtained

123

TABLE 1. Immunoreactivities of mouse monoclonal antibodies against melanoma

Reactivity Group	No. of Antibodies Available	Prototype	Isotype	Antigen Identified	Binding to: Melanoma	Nevi	Melanocytes	Cross-Reactivity
A	3	ME 77-71 ME 20.11	γ1 γ1	N.D.[a] p28 K	15/31[b] 7/11	16/46 1/8	0/15 0/2	
B	12 1	ME 95-45 Nu4B	γ1 γ2a	proteoglycan p130 K p105 K	37/42 81/89	27/35 42/49	0/4 0/4	Fetal cells, tumors; of neural crest origin
C	11 1	ME 82-11 ME 31.1	γ1 γ3	p75 K ganglioside	38/42 4/15	36/41 0/12	13/15 0/4	Cells expressing NGF[c] receptor
D	2	ME 11-11	γ1	p84 K	10/17	8/12	0/4	
E	12 1 1	ME 9-61 ME 75-29 ME 36.1	γ2b γ1 γ3	p97 K p120 K ganglioside	26/29 19/19 4/15	12/14 7/8 0/2	0/6 0/8 0/4	Various carcinomas
F	15	ME 5073	γ2b	N.D.[a]	15/15	6/6	4/4	Various normal and malignant cells
G	24	13-17	γ1	HLA-DR	29/38	39/47	0/15	B-lymphocytes

[a] N.D. - not detected.
[b] Ratio of numbers of cultured binding MAb to number of cultures examined.
[c] Nerve growth factor.

from lesions at various stages of the malignant process. Most of the MAbs, regardless of whether they are specific for melanoma-associated antigens or cross-react with other tumor types, react with 90% of either fresh or cultured melanomas obtained from different donors. Most of the MAbs define protein antigens, except for three (one not shown) which define carbohydrate determinants of glycolipids. Many MAbs are directed against the same proteoglycan antigen (24) or the DR antigen, both of which are strongly expressed by melanoma cells. One group of MAbs (Group C) was found to define the nerve growth factor (NGF) receptor (25) (see below).

It is also apparent that this panel of MAbs cannot distinguish between antigen(s) expressed by melanoma cells vis-a-vis antigen(s) expressed by nevus cells maintained in culture (16). However, normal human melanocytes do not bind most MAbs defining melanoma associated antigens. On the other hand, after immunization of mice with nevus cells, the hybridomas generated secrete antibodies that bind to nevus cells and, to a lesser extent, to normal melanocytes but do not react with cells of melanomas. If antigen(s) defined by this group of MAbs is not expressed by cells undergoing malignant transformation, this category of MAbs might be useful for the "negative selection" of nevus cells exposed to various transforming factors.

MAbs that can be used in immunoperoxidase (IP) staining of fixed tissue[1] also do not distinguish between nevus and melanoma cells, but again permit a clear distinction between these lesions and cells of normal skin including melanocytes (Figure 1).

CHROMOSOMAL ABNORMALITIES IN MELANOMAS

As demonstrated conclusively by Balaban et al. (5), cells of malignant melanoma show non-random chromosomal aberrations, which involve in almost all cases chromosome 1 (deletion or translocation of a portion of the short arm) and in many cases, polysomy of chromosome 7. These lesions seem to be characteristic for melanomas since they are rather infrequently encountered in other human malignancies (5). Lesions of chromosome 6 may also be involved in cases of melanoma but probably less frequently than those involving chromosomes 1 and 7. So far no chromosomal abnormalities have been associated with benign nevus cells.

GROWTH FACTORS AND MELANOMAS

The identity of the antigen recognized by the seven MAbs that immunoprecipitated a melanoma-associated antigen of M_r 75,000 (see Table 1) has been confirmed by inhibition of binding of ^{125}I-labeled nerve growth factor (NGF) to melanoma

---

[1]Barbara Atkinson, unpublished observation.

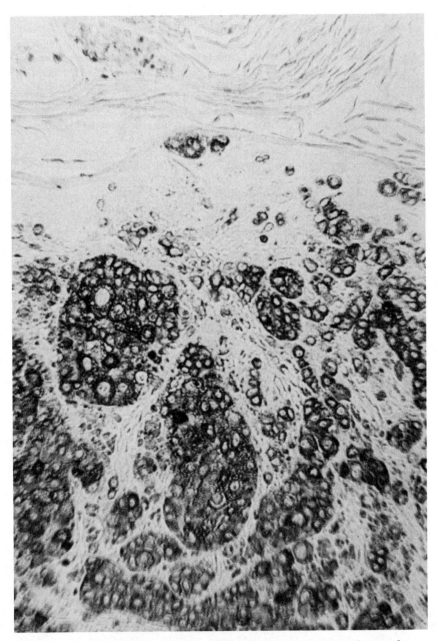

FIG. 1. Paraffin block section of superficial spreading melanoma (SSM) of the skin, level III, with invasion to 0.72 mm.
Melanoma cells both within the epidermis and invasive into the
dermis are strongly reactive with ME492 antibody (MAG antigen)
in the biotin-avidin IP reaction using DAB as the chromagen
(counterstained with hematoxylin, magnification 40X).

TABLE 2. Binding of MAb ME 82-11 (anti-NGF receptor) to melanocytic cells in mixed hemadsorption assay

Melanocytic Cells of:	No. of Cultures Tested	No. positive[a]				
		++++	+++	++	+	-
Metastatic melanoma	27	12	7	6	0	2
Primary melanoma	11	9	1	0	0	1
VGP[b] RGP	2	2	0	0	0	0
Nevi	26	1	11	1	3	10
Normal skin	15	0	2	4	7	2

[a]++++ >80% of cells positive; +++ 40-80% positive; ++ 20-40% positive; and + 5-20% positive
[b]VGP = Vertical growth phase; RGP = radial growth phase.

Since the locus for the epidermal growth factor (EGF) receptor is on human chromosome 7 (17) and since melanoma cells more often than not display polysomy of this chromosome, it was of interest to determine whether EGF receptors were expressed by melanoma cells showing trisomy of chromosome 7. The results in Table 3 indicate that this is the case. EGF receptors were expressed only by cells of those melanomas that showed trisomy of chromosome 7 and that had originated either from vertical growth phase melanoma or from metastatic melanoma, lesions often obtained from different sites of the same patient.

cells by each of the respective MAbs (25). The NGF receptor seems to be expressed by all normal and neoplastic pigmented cells, but its concentration on the cell surface seems to be related to the stage of neoplastic transformation. As shown in Table 2, NGF receptor is present at high concentration on the melanoma cell surface and at low concentration on the surface of normal melanocytes. Although cells of pigmented lesions express the NGF receptor, there is no evidence that these cells actually produce NGF regardless of their stage of malignant transformation. On the other hand, there is good evidence that melanoma cells in culture produce growth factors, as demonstrated by the mitogenic effect of tissue culture media

TABLE 3. <u>EGF-Receptor expression by melanocytic cells</u>

Origin of cells		Chromosomal abnormality involving chromosome 7	Presence of EGF Receptor
Normal skin	FM47	None	No
	FM48	None	No
	FM49	None	No
Congenital nevus	WML938	None	No
	WML941	None	No
Primary radial growth phase melanoma	WM245	None	No
	WM35	None	No
Primary vertical growth phase melanoma	WM75**	-7	No
	WM902B		No
	WM278	Normal	No
	WM-853-2	Normal	No
	WM793	+7;7p+	Yes
	WM115*	+7	Yes
Metastatic melanoma	WM373**	del(7)(q22)	No
	WM46	Normal	No
	SKMEL23	7q+(q36)	No
	SKMEL37	7p+q+(p22q36)	No
	WM918	t1;7(p;q)+7;1(p;q)	No
	WM239A*	+7	Yes
	WM-266-4*	+7	Yes
	WM873-1***	+7	Yes
	WM873-2***	+7	Yes
	WM873-3***	+7	Yes
	WM858***	+7	Yes

Asterisks indicate samples obtained from tumors at different sites of the same patient.

from these cells on normal human fibroblasts, and that one of the growth factors produced is closely related to or identical with platelet-derived growth factor (PDGF)[2].

ONC GENE(S)

No significant results have been obtained so far to indicate the presence of <u>onc</u> gene(s) in human melanoma. The

[2]Bengt Westermark, unpublished observation.

TABLE 4. <u>Characteristics of melanocytic cells in culture</u>

Characteristics	Origin of Cells			
	Skin melanocytes	Nevus	Radial growth phase	Vertical growth phase and metastases
Growth in culture:				
Promoter required	Yes[a]	No	No	No
Anchorage independence	No	Yes	Yes	Yes
Growth factor production	No	No	No	Yes
NGF receptor	Yes[b]	Yes[b]	Yes[b]	Yes[b]
EGF receptor	No	No	No	Yes[c]
Finite lifetime	Yes	Yes	?	No
Chromosomal abnormalities	No	No	Yes	Yes
Tumors in nude mice	No	No	No	Yes
Antigens expressed[d]				
MAA	No	Yes	Yes	Yes
NAA	Yes	Yes	Yes	No

[a]Phorbol ester or bovine brain extract
[b]In increasing concentration for malignant cells
[c]Only in tumors with chromosome 7 trisomy
[d]MAA = Melanoma-associated antigen;
   NAA = Nevus-associated antigen.

break in the segment of chromosome 1 occurs at the loci for
the N-<u>ras onc</u> gene (3) and for the beta chain of NGF (9).
However, there is as yet no evidence for involvement of N-
<u>ras</u>, and no data are available on the homology of NGF
sequences with any known <u>onc</u> gene. Thus, this line of
investigation awaits further experimentation. On the other
hand, expression of EGF receptor by cells of metastatic
melanoma (Table 3) makes it interesting to study amplification of the <u>erb</u>-b gene by the same cells in light of the

sequence homology between the EGF receptor and the erb-b
gene (8). If the growth factor produced by melanoma cells
is PDGF, one can consider screening melanoma cells for the
presence of the c-sis gene, considering the sequence homology between PDGF and Simian sarcoma virus (SSV) (29). It
should be pointed out, however, that the locus for PDGF is
on chromosome 22 (28) and there are no indications that this
chromosome is involved in melanomas.

CHARACTERISTICS OF MELANOCYTIC CELLS IN CULTURE

These are summarized in Table 4. Normal melanocytes
require the addition of either phorbol ester or bovine brain
extract to the culture medium as promoters. Cells obtained
from nevi and melanomas require no exogenous factors for
growth and, unlike melanocytes, are anchorage-independent.

As mentioned before, only cells originating from either
primary or vertical growth phase melanoma or from metastases
of the tumor produce growth factor (PDGF?), and those cells
that show trisomy of chromosome 7 express EGF receptors.
The NGF receptor is expressed in increasing concentrations
by the more malignant cells of the melanocytic series.
Cultures of nevi, like those of normal human cells, have a
finite lifetime. It is often difficult to establish
cultures originating from radial growth phase melanoma but,
once established, the cultures can be maintained for prolonged periods of time, perhaps even indefinitely. Only
cultures of primary vertical growth phase melanoma and
metastatic melanomas can be maintained indefinitely and also
produce tumors in nude mice.

Analysis of the data presented in Table 4 shows a
striking contrast between the characteristics of cultures of
skin melanocytes and those of primary vertical growth phase
and metastatic melanomas. The differences in culture
characteristics between nevi and radial growth phase melanoma cells, on the one hand, and between those cultures and
normal melanocytes and metastatic melanoma, respectively,
are slightly blurred. For example, cells derived from nevi
and skin melanocytes have a finite lifetime in culture and
express the nevus-associated antigen (NAA). However, unlike
melanocytes, cultures of nevi do not require exogenous factors for growth and share this characteristic and also
anchorage independence with malignant cells. Antigens
expressed by melanomas are also expressed by cells derived
from nevi. Some of these characteristics may be attributed
to the preselection for cells from each tissue that will
grow in culture, and to the heterogeneity of cells maintained in culture. However, progeny cultures of single cell
clones of melanoma cultures show remarkable homogeneity
(13), and identical characteristics are displayed by

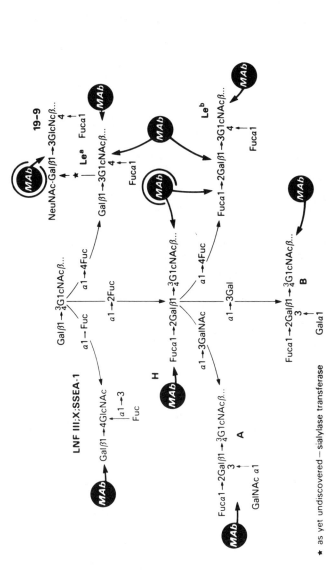

FIG. 2. Monoclonal antibodies (MAb) that bind to carbohydrate moieties of antigen representing major and minor blood groups. The precursor is lactotetraosylceramide when galactose is linked β1-3 to glucosamine, or paragloboside when galactose is linked β1-4 to glucosamine. Arrows indicate the glucosyltransferases that produce the antigens from the two precursors. The sialylase which transfers sialic acid to Le[a] carbohydrate to synthesize antigen 19-9 is unknown. (Reprinted with permission of Grune and Stratton.)

cultures derived from lesions of the same donors at different stages of tumor progression.

ADENOCARCINOMAS OF GASTROINTESTINAL TRACT

Most of the antigen(s) defined by MAbs against melanoma are proteins (Table 1). However, immunization of mice with cells of gastrointestinal cancers results in the production of hybridomas that secrete MAbs binding to glycolipids (14). Figure 2 shows the carbohydrate determinants of glycolipids (14) recognized by these MAbs. Either of the carbohydrate compounds lactotetraosylceramide (Galβ1$\rightarrow$3GlcNAcβ...) or paragloboside (Galβ1$\rightarrow$4GlcNAcβ...) or both are precursors for carbohydrate moieties of glycolipids representing major (H and AB) or minor (Lewis A and B) blood groups. The lacto-N-fucopentaose III, also defined by MAbs against gastrointestinal cancers, has been described elsewhere (10) as stage-specific embryonic antigen (SSEA) and is one of the very few antigens shared by humans and other species (mouse), as detected by MAbs against human tumors.

As shown in Figure 2, one MAb recognizes determinants shared by Lewis B and H carbohydrates, and another MAb, determinants shared by Lewis A and B carbohydrates (14). The remaining MAbs are specific for a given glycolipid.

GASTROINTESTINAL CANCER ANTIGEN (GICA or 19-9)

The antigen recognized by MAb 19-9 (Figure 2) is a ganglioside with a sialylated Lewis A carbohydrate (22). This antigen is expressed by cells of adenocarcinomas of the gastrointestinal tract (stomach, pancreas, colon and rectum) and is also found in meconium, probably because of the presence of shed fetal intestinal cells. Except for its expression by one layer of epithelial cells lining the secretory ducts of normal pancreas, bronchi, etc., and its secretion in saliva of individuals phenotypically Le^{a+b-} and Le^{a-b+}, it is not found in any other tissue of normal individuals. Its presence in the sera of patients with gastrointestinal cancer has been exploited in the diagnosis of cancer. GICA is expressed in cells of intestinal polyps (adenomas) and current investigations are aimed at determining whether the presence of GICA in sera of subjects with familial polyposis correlates with malignant transformation of the polyps[3].

Radiolabeled MAb 19-9 can be used either alone or in combination with MAbs defining carcinoembryonic antigen (CEA) (6) for the imaging of gastrointestinal tract cancers in patients. In some cases, immunoscintigraphy with an MAb is the only method to localize these types of cancer in the human body (23).

---

[3]Carol Makin, personal communication.

DESTRUCTION OF GASTROINTESTINAL CANCERS

Human tumors xenotransplanted to nude mice are destroyed by MAb (11). As shown in Table 5, MAbs with tumoricidal ability were, with the exception of one MAb, all of IgG2a isotype. MAbs mediated this tumoricidal effect through interaction with macrophages. This specific destruction of tumor cells was also demonstrated in vitro by "arming" peritoneal mouse macrophages with a tumor-binding IgG2a MAb. The expression of Fc receptors that bind IgG2a mouse MAb was induced in macrophages by injecting mice in the peritoneal cavity with thioglycolate broth (1) or by contact of the macrophages with tumor tissue. Destruction of the tumor does not occur through phagocytosis, but by secretion of H_2O_2 by the "induced" macrophages (1). The successful destruction of tumor cells does not depend on the affinity of a given MAb for either Fc receptor of macrophages or for tumor cells, but instead on the concentration of antigenic sites on the surface of the tumor cell binding the MAb (18,12).

TABLE 5. <u>Inhibition of human tumor growth by mouse</u>
<u>monoclonal antibodies</u>

	Monoclonal antibody isotype					
	IgG1	IgG2a	IgG2b	IgG3	IgM	IgA
Number of antibodies tested	16	18	3	2	4	1
Number of tumor growth-inhibiting antibodies	0	9	0	1	0	0

Human macrophages either isolated from tumor tissue or obtained after stimulation of peripheral blood monocytes with γ-interferon (2) or obtained after prolonged cultivation in vitro (27) express Fc receptors for mouse IgG2a MAb and destroy tumor cells which bind the respective MAb. Human γ1 seems to bind to the same Fc receptor on human macrophages as mouse IgG2a (Figure 3).

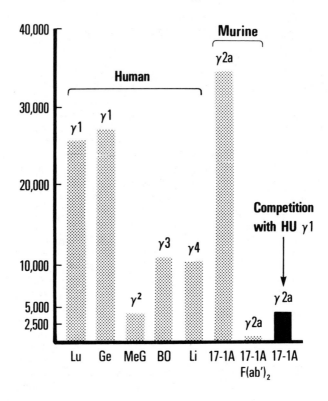

COMPARATIVE BINDING OF ^{125}I–HUMAN
IMMUNOGLOBULIN AND MOUSE 17-1A TO
HUMAN MACROPHAGES

FIG. 3. Human peripheral blood monocytes maintained in
culture for 30 days were expressed to either ^{125}I-labeled
mouse IgG2a or ^{125}I-labeled fractions of human IgG (kindly
provided by Dr. Keith Dorrington, Toronto, Canada).
Although binding values were highest for mouse IgG2a, human
γ1 bound almost as well to macrophages. When macrophages
were first exposed to mouse IgG2a (17-1A MAb) and then to
labeled human γ1, the presence of the mouse IgG2a effectively blocked binding of the human γ1 (solid bar). As
expected, F(ab')$_2$ fragments of mouse 17-1A MAb do not
bind to the Fc receptor of human macrophages (Lubeck, M.,
and Steplewski, Z., personal communication).

IMMUNOREACTIVITY OF HUMAN SUBJECTS TO INJECTION OF
TUMORICIDAL MOUSE MAB

Following intravenous administration of 15-1000 mg of MAb, mouse globulin circulated in the blood of patients for 1-50 days, depending on the dose administered (19,26). Patients injected with less than 250 mg of MAb developed anti-murine antibody. The response of patients who received larger doses of MAb varied. In some patients, administration of 700 mg of MAb followed by 100 mg of MAb at weekly intervals resulted in "tolerance" to mouse globulin maintained by a high T suppressor to T helper cell ratio[4].

All patients with an anti-murine antibody response also developed an anti-idiotype response directed to a specific idiotype of the mouse MAb they received (20). Anti-idiotype can be produced in vitro by stimulation with idiotype (MAb) of B cells obtained from cancer patients injected with MAb[4].

Since specific tumor extracts inhibit binding of anti-idiotype to the idiotype and, at the same time, do not bind to the anti-idiotype, it is possible that the anti-idiotype contains an internal image of the cancer antigen (20). This, in turn, may produce in the patient a reconstructed idiotype (Ab3) which may react to the patient's own tumor. Verification of this hypothesis will require identification of tumor-binding antibodies in the sera of patients who developed anti-idiotype after MAb injection or in the sera of patients who will be immunized with a preformed anti-idiotype of human or animal origin.

ENVOI

Knowledge of human tumor antigens has advanced to the point that identification of the antigen as either protein or carbohydrate is within the capabilities of present-day techniques. MAbs defining these antigens are in use today for diagnosis of human cancer by serological, immunohistological or immunoscintigraphic procedures.

The mechanisms of suppression of human tumor growth by MAbs has been elucidated in experimental models and knowledge of this phenomenon and of the immune response of cancer patients to MAb may ultimately lead to the successful immunotherapy of cancer in man.

Acknowledgement

Work reported here was supported in part by grants CA-25874, CA-21124, CA-33491, and CA-10815 and awarded by the National Cancer Institute, Department of Health and Human Resources.

---

[4]Elaine DeFreitas, personal communication.

REFERENCES

1. Adams, D.O., Hall, T., Steplewski, Z., and Koprowski, H. (1984): Proc. Natl. Acad. Sci. USA, (in press).

2. Akiyama, Y., Lubeck, M.D., Steplewski, Z., and Koprowski, H. (1984): Submitted to Cancer Res.

3. Albino, A.P., Le Strange, R., Oliff, A.I., Furth, M.E., and Old, L.J. (1984): Nature, 308:69-72.

4. Atkinson, B., Ernst, C.S., Herlyn, M., Steplewski, Z., Sears, H.F., and Koprowski, H. (1982): Cancer Res., 42:4820-4823.

5. Balaban, G., Herlyn, M., Guerry, D., Bartolo, R., Koprowski, H., Clark, W.H., and Nowell, P.C. (1984): Cancer Genet. Cytogenet. 11:429-439.

6. Chatal, J-F, Saccavini, J-C, Fumoleau, P., Douillard, J-Y, Curtet, C., Kremer, M., LeMevel, B., and Koprowski, H. (1984): J. Nuclear Med., 25:307-314.

7. Clark, W.H., Elder, D., Guerry, D., Epstein, M.N., Greene, M.H., and Van Horn, M. (1984): Human Pathol. (in press).

8. Downward, J., Yarden, Y., Mayes, E., Scrace, G., Totty, N., Stockwell, P., Ullrich, A., Schlessinger, J., and Waterfield, M.D. (1984): Nature, 307:521-527.

9. Francke, U., De Martinville, B., Coussens, L., and Ullrich, A. (1983): Science, 222:1248-1250.

10. Hakomori, S.I. and Kannagi, R. (1983): J. Natl. Cancer Inst., 71:231-251.

11. Herlyn, D.H. and Koprowski, H. (1982): Proc. Natl. Acad. Sci. USA, 79:4761-4765.

12. Herlyn, D., Herlyn, M., Steplewski, Z., and Koprowski, H. (1984): Submitted to J. Immunol.

13. Herlyn, M., Clark, W.H., Mastrangelo, M.J., Guerry, D., Elder, D.E., LaRossa, D., Hamilton, R., Bondi, E., Tuthill, R., Steplewski, Z., and Koprowski, H. (1980): Cancer Res., 40:3602-3609.

14. Herlyn, M. and Koprowski, H. (1984): In: Clinical Laboratory Molecular Analyses: New Strategies in Autoimmunity, Cancer and Virology, edited by R. Nakamura, W.R. Vito and E.S. Tucker, III. Grune and Stratton, San Diego. (in press).

15. Herlyn, M., Steplewski, Z., Herlyn, D., Clark, W.H., Ross, A.H., Blaszczyk, M., Pak, K.Y., and Koprowski, H. (1983): Cancer Invest. 1:215-224.

16. Herlyn, M., Herlyn, D., Elder, D.E., Bondi, E., LaRossa, D., Hamilton, R., Sears, H.F., Balaban, G., Guerry, D., Clark, W.H., and Koprowski, H. (1983): Cancer Res., 43:5502-5508.

17. Kondo, I. and Shimizu, N. (1983): Cytogenet. Cell Genet., 35:9-14.

18. Koprowski, H. (1984): In: Cancer Cells 1, The Transformed Phenotype, pp.293-297. Cold Spring Harbor Laboratory, New York.

19. Koprowski, H. (1983) In: Monoclonal Antibodies in Cancer - Proceedings of the IV Armand Hammer Cancer Symposium, pp. 17-38. Academic Press, New York.

20. Koprowski, H., Herlyn, D., Lubeck, M., DeFreitas, E., and Sears, H.F. (1984): Proc. Natl. Acad. Sci. USA, 81:216-219.

21. Koprowski, H., Steplewski, Z., Herlyn, D., and Herlyn, M. (1978): Proc. Natl. Acad. Sci. USA, 75:3405-3409.

22. Magnani, J.L., Nilsson, B.L., Brockhaus, M., Zopf, D., Steplewski, Z., Koprowski, H., and Ginsburg, V. (1982): J. Biol. Chem. 257:14365-14369.

23. Moldofsky, P.J., Sears, H.F., Mulhern, C.B., Hammond, N.D., Powe, J., Gatenby, R.A., Steplewski, Z., and Koprowski, H. (1984): New Eng. J. Med. (in press).

24. Ross, A.H., Cossu, G., Herlyn, M., Bell, J.R., Steplewski, Z., and Koprowski, H. (1983): Arch. Biochem. Biophys. 225:370-383.

25. Ross, A.H., Grob, P., Bothwell, M., Elder, D.E., Ernst, C.S., Marano, N., Ghrist, B.F.D., Slemp, C.C., Herlyn, M., Atkinson, B., and Koprowski, H. (1984): Proc. Natl. Acad. Sci. USA (in press).

26. Sears, H.F., Herlyn, D., Steplewski, Z., and Koprowski,
     H. (1984): <u>J. Biological Response Modifiers</u> 3:138-150.

27. Steplewski, Z., Lubeck, M.D., and Koprowski, H.
     (1983): <u>Science,</u> 221:865-867.

28. Swan, D.C., McBride, O.W., Robbins, K.C., Keithley,
     D.A., Reddy, E.P., and Aaronson, S.A. (1982): <u>Proc.
     Natl. Acad. Sci. USA</u>, 79:4691-4695.

29. Waterfield, M.D., Serace, G.T., Whittle, N., Stroolant,
     P., Johnsson, A., Wasteson, A., Westermark, B., Heldin,
     C-H., Huang, J.S., and Deuel, T.F. (1983): <u>Nature</u>
     304:35-39.

Molecular Biology of Tumor Cells, edited by
B. Wahren et al. Raven Press, New York © 1985.

Glycosphingolipids as Differentiation and Tumor Markers and as Regulators of Cell Proliferation

Sen-itiroh Hakomori

Program of Biochemical Oncology/Membrane Research, Fred Hutchinson Cancer Research Center, Seattle, Washington 98104

SIGNIFICANCE OF GLYCOSYLATION

Cells undergo functional modulation by two major chemical modifications, one of which is phosphorylation and another, glycosylation of regulatory proteins, enzymes, and membrane lipids. In addition, less frequent modifications such as methylation, acetylation, and sulfation of enzymes, lipids, regulatory proteins, and pericellular components have been known to occur. Currently, a great deal of interest has been focused on phosphorylation as a ubiquitous and essential modulatory mechanism of cellular function. This idea has been greatly reinforced by the fact that many transforming genes (oncogenes) encode phosphoproteins which by themselves are protein kinases, as extensively discussed in this symposium.

Although less attention has been paid to the process of glycosylation than to phosphorylation, the changes in glycosylation of proteins and membrane lipids occur as quickly and dramatically as the process of phosphorylation at all stages of differentiation, development, and oncogenesis. While phosphorylation patterns are few, the patterns of glycosylation are numerous; over 100 types of glycosylated structures have been identified and characterized among those bound to lipids (glycolipids). Such variation can also be found in the peripheral region of carbohydrates in glycoproteins, in addition to the structural variation in the core region bound to N- or O-glycoside.

In contrast to phosphorylation, which directly regulates protein function, glycosylation affects the conformation, localization, and organization of proteins and lipids in membranes, particularly cell surface membranes, and offers cell recognition sites for cell social events (Table I). With this functional significance of glycosylation in mind, our studies have been directed to i) characterization of glycosylation patterns associated with development, differentiation, and oncogenesis; ii) chemical identification of carbohydrate tumor antigens; iii) a possible regulation of cell growth by gangliosides. These topics have been reviewed extensively (1,2).

THE MAJOR CARBOHYDRATE CHANGES ASSOCIATED WITH DIFFERENTIATION IN EARLY EMBRYO AND IN MOUSE MYELOGENEOUS LEUKEMIA M1 CELLS

Perhaps the most remarkable examples of cell social changes mediated by the change of cell surface membranes have been found in the processes of embryonic development and cellular differentiation. Such membrane changes have been described through the orderly appearance or disappearance of cell surface markers detected by various antibodies, such as blood group ABH, Forssman, and blood group Ii (for a review, see 3,4). The monoclonal antibodies directed to embryonal carcinoma F9 cells and those directed to 4-8 cell stage mouse embryos have been shown to define clear stage-specific changes in certain carbohydrate molecules in the preimplantation embryo (5,6). The antigen defined by the former antibody is called stage-specific embryonic antigen 1 (SSEA-1), which is expressed maximally at the morula and in the inner cell mass of blastocysts, and declines at later stages of differentiation (see Fig. 1). The molecule defined by the latter antibody is expressed maximally at 4-8 cell stage mouse embryos, disappears at later stages of differentiation, and is called stage-specific embryonic antigen 3 (SSEA-3) (see Fig. 1). A monoclonal antibody directed to human teratocarcinoma 2102 defines a similar molecule expressed maximally at 4-8 cell stage embryos, which is called stage-specific embryonic antigen 4 (SSEA-4) (7).

We and others have characterized the chemical structure of the molecules that are defined by these antibodies, as shown in the footnote to Fig. 1. SSEA-1 has been identified as having X-hapten structure (8,9). A series of glycolipid antigens in erythrocyte membranes that are reactive with anti-SSEA-1 antibody have been isolated and characterized as y_2, z_1, and z_2 molecules, as shown in Table II (9). The glycolipid antigens reactive with anti-SSEA-3 antibody have been isolated and characterized from a large quantity (more than 100 ml of cultured packed cells) of human teratocarcinoma 2102. Interestingly, the glycolipids

TABLE I. Biological significance of glycosylation.

Lipid glycosylation:

1) Confers membrane rigidity
2) Regulates membrane protein function (receptors, adhesive proteins, etc.)
3) Determines cell social events, interaction with various ligands (antibodies, toxins, bacterial, viral and cellular lectins)

Protein glycosylation:

1) Maintains protein conformation
2) Affects the rate of protein degradation (regulates turnover)
3) Determines the localization, mobility and organization of proteins
4) Determines cell social events (the same as lipid glycosylation, but more indirectly)

Stage Specific Expression of Two Carbohydrate Epitopes

in Early Mouse Embryo

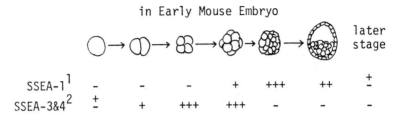

						later stage
SSEA-1[1]	-	-	-	+	+++	++	±
SSEA-3&4[2]	±	+	+++	+++	-	-	-

1. Structure: X-hapten/or LFP III (See Ref. 9,10)

$$Gal\beta1\rightarrow4GlcNAc\beta1\rightarrow R$$
$$\overset{3}{\underset{\uparrow}{}}$$
$$Fuc\alpha1$$

2. Structure: Extended globo-series (See Ref. 11,12)

$$NeuAc\alpha2\rightarrow3\underbrace{Gal\beta1\rightarrow3\underbrace{GalNAc\beta1\rightarrow3Gal\alpha1\rightarrow4Gal}_{3}}_{4}$$

Figure 1. Two major carbohydrate determinants, SSEA-1 and SSEA-3, expressed at different stages of preimplantation mouse embryo. SSEA-3 is maximally expressed at the 2-4 cell stage, in contrast to SSEA-1, which is expressed maximally at the morula and the inner cell mass of the blastocyst. A third antigen, SSEA-4, defined by its monoclonal antibody, constitutes the terminal structure of the same molecule as SSEA-3. The structure defined by the anti-SSEA-4 antibody is NeuAcα2→3Galβ1→3GalNAc (see footnote).

reactive with anti-SSEA-3 antibody belong to a new class of extended globoseries[1], as shown in Table II (10), and the epitope structure is located at the internal GalNAcβ1→3Galα1→4Gal chain. Galβ1→3 substitution to the GalNAc residue of globoside is essential to enhance the reactivity of the SSEA-3 antibody. The antibody to SSEA-4 has been identified as recognizing the terminal NeuAcα2→3Galβ1→3GalNAc residue (7). Thus, a new globoseries ganglioside (GL-7) can be defined by the antibodies to SSEA-3 and SSEA-4.

---

[1] Three series of glycolipids are defined as follows: ganglioseries contain Galβ1→3GalNAcβ1→4Galβ1→4Glc, lactoseries contain Galβ1→4GlcNAcβ1→3Galβ1→4Glc, and globoseries contain GalNAcβ1→3Galα1→4Galβ1→4Glc as the core structure (1).

TABLE II. <u>Carbohydrate structures defined by SSEA-1, 3, and 4</u>

<u>SSEA-1</u> (from 7,9,10)

y_2 Galβ1→4GlcNAcβ1→3Galβ1→4GlcNAcβ1→3LacCer
           3
           ↑
        Fucα1

z_1 Galβ1→4GlcNAcβ1→3Galβ1→4GlcNAcβ1→3Galβ1→4GlcNAcβ1→3LacCer
           3
           ↑
        Fucα1

z_2 Galβ1→4GlcNAcβ1→3Galβ1→4GlcNAcβ1→3Galβ1→4GlcNAcβ1→3LacCer
           3   3
           ↑   ↑
        Fucα1   Fucα1

<u>SSEA-3</u> (Extended globoseries)

GL4   GalNAcβ1→3Galα1→4Galβ1→4Glcβ1→1Cer

GL5   <u>Galβ1→3GalNAcβ1</u>→3Galα1→4Galβ1→4Glcβ1→1Cer

GL7   <u>NeuAcα2→3Galβ1→3GalNAcβ1</u>→3Galα1→4Galβ1→4Glcβ1→1Cer

<u>SSEA-4</u>

Since SSEA-3 defines an earlier stage in early mouse embryos than SSEA-1, a drastic shift from globo- to lactoseries may take place during the process of differentiation from the 4-8 cell stage embryo, through morula, to blastocyst (see Fig. 2). Since undifferentiated human teratocarcinoma 2102 cells express SSEA-3 and 4, but not SSEA-1, and differentiated cells express SSEA-1, but a lower quantity of SSEA-3 and 4, a similar shifting from globo- to lactoseries structures may take place during differentiation of human teratocarcinoma, and perhaps in human embryos as well (7).

A similar change of glycolipids from ganglio- through lacto- to globoseries has been noticed during differentiation of mouse myelogeneous leukemia M1 cells. The major glycolipids in undifferentiated myelogeneous leukemia M1 cells have been characterized as gangliotriaosylceramide (Gg3) and i-active lacto-<u>nor</u>octaosylceramide (nLc$_6$). On differentiation, synthesis

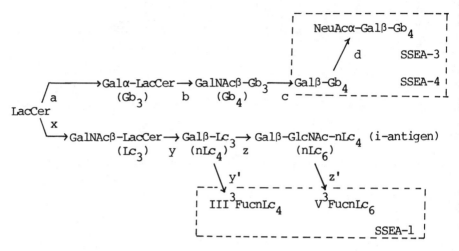

Figure 2. Shifting of glycolipid expression from
extended globoseries (SSEA-3 and 4) to lactoseries with
fucosyl substitution (SSEA-1), which occurs associated with
early embryogenesis. Globoseries synthesis as in route
a→b→c→d leads to the expression of SSEA-3 and 4 antigens and
declines at the morula stage. In turn, synthesis of
lactoseries as in route x→y→z and y→y', z→z' is greatly
enhanced, which leads to the expression of i antigen and
SSEA-1.

of ganglioseries glycolipids declines and lactoseries synthesis
is enhanced, which leads to the synthesis of I-active branched
lacto-isooctaosyl structure. On further differentiation into
macrophage-like Ml$^+$ cells, synthesis of globoseries is initiated,
which leads to the formation of P^k positive cells (Fig. 3)(11).

At present, the biological significance of such a drastic
change from one series to another series of carbohydrate structure during the processes of differentiation and development is
not well known. The process of cell recognition may be dramatically altered and cell adhesion may be greatly modified, which is
an important basis for cell differentiation and development.
Recently we have observed that the compaction of the morulae was
inhibited by liposomes containing monofucosylated X-hapten, i.e.,
y_2 glycolipid (V^{3}FucnLc$_6$) or z_1 glycolipid (VII^{3}FucnLc$_8$) (see
Table II) (Fenderson, B., and Hakomori, S., unpublished observation). The compaction was not inhibited by lactofucopentaose III
or II even at 2 mM concentration. However, the compaction was
inhibited by synthetic lactofucopentaosyl(III) di-lysine
conjugates (Fenderson, B., Zehavi, U., and Hakomori, S.,
unpublished observation). Thus, cell recognition through the
X-hapten having a long chain arm and a multi-valency are
essential to accomplish the process of compaction of morulae, a
key step for the development of the preimplantation embryo.

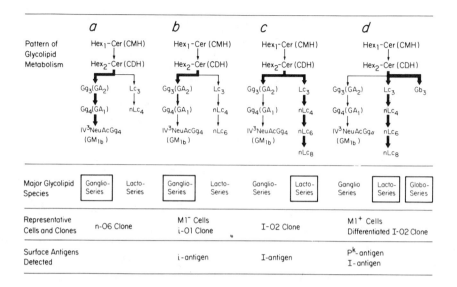

Figure 3. Shifting of glycolipid synthesis from
ganglioseries (a,b) in undifferentiated murine leukemia Ml⁻
cells thorugh lactoseries (b,c) to globoseries (d) associated
with differentiation into macrophage (Ml⁺ cells). Major
synthetic pathway (bold arrow) from Gg_3 to GM_{1b} (stage a) in
undifferentiated cells declines, which leads to a decrease of
GM_{1b}, and an increase of Gg_3 at the initial stage of
differentiation (stage b). Further progress of
differentiation results in enhanced synthesis of nLc_4, nLc_6,
and iLc_8, which leads to conversion from i to I antigen
(stage c). In the terminal stage of differentiation with the
clear appearance of macrophage phenotypes, synthesis of
globoseries is initiated and Gb_3 (P^k antigen) is clearly
expressed. I antigen (iLc_8) is continuously expressed (from
Kannagi et al., 11).

GLYCOLIPID CHANGES ASSOCIATED WITH ONCOGENIC TRANSFORMATION AND TUMOR-ASSOCIATED GLYCOLIPID ANTIGENS

The glycolipid changes observed in a number of transformed
cells in vitro and tumor cells in vivo can be classified into two
types: 1) incomplete synthesis with a frequent accumulation of
precursor glycolipids, and 2) activation of the synthesis of a
new glycolipid which is absent in progenitor cells. In addition,
glycolipids in tumor cells are more exposed than in normal cells
due to organizational changes of tumor cell membranes (for a
review see 2). Either of these processes or a combination of

TABLE III. Types of changes in glycolipids associated with oncogenic transformation.

1. Incomplete synthesis with or without precursor accumulation due to a blocked glycosyltransferase.

   e.g. blocked synthesis of GM_3, GM_1, GT, Gb_4, Gb_5, etc. and accumulation of LacCer, Gg_3, Lc_3, GD_3, GD_2, etc.

2. Neosynthesis due to a de novo activation of glycosyltransferase.

   e.g. synthesis of various fucolipids and sialosyl fucolipids

3. Organizational change of glycolipids in membrane ⟶ loss of crypticity.

mechanisms leads to the formation of tumor-associated antigens (see Table III). With systematic chemical analysis using polyclonal antibodies, glycolipid tumor antigens have been well established in a few experimental tumor systems, such as gangliotriaosylceramide in Kirsten sarcoma in Balb/c mice or in mouse lymphoma L5178 (12,13). The incompatible blood group antigens in some human cancers may represent human cancer-associated antigens (for a review see 2). Since the monoclonal antibody approach was introduced in tumor immunology, a number of "tumor-specific" monoclonal antibodies have been described which define certain glycolipids. Some of them define the precursor glycolipids accumulating in certain types of human cancer, as shown in Table IV. Others define "neoglycolipids", which are essentially absent in normal cells or tissues and are newly synthesized in neoplastic cells and tissues. Typical examples of neoglycolipids are the sialosyl-Le[a] antigen defined by the antibody N-19-9 (17-19), and the poly-X antigen (20-23), as shown in Table V. Particular interest has been aroused by an accumulation of di- or trifucosylated type 2 chain and their sialylated forms (23). Only tumors which accumulate lacto-fucopentaosyl-(III)ceramide accumulate the di- and tri-fucosylated derivatives. A few monoclonal antibodies have been isolated which define these structures (22,23). Some of these monoclonal antibodies, such as FH4 which recognizes internal difucosyl structure (see Fig. 4), show higher specificity and more restricted reactivity for certain types of human cancer cells (24). Application of these monoclonal antibodies, which define specific cell surface carbohydrates, to diagnosis and treatment of human cancer is promising, but further extensive studies are needed.

TABLE IV. <u>Precursor glycolipids accumulating in some human</u>
<u>cancers recognized by monoclonal "tumor-specific" antibodies</u>

1. Globotriaosylceramide (Gb3) in Burkitt lymphoma (14)

Structure: Galα1→4Galβ1→4Glcβ1→1Cer

Observation: a) Rat hybridoma IgM antibody (38-13) was
                 selected for specific reactivity to Burkitt
                 lymphoma.

                 b)$_k$ The antibody defined globotriaosylceramide
                 (P^k antigen).

2. GD$_3$ ganglioside in human melanoma (15,16)

Structure: NeuAcα2→8NeuAcα2→3Galβ1→4Glcβ1→1Cer (GD$_3$)

Observation: Mouse hybridoma antibodies (R24, 4.2) selected
                 by specific reactivity with human melanoma.

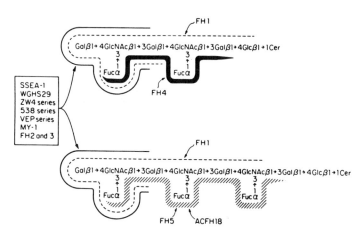

Figure 4. The epitope structure of various antibodies
directed to fucosylated type 2 chain. A number of monoclonal
antibodies to teratocarcinoma and various human cancers such
as WGHS and ZW series (gastrointestinal tumors), 538 series
(lung cancer), and VEP series and My-1 (myelogeneous leukemia) are directed to X-hapten (terminal structure above). In
contrast, FH4, prepared by immunization with a pure difucosyl
type 2 chain (upper structure), is directed towards difucosyl
structure. A possible epitope structure of FH4 is shown by a
bold solid line. Other monoclonal antibodies (FH5, ACFH18)
are directed towards a trifucosylated structure (shown by a
shadow).

TABLE V. <u>Complex glycolipids accumulating in human cancer</u>
<u>defined by monoclonal antibodies</u>

1. Poly-X antigen in various human adenocarcinoma (20,21) as
defined by monoclonal antibody "FH4" (22)

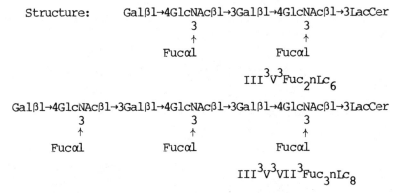

Structure: Galβ1→4GlcNAcβ1→3Galβ1→4GlcNAcβ1→3LacCer
                       3   3
                       ↑   ↑
                     Fucα1   Fucα1

$$III^3V^3Fuc_2nLc_6$$

Galβ1→4GlcNAcβ1→3Galβ1→4GlcNAcβ1→3Galβ1→4GlcNAcβ1→3LacCer
     3   3   3
     ↑   ↑   ↑
   Fucα1   Fucα1   Fucα1

$$III^3V^3VII^3Fuc_3nLc_8$$

2. A novel fucoganglioside of human colonic cancer defined by
monoclonal antibody (IB9) (32)

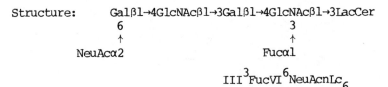

Structure: Galβ1→4GlcNAcβ1→3Galβ1→4GlcNAcβ1→3LacCer
                       6   3
                       ↑   ↑
                   NeuAcα2   Fucα1

$$III^3FucVI^6NeuAcnLc_6$$

3. A novel fucoganglioside of human colonic cancer 6B defined by
monoclonal antibody (FH6) (23)

Structure: Galβ1→4GlcNAcβ1→3Galβ1→4GlcNAcβ1→3LacCer
                       3   4   4
                       ↑   ↑   ↑
                   NeuAcα2   Fucα1   Fucα1

$$III^3V^3FucVI^3NeuAcnLc_6$$

FACTORS AFFECTING EXPRESSION OF GLYCOLIPID TUMOR ANTIGENS
AND SIGNIFICANCE OF GLYCOLIPID MARKERS IN TUMOR IMMUNOLOGY

Many tumor cells are capable of synthesizing certain
glycolipids which are not detectable at the cell surface by
antibodies and exogenous ligands. The chemical quantity of

glycolipids assembled at the cell surface and various other
factors affecting the crypticity of glycolipids in membranes are
important to determine the glycolipid expression at the cell
surface. The exact mechanism controlling glycolipid crypticity
is still unknown, but coexisting longer-chain glycolipids and
glycoproteins may mask shorter chain glycolipids, which are tumor
antigens (33). For some cells, sialidase treatment greatly
enhances glycolipid exposure at the cell surface (34).

Antigenicity as well as immunogenicity of glycolipids may
well be controlled by ceramide composition. Glycolipids having
ceramides with shorter chain fatty acids are less active than
those with longer chain fatty acids or with α-hydroxylated fatty
acids (33). The reactivity of lactosylceramide with longer chain
α-hydroxylated fatty acids to its monoclonal antibody was
significantly greater than that of lactosylceramide with shorter
chain fatty acids (35). The factors affecting glycolipid
expression were previously reviewed (2) and are hereby summarized
in the scheme shown in Fig. 5.

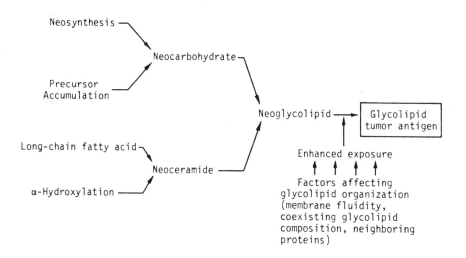

Figure 5. Mechanism for expression of tumor-associated
glycolipid antigens. Either neosynthesis or precursor
accumulation due to a block of glycosyltransferase results in
accumulation of a neoglycolipid which is absent or present in
small quantity in normal cells. Often neoglycolipids have
unusual ceramide composition (neoceramide). Synthesis of a
neoglycolipid alone is not sufficient to express the
glycolipid antigen at the cell surface. Various factors
affecting glycolipid organization, as discussed in the text,
are essential.

Tumor-associated glycolipid markers are, in general, poorly immunogenic in syngeneic hosts and may have been overlooked by the classical techniques of tumor immunology. A number of glycolipid antigens, however, have been discovered and characterized using monoclonal antibody techniques. In contrast to protein antigens, their epitope structures are well-defined, and the abnormal enzymes involved in synthesis of a specific structure can be predicted. The isolation and a search for mechanism of specific glycosyltransferases are being actively pursued.

BIOLOGICAL SIGNIFICANCE OF GLYCOLIPID CHANGES IN TUMORS

The biological significance of glycolipid changes associated with oncogenic transformation has been ambiguous, although a strong possibility exists that the changes in transformed cells may be associated with a decrease in cell adhesiveness, aberrant cell recognition, and loss of growth regulation (1,25).

Loss of cell adhesiveness and glycolipid changes: GM_3 is present in the cell adhesion matrix of both normal and transformed hamster fibroblasts (BHK C21). Although the chemical quantity of GM_3 in whole cells is much lower in transformed cells than in normal cells, its metabolic labeling activity is much higher in transformed cells, and cell adhesion is inhibited in the presence of GM_3 (25). These data suggest that cell adhesion is regulated by GM_3 through different mechanisms in normal and transformed cells.

Loss of cell growth regulation and glycolipid changes: The loss of a particular ganglioside, which occurs in some transformed cell lines, can be correlated with a loss of growth control, as shown in Table VI, in which some evidence for such an association is listed. All these phenomena are, however, indirect evidence. Glycolipids exogenously added in cell culture are slowly incorporated into plasma membranes, inhibit cell growth, and modify growth behavior (26,27). With the availability of purified growth factors and serum-free culture conditions in recent years (28), we have been able to examine this phenomenon in mouse Swiss 3T3 cells in greater detail with the following results (29,30): 1) Cell growth (cell number increase) in serum-free medium was specifically inhibited by the presence of GM_1 and to a lesser extent by GM_3, but not by $NeuAcnLc_4$, although the gangliosides were incorporated equally well into cell membranes. GM_3 inhibited both PDGF- and EGF-stimulated mitogenesis determined by thymidine incorporation, while GM_1 could only inhibit PDGF-stimulated mitogenesis. $NeuAcnLc_4$ had no effect on mitogen-stimulated thymidine incorporation. Both GM_1 and GM_3 inhibited PDGF-dependent DNA synthesis. 2) The concentration-dependent binding of $[^{125}I]$-PDGF to cells indicated that cells whose growth was inhibited by GM_1

or GM_3 showed an increased affinity for PDGF as compared to cells grown without addition of ganglioside, while the total number of receptors stayed the same. This indicates that gangliosides that induce growth inhibition alter the affinity of the receptor to PDGF. Addition of ganglioside did not affect the binding of [^{125}I]-EGF. 3) No direct interaction was observed between gangliosides and growth factors, as evidenced by the lack of competition by ganglioside-containing liposomes for cellular binding of [^{125}I] growth factors (data not shown). 4) GM_1 and GM_3, but neither $NeuAcnLc_4$ nor Gb_4, inhibited the PDGF-stimulated tyrosine phosphorylation by membrane preparations of a 170,000 molecular weight protein, which was identified as the PDGF receptor (see Fig. 6). Thus, the level of gangliosides GM_1 and GM_3 in membranes may modulate PDGF receptor function by affecting the degree of tyrosine-phosphorylation and may alter the affinity of the receptor for PDGF (30).

TABLE VI. Evidence that glycolipids may regulate cell proliferation (for a review of each item, see 1)

1. Contact inhibition of cell growth accompanies change of glycolipid synthesis.

2. Various glycolipids are more highly exposed at Gl phase, and some at G2 phase.

3. Butyrate induces cell growth inhibition and enhances GM_3 synthesis.

4. Retinoids induce contact inhibition, enhance GM_3 synthesis and glycolipid response.

5. Antibodies to GM_3, but not to globoside, inhibit 3T3 and NIL cell growth and enhance GM_3 synthesis.

6. Exogenous addition of glycolipids incorporated into cell membranes inhibits cell growth through extension of Gl phase.

An "allosteric regulator" model for the EGF receptor in which several binding sites on the receptor protein in addition to the EGF binding site were postulated. Since the chemical level and organization of gangliosides in plasma membranes may affect the allosteric configuration of the receptor, it is possible that one of the additional sites on the growth hormone receptor may bind GM_1 or GM_3 either directly or through an intermediate gangliophilic protein (see Fig. 7). Organization of gangliosides with such receptors may alter the receptor-receptor interaction which is necessary for internalization of the receptor-growth

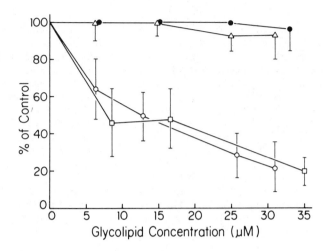

<u>Figure 6</u>. The inhibition of PDGF-dependent tyrosine-
phosphorylation in Mr-170,000 phosphoprotein by gangliosides.
Swiss 3T3 cell membranes were incubated with 10 nM [^{32}]-ATP
and 60 nmoles of PDGF with various concentrations of
glycolipids as indicated for 30 min at 30°C. Proteins were
separated by polyacrylamide gel electrophoresis base-treated
to eliminate serine or threonine phosphates. After
visualization of [32]-labeled proteins by autoradiography,
the receptor Mr-170,000 protein was cut from the gel and
counted in a scintillation counter. Results are expressed as
percent of maximum PDGF-dependent response. The results
shown are the average of at least three determinations. **O** ,
GM_1; **◻** , GM_3; **●** , globoside; **△** , sialosyl paragloboside.

hormone complex. The model may be useful for further studies of
cell growth regulation through membrane gangliosides. A loss or
reduction of GM_3 or GM_1 due to a blocked synthesis in various
oncogenic transformants may cause a loss of allosteric regulation
through the growth factor receptor on one hand, and may induce
precursor accumulation and cause enchanced antigenicity of the
precursor glycolipid antigen on the other hand. The growth
factor requirement of each normal and transformed cell is
different. The mechanisms by which glycolipids regulate growth
factor receptors may also be different. The model described
above represents only one example. A large variety of growth
factor requirements may be associated with a number of regulator
glycolipids which are also "sensors" of the external environment.
I believe this model will eventually fill the gap in our
knowledge on how glycolipids regulate cell growth adapted to
external environments. A possible consequence of a blocked
synthesis of gangliosides is shown in Fig. 8.

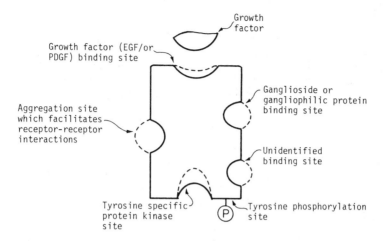

Figure 7. "Allosteric regulator" model of growth factor receptor adapted from Schlessinger et al. (31). The binding of the growth factor to the receptor may affect i) tyrosine-specific protein kinase, which is independent of cyclic AMP-dependent kinase, ii) receptor-receptor aggregation, which facilitates clustering and internaliztion of the receptor-growth factor complex, and iii) direct binding to gangliosides or indirect binding through a gangliophilic protein. This model is based on the fact that PDGF-dependent tyrosine-phosphorylation of the receptor protein (Mr-170,000) as well as PDGF-dependent cell growth and mitogenesis were inhibited by exogenous enrichment of membrane gangliosides. This model also explains how ganglioside enrichment of membranes alters the affinity of cells to growth factors.

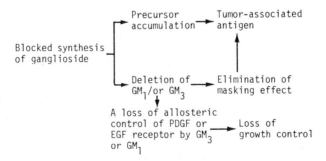

Figure 8. A possible sequence of events in mouse cells following a blocked synthesis of ganglioside.

Acknowledgements

The authors thank for general support the National Institutes of Health (Grants CA20026, CA19224, GM23100), the American Cancer Society (BC9M), and the Otsuka Research Foundation. This work has been accomplished in collaboration with Drs. Reiji Kannagi, Eric G. Bremer, Eric Holmes, Ed Nudelman, Steven B. Levery, Nancy Cochran, William W. Young, Jr., Davor Solter, and Barbara B. Knowles.

REFERENCES

1. Hakomori, S. (1981). Ann. Rev. Biochem. 50, 733-764.

2. Hakomori, S. and Kannagi, R. (1983). J. Natl. Cancer Inst. 71, 231-251.

3. Feizi, T. (1983). Biochem. Society Transactions, 2, 263-266.

4. Hakomori, S., Fukuda, M. and Nudelman, E. (1982). In "Teratocarcinoma and Embryonic Cell Interactions" (Ed. T. Muramatsu, G. Gachelin, A.A. Moscona and Y. Ikawa) Proceedings of First Hiei Symposium on Teratocarcinoma, pp. 179-200. Springer-Verlag, Heidelberg and New York.

5. Solter, D. and Knowles, B.B. (1978). Proc. Natl. Acad. Sci. USA 75, 5565-5569.

6. Shevinsky, L.H., Knowles, B.B., Damjanov, I. and Solter, D. (1982). Cell 30, 697-705.

7. Kannagi, R., Cochran, N.A., Ishigami, F., Hakomori, S., Andrews, P.W., Knowles, B.B. and Solter, D. (1983). EMBO Journal 2, 2355-2361.

8. Gooi, H.C., Feizi, T., Kapadia, A., Knowles, B.B., Solter, D. and Evans, J.M. (1981). Nature 292, 156-158.

9. Kannagi, R., Nudelman, E., Levery, S.B. and Hakomori, S. (1982). J. Biol. Chem. 257, 14865-14874.

10. Kannagi, R., Levery, S.B., Ishigami, F., Hakomori, S., Shevinsky, L.H., Knowles, B.B. and Solter D. (1983). J. Biol. Chem. 258, 8934-8942.

11. Kannagi, R., Levery, S.B. and Hakomori, S. (1983). Proc. Natl. Acad. Sci. USA 80, 2844-2848.

12. Rosenfelder, G., Young, W.W. Jr. and Hakomori, S. (1977). Cancer Res. 37, 1333-1339.

13. Young, W.W. Jr. and Hakomori, S. (1981). Science 211, 487-489.

14. Nudelman, E., Kannagi, R., Hakomori, S., Parsons, M., Lipinski, M., Wiels, J., Fellous, M., and Tursz, T. (1983) Science 220, 509-511.

15. Nudelman, E., Hakomori, S., Kannagi, R., Levery, S., Yeh, M.-Y., Hellstrom, K.E. and Hellstrom, I. (1982). J. Biol. Chem. 257, 12752-12756.

16. Pukel, C.S., Lloyd, K.O., Trabassos, L.R., Dippold, W.G., Oettgen, H.F. and Old, L.J. (1982). J. Exp. Med. 155, 1133-1147.

17. Koprowski , H., Herlyn, M., Steplewski, Z. and Sears, H.F. (1981). Science 212, 53-54.

18. Magnani, J.L., Nilsson, B., Brockhaus, M., Zopf, D., Steplewski, S., Koprowski, H. and Ginsvurg, V. (1982). J. Biol. Chem. 257, 14365-14369.

19. Falk, K.-E., Karlsson, K.-A., Larson, G., Thurin, J., Blaszczyk, M., Steplewski, Z., and Koprowski, H. (1983). Biochem. Biophys. Res. Commun. 110, 383-391.

20. Hakomori, S., Nudelman, E., Kannagi, R. and Levery, S.B. (1982). Biochem. Biophys. Res. Commun. 109, 36-44.

21. Hakomori, S., Nudelman, E., Levery, S.B. and Kannagi, R. (1984). J. Biol. Chem. 259, 4672-4680.

22. Fukushi, Y., Hakomori, S., Nudelman, E. and Cochran, N. (1984). J. Biol. Chem. 259, 4681-4685.

23. Fukushi,Y., Nudelman, E., Levery, S.B., Rauvala, H. and Hakomori, S. (1984). J. Biol. Chem., in press.

24. Fukushi, Y., Hakomori, S. and Shepard, T. (1984). J. Exp. Med., in press.

25. Okada, Y., Bremer, E.G., Mugnai, G. and Hakomori, S. (1984). Exp. Cell Res., in press.

26. Laine, R.A. and Hakomori, S. (1973). Biochem. Biophys. Res. Commun. 54: 1039-1045.

27. Keenan, T.W., Schmid, E., Franke, W.W. and Wiegandt, H. (1975). Exp. Cell Res. 92, 259-270.

28. Barnes, D. and Sato, G. (1980). Anal. Biochem. 102, 255-270.

29. Bremer, E.G. and Hakomori, S. (1982). Biochem. Biophys. Res. Commun. 106, 711-718.

30. Bremer, E.G., Hakomori, S., Bowen-Pope, D.F., Raines, E. and Ross, R. (1984). J. Biol. Chem., in press..

31. Schlessinger, J., Schreiber, A.B., Levi, A., Lax, I., Liberman, T. and Yarden, Y. (1983). CRC Reviews in Biochemistry 14, 93-111

32. Hakomori, S., Nudelman, E., Levery, S.B. and Patterson, C.M. (1983). Biochem. Biophys. Res. Commun. 113, 791-798.

33. Kannagi, R., Stroup, R., Cochran, N.A., Urdal, D.L., Young, W.W., Jr., and Hakomori, S. (1983). Cancer Res. 43, 4997-5005.

34. Urdal, D.L., and Hakomori, S. (1983). J. Biol. Chem. 258, 6869-6874.

35. Symington, F.W., Bernstein, I.D., and Hakomori, S. (1984) J. Biol. Chem. 259, 6008-6012.

Molecular Biology of Tumor Cells, edited by
B. Wahren et al. Raven Press, New York © 1985.

Isolation of a cDNA Clone for Human Melanoma-Associated Antigen p97

*,†Joseph P. Brown, *Timothy M. Rose, *John W. Forstrom,
*,‡Ingegerd Hellström, and *,†Karl Erik Hellström

*Program in Tumor Immunology, Fred Hutchinson Cancer Research Center, Seattle,
Washington 98104; Departments of †Pathology and ‡Microbiology/Immunology, University of
Washington, Seattle, Washington 98195*

ABSTRACT

Polysomes bearing nascent chains of human melanoma-associated antigen p97 were purified by affinity chromatography with monoclonal antibodies specific for p97. Translation of mRNA from the purified polysomes both in Xenopus laevis oocytes and in the reticulocyte lysate system showed that p97 mRNA activity had been enriched approximately 200-fold, p97 being the major translation product. A melanoma cDNA library was screened by differential hybridization with p97-enriched and unenriched cDNA probes and by hybrid-selected translation, leading to the identification of a plasmid containing a 300 base pair cDNA insert derived from p97 mRNA. The cloned cDNA was used as a hybridization probe to confirm the enrichment obtained by polysome immunopurification and to show that p97 mRNA is present in much larger amounts in melanoma cells than in fibroblasts.

INTRODUCTION

p97 is a 97,000 molecular weight (MW) cell-surface glycoprotein, which was identified by using monoclonal antibodies (6,8,26). It is present in most human melanomas but in only trace amounts in normal adult tissues (4,5,10). The N-terminal amino acid sequence of p97 is homologous to that of transferrin, and like transferrin p97 binds iron (3). Analysis of somatic cell hybrids has shown that the p97 gene, like the genes for transferrin and transferrin receptor, is located on chromosome 3 (19). Taken together these observations suggest that p97 plays a role in iron metabolism.

In order to identify functional domains and antigenic determinants of p97, we propose to determine its
complete amino acid sequence. Direct determination of
the entire sequence is impractical because of the small
amounts of the protein available and its large size
(3). In contrast, it would be quite feasible to sequence cDNA clones coding for p97. In this paper, we describe the purification and in vitro translation of
p97 mRNA, identification of a p97 cDNA clone, and use
of the cloned cDNA as a hybridization probe to analyze
p97 mRNA.

MATERIALS AND METHODS

Polysome immunopurification

Polysomes (100 to 200 E_{260} units) prepared from SK-
MEL 28 melanoma cells (7) by magnesium precipitation
(16) were incubated with monoclonal IgG2a antibodies
specific for p97 (5 mg) and passed through a 5 ml protein A-Sepharose CL-2B column as described (12). p97-
enriched mRNA was purified from the adsorbed polysomes
by elution with EDTA and affinity chromatography on
oligo (dT)-cellulose.

Translation in oocytes

mRNA was injected into Xenopus laevis oocytes (11),
which were incubated at 20°C for 20 hours and homoge-
nized in 5 volumes 20 mM Tris-HCl pH 8.0, 100 mM NaCl,
1 mM EDTA, 0.5% Nonidet p-40, 1 mM phenylmethyl sulfo-
nyl fluoride. The lysate was centrifuged at 30,000 x g
for 30 min. at 0°C, and the supernatant was assayed for
p97 by double determinant immunoassay (5,19).

Cell-free translation

mRNA was translated in the micrococcal nuclease-
treated rabbit reticulocyte lysate system (18), and
the methionine-labelled translation products were analyzed by sodium dodecyl sulfate-8% polyacrylamide gel
electrophoresis (SDS-PAGE; 13), either directly or
after immunoprecipitation with mouse antiserum specific for denatured p97 (3) as described (4). The gel
was treated with ENHANCE (New England Nuclear, Boston,
MA) and autoradiographed with preflashed Kodak AR film
at -70°C.

cDNA cloning

For first strand cDNA synthesis, 500 ng mRNA template and 1 µg oligo (dT)$_{12-18}$ primer (Collaborative Research, Waltham, MA) were incubated with 20 units reverse transcriptase (Life Sciences, Inc., St. Petersburg, FL) in 10 µl 100 mM Tris-HCl pH 8.3, 10 mM MgCl$_2$,140 mM NaCl, 20 mM 2-mercaptoethanol, 1 mM dNTP, 10 µCi ^{32}P-TTP, and 2,000 units/ml placental ribonuclease inhibitor (Biotec, Madison, WI) for 1 hour at 45°C. EDTA (10 mM) and NaOH (300 mM) were added, and the mixture was incubated at 65°C for 10 min and then neutralized. After this and each of the three subsequent enzymic steps, the cDNA was phenol-extracted, chromatographed on a column of BioGel A 1.5m (BioRad, Richmond, CA) equilibrated with TNE (10 mM Tris-HCl pH 8.0, 100 mM NaCl, 1 mM EDTA), and recovered by ethanol precipitation with 20 µg carrier tRNA. The second strand was synthesized by incubation with 7 units of the large fragment of E. coli DNA polymerase (BRL) in 10 µl 100 mM HEPES pH 6.9, 10 mM MgCl$_2$, 2.5 mM dithiothreitol, 70 mM KCl, 1 mM each dNTP for 4 hours at 12.5°C. The double stranded cDNA was digested with 2 units S1 nuclease in 50 µl 50 mM sodium acetate pH 4.5, 300 mM NaCl, 3 mM zinc acetate for 1 hour at 37°C, and then dC-tailed with 18 units terminal deoxylnucleotidyl transferase (BRL) in 10 µl 200 mM potassium cacodylate pH 7.3, 1 mM CoCl$_2$, 0.2 mM dithiothreitol , 100 mM ^{3}H-dCTP (specific activity 25 Ci/mmol) for 1 hour at 37°C. Tailed cDNA (10 ng) was annealed with 100 ng Pst I-digested, dG-tailed pBR322 (BRL) in 100 µl TNE (9,23) and used to transform CaCl$_2$-treated E. coli RR1.

Colony screening

DNA from colonies of transformed bacteria was bound to paper as described (22). The filters were incubated with ^{32}P-labelled cDNA probe (2 to 5 x 10^5 dpm/ml) in 5X NaCl/Cit (IX NaCl/Cit is 150 mM NaCl, 15 mM citrate pH 7.0) containing 50% formamide, 25 mM sodium phosphate, and 0.02% bovine serum albumin, Ficoll, polyvinylpyrrolidone and herring sperm DNA for 1 to 2 days at 42°C, washed at 50°C in 2X NaCl/Cit and autoradiographed for 1 to 3 days at -70°C with an intensifying screen.

Hybrid-selection

Plasmids were purified as described (2) and 1 to 5 µg were dissolved in 6 µl 2 M NaCl containing 0.2 M

NH_4OH, incubated at 100°C for 1 min and spotted on to
9 mm diameter semicircles of BA85 nitrocellulose
(Schleicher and Schuell, Keene, NH), which were incubated overnight at 80°C in vacuo and washed as described (20). p97-enriched mRNA (200 ng) was dissolved in
30 µl 65% formamide, 400 mM NaCl, 10 mM PIPES pH 6.4,
0.1% SDS, heated at 70°C for 10 min, and 4 µl were
spotted on to each filter. The filters were sandwiched
between siliconized glass slides and incubated at 48°C
for 2 hours. The filters were washed and bound mRNA
was recovered as described (17).

RNA dot blot hybridization

mRNA was denatured with formaldehyde and transferred
to nitrocellulose as described (25). The filter was
hybridized as described above with a ^{32}P-labelled probe (4 x 10^6 dpm/ml) prepared by nick translation (20)
of the p97-1 cDNA insert, washed at 50°C with 0.1X
NaCl/Cit and autoradiographed at -70°C with an intensifying screen.

RESULTS

Purification of p97 mRNA

Polysomes bearing p97 nascent chains were purified
by incubation with a mixture of 3 IgG2a monoclonal
antibodies (96.5, 118.1, 133.2) specific for distinct
epitopes of p97 (4,5,6,19) followed by affinity chromatography on a protein A column, and used as a source
of p97-enriched mRNA. In a typical experiment, 4 g
melanoma cells (from 24 roller bottles) yielded 150
E_{260} units of polysomes, from which we obtained 260 ng
p97-enriched mRNA, 0.23% of the total mRNA. We found
it necessary to add carrier tRNA (20 µg) to allow us
to recover this small amount of mRNA by ethanol precipitation. Submicrogram amounts of mRNA mixed with much
longer amounts of carrier tRNA were quantitated by
measuring oligo(dT)-primed synthesis of cDNA, essentially as described under "cDNA cloning" in Methods.
p97-enriched and unenriched mRNA were translated in
Xenopus oocytes, lysates of which were subsequently
assayed for p97. A highly specific double determinant
immunoassay (DDIA), which utilizes monoclonal antibodies specific for two distinct epitopes of p97 (5,
19), was used for this purpose. In a typical experiment oocytes synthesized 80 pg p97 per ng p97-enriched
mRNA, but only 0.44 pg p97 per ng unenriched mRNA,
showing that p97 mRNA activity had been enriched 180-
fold. The yield of p97 mRNA activity was 42%.
Translation in the reticulocyte lysate system was

used to allow biochemical characterization of the translation product and assessment of the degree of contamination of p97-enriched mRNA with other mRNA species. p97-enriched mRNA was found to code for a major polypeptide with an apparent MW on SDS-PAGE of 84,000, which was not detectable in the translation products of unenriched mRNA (Fig. 1A). The 84,000 MW polypeptide was immunoprecipitated by antiserum specific for p97 (Fig. 1B), and we conclude that it was the

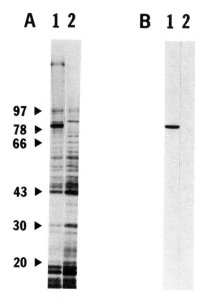

FIG. 1. Cell-free translation of p97 mRNA. 5 ng mRNA was translated in the reticulocyte lysate system, and the translation products were analyzed by SDS-PAGE and autoradiography. A, 0.5 ul total translation products, 6-day exposure; B, 5 ul translation products immunoprecipitated with anti-p97 serum, 1-day exposure. 1, p97-enriched mRNA; 2, unenriched mRNA. MW markers: phosphorylase b, 97,000; conalbumin preprotein, 78,000; serum albumin, 66,000; ovalbumin, 43,000; carbonic anhydrase 30,000; soybean trypsin inhibitor, 20,000.

unglycosylated precursor of p97. It was not, however, immunoprecipitated by any of the 3 monoclonal antibodies specific for p97 (data not shown). The 84,000 MW polypeptide constituted, we estimated, approximately 10% of the translation products, suggesting that p97 mRNA comprised a similar proportion of the p97-enriched mRNA.

cDNA cloning

p97-enriched mRNA (50 ng) was mixed with a 10-fold
excess of unenriched mRNA, so that there would be
enough cDNA to allow each step of the synthesis to be
monitored by gel electrophoresis, and converted to
double-stranded cDNA, the yield of which was 40 ng,
ranging in size from 200 to 1,400 base pairs. The cDNA
was dC-tailed and 10 ng was annealed with 100 ng dG-
tailed, PstI-digested pBR322 (23). Transformation of
E. coli RR1 yielded 19,000 tetracycline-resistant
transformants. The colonies were screened by differential hybridization with cDNA probes synthesized on unenriched and p97-enriched mRNA templates. Those that
hybridized at least 10-fold more strongly to the enriched probe were tested by hybrid-selection and cell-
free translation, first as pools of six and then in-
dividually. One plasmid which hybridized to p97-en-
riched cDNA but not detectably to unenriched cDNA and
also selected p97 mRNA in hybrid-selected translation
experiments (Fig. 2) was chosen for further study and
was shown by PstI-digestion and 2% agarose gel electrophoresis to contain a 300 bp insert.

Analysis of p97 mRNA by hybridization with cloned p97 cDNA

mRNA was denatured with formaldehyde, bound to
nitrocellulose, and hybridized with nick-translated
p97 cDNA. The probe hybridized more strongly to 5 ng
of p97-enriched mRNA than to 500 ng of unenriched mRNA
(Fig. 3), consistent with their respective p97 mRNA
activities in translation assays. Hybridization to 500
ng fibroblast mRNA was barely detectable, being at
least 20-fold weaker than to unenriched melanoma mRNA
(Fig. 3).

DISCUSSION

Cell surface proteins such as p97 generally comprise less than 0.05% of cell protein, and their mRNAs
are of similarly low abundance (3,12,17). Consequently,
to obtain a cDNA clone for a particular cell surface
protein, one must screen at least several thousand
cDNA clones, assuming that the library is prepared
from unenriched mRNA. Although hybrid-selected translation has been used for primary screening of cDNA
libraries (17,24), in situ hybridization with synthetic oligo-nucleotides (21) or cDNA probes (12) has
found more general application.
    In the case of p97 we felt that the best way to ob-
tain a cDNA probe was to use monoclonal antibodies,

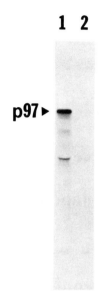

FIG. 2. Hybrid selection of p97 mRNA. Plasmids were bound to nitrocellulose and incubated with p97-enriched mRNA. Hybridized mRNA was recovered and translated in the reticulocyte lysate system, and the translation products were immunoprecipitated with anti-p97 serum and analyzed by SDS-PAGE and autoradiography for 14 days. 1, plasmid containing p97 cDNA insert; 2, negative control plasmid.

which were already available, to purify polysomes bearing p97 nascent chains as a source of p97 mRNA (15). This technique, known as polysome immunopurification, has been used to purify HLA-DR mRNA more than 1,000 fold (12).

A potential problem with using monoclonal antibodies for polysome purification is that antibodies obtained by immunization with the native protein may not recognize nascent chains. In the case of HLA-DR, for example, the monoclonal antibody used successfully was obtained by immunizing with dissociated HLA-DR heavy chain; it showed no reactivity with the native molecule, although it did bind the cell-free translation product. In contrast, we used antibodies obtained by immunization with native p97. These antibodies recognize epitopes present on the 40,000 MW N-terminal domain of native p97 but absent from denatured p97 and from the reticulocyte lysate translation product (4, and J.P.B., unpublished work). Our results show that at least one of the antibodies binds p97 nascent chains, and we conclude that

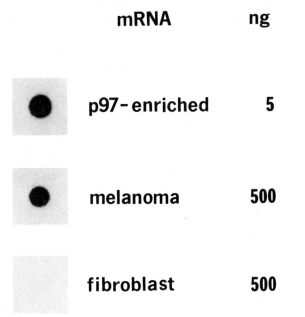

mRNA   **ng**

p97-enriched   **5**

melanoma   **500**

fibroblast   **500**

FIG. 3. Dot blot of p97 mRNA. mRNA was denatured with formaldehyde, bound to nitrocellulose, and hybridized for 1 day with ^{32}P-labelled cloned p97 cDNA. The filter was washed and auroradiographed for 1 day.

the N-terminal domain of p97 adopts (at least in part) its native conformation before the p97 molecule is completely synthesized. We can draw two general conclusions from these observations: First, monoclonal antibodies specific for native proteins (which are more readily available than antibodies specific for denatured proteins) may be of general value for polysome immunopurification. Second, failure of an antibody to immunoprecipitate a cell-free translation product does not preclude its use for polysome immunopurification.

Translation of mRNA from the immunopurified polysomes both in oocytes and in a cell-free system showed that a 180-fold purification had been achieved and suggested that p97 mRNA was a major component of the enriched mRNA. We found that the oocyte assay was by far the more sensitive of the two, possibly because of the longer incubation time and the highly sensitive DDIA used to assay the translation products. The cell-free translation product, which had a MW of 84,000, was precipitated by an antiserum specific for denatured p97 but by none of the monoclonal antibodies.

The difference in MW between the cell-free translation product and the protein present at the surface of melanoma cells is probably due to glycosylation of the latter (5,8), and the difference in antigenicity can be ascribed to lack of appropriate post-translational modification in the cell-free system. It is interesting to note that the cell-free translation product of p97 is significantly larger than transferrin, which has a MW of 75,000 (14). This may be due to the presence in p97 of a signal peptide and transmembranous and cytoplasmic domains.

A recombinant plasmid which was identified by screening a cDNA library by differential hybridization and hybrid-selected translation, contained a 300 bp cDNA insert derived from p97 mRNA. Since the cDNA library was obtained by priming with oligo (dT), we expected that cloned sequence would prove to be derived from the 3' end of the mRNA. This was confirmed by sequence analysis (data not shown).

Use of the cloned cDNA as a hybridization probe confirmed the greater than 100-fold enrichment of p97 obtained by polysome immunopurification, and also established that fibroblasts contain much smaller amounts of p97 mRNA than do melanoma cells. The latter observation is consistent with the much lower levels of p97 in fibroblasts (5).

Sucrose gradient centrifugation and agarose gel electrophoresis under denaturing conditions showed that p97 mRNA comprises approximately 4.4 kilobases, considerably larger than the minimum of 2.3 kilobases required to code for the 84,000 MW translation product (data not shown). We propose to use the partial p97 cDNA clone to screen a cDNA library for a full-length clone. This will enable us to obtain the complete amino acid sequence of p97. Comparison of the p97 sequence with that of transferrin (14) should help elucidate the evolutionary and functional relationship between these two proteins and allow us to identify putative transmembranous and cytoplasm domains of p97. Knowledge of the amino acid sequence of p97 will also make it possible to identify antigenic sites, which might be mimicked by synthetic peptides.

The cloned cDNA will also be used to screen a genomic library for clones containing the p97 structural gene. One of our goals is to express the p97 gene in mouse cells, as has been done for human major histocompatibility antigen genes (1). This should facilitate studies of the function of p97 and provide a mouse model system in which p97-targeted immunotherapy can be evaluated prior to testing in humans.

ACKNOWLEDGEMENTS

We are grateful to Drs. Stanley McKnight, Richard
Gelinas, Steve McKnight, James Lewis, and Diane Durnam
for their unstinting advice and encouragement, and to
Cynthia Green for her excellent technical assistance.
This investigation was supported by PHS grants numbers
19148, 19149, CA 27841, 34777, 37440 and 36883, awarded by the National Cancer Institute, DHHS.

REFERENCES

1. Barbosa, J.A., Kamarack, M.E., Biro, P.A.,
      Weissman, S.M., and Ruddle, T.H. (1982): Proc.
      Natl. Acad. Sci. USA 79:6327-6331
2. Birnboim, H.C., and Doly, J. (1979): Nucleic Acids
      Res. 7:1513-1523
3. Brown, J.P., Hewick, R.M., Hellström, I., Hellström,
      K.E., Doolittle, R.F., and Dreyer, W.J. (1982):
      Nature 296:171-173
4. Brown, J.P., Nishiyama, K., Hellström, I., and
      Hellström, K.E. (1981): J. Immunol. 127:539-546
5. Brown, J.P., Woodbury, R.G., Hart, C.E., Hellström,
      I., and Hellström, K.E. (1981): Proc. Natl.
      Acad. Sci. USA 78:539-543
6. Brown, J.P., Wright, P.W., Hart, C.E., Woodbury,
      R.G., Hellström, K.E., and Hellström, I. (1980):
      J. Biol. Chem. 255:4980-4983
7. Carey, T.E., Takahashi, T., Resnick, L.A., Oettgen,
      H.F., and Old, L.J. (1976): Proc. Natl. Acad.
      Sci. USA 73:3278-3282
8. Dippold, W.G., Lloyd, K.O., Li, L.T., Ikeda, H.,
      Oettgen, H.F., and Old, L.J. (1980): Proc. Natl.
      Acad. Sci. USA 77:6114-6118
9. Efstratiadis, A., and Villa-Komaroff, L. (1979):
      In: Genetic Engineering, edited by J.K. Stelow,
      and A. Hollaender, Vol. 1, pp. 15-36, Plenum
      Press, New York
10. Garrigues, H.J., Tilgen, W., Hellström, I., Franke,
      W., and Hellström, K.E. (1982): Int. J. Cancer
      29:511-515
11. Gurdon, J.B. (1974): The Control of Gene Expression
      in Animal Development. Harvard University Press,
      Cambridge, MA.
12. Korman, A.J., Knudsen, P.J., Kaufman, J.F., and
      Strominger, J.L. (1982): Proc. Natl. Acad. Sci.
      USA 79:1844-1848
13. Laemmli, U.K. (1970): Nature 227:680-685.
14. McGillivray, R.T.A., Mendex, E., Sinha, S.K.,
      Sutton, M.R., Lindeback-Zins, J., and Brew, K.
      (1982): Proc. Natl. Acad. Sci. USA 79:2504-2508

15. Palacios, R., Palmiter, R.D., and Schimke, R.T. (1972): J. Biol. Chem. 247:2316-2321
16. Palmiter, R.D. (1974): Biochem. 13:3606-3615
17. Parnes, J.R., Velan, B., Felsenfeld, A., Pamanathan, L., Ferrini, U., Appella, E., and Seidman, J.G. (1981): Proc. Natl. Acad. Sci. USA 78:2253-2257
18. Pelham, H.R., and Jackson, R.J. (1976): Eur. J. Biochem. 67:247-256
19. Plowman, G.D., Brown, J.P., Enns, C.A., Schröder, J., Nikinmaa, B., Sussman, H.H., Hellström, K. E., and Hellström, I. (1983): Nature 303:70-72
20. Rigby, P.W.J., Dieckman, M., Rhodes, C., and Berg, P. (1977): J. Mol. Biol. 113:237-251
21. Stetler, D., Das, H., Nunberg, J.H., Saiki, R., Shen-Dong, R., Mullis, K.B., Weissman, S.M., and Erlich, H.A. (1982): Proc. Natl. Acad. Sci. USA 79:5966-5970
22. Taub, F., and Thompson, B. (1982): Anal. Biochem. 126:222-230
23. Villa-Komaroff, L., Efstratiadis, A., Broome, S., Lomedico, P., Tizard, R., Nabaer, S.P., Chick, W.L., and Gilbert, W. (1978): Proc. Natl. Acad. Sci. USA 75:3727-3731
24. Wake, C.T., Long, E.O., Strubin, M., Gross, N., Accola, R., Carrel, S., and Mach, B. (1982): Proc. Natl. Acad. Sci. USA 79:6979-6983
25. White, B.A., and Bancroft, F.C. (1982): J. Biol. Chem. 257:8569-8572
26. Woodbury, R.G., Brown, J.P., Yeh, M.-Y., Hellström, I., and Hellström, K.E. (1980): Proc. Natl. Acad. Sci. USA 77:2183-2187.

Molecular Biology of Tumor Cells, edited by
B. Wahren et al. Raven Press, New York © 1985.

Molecular and Biological Profiles of Two Unique Antigens Associated with Human Melanoma

Ralph A. Reisfeld, Gregor Schulz, David A. Cheresh, and
John R. Harper

*Department of Immunology, Scripps Clinic and Research Foundation,
La Jolla, California 92037*

It is now well established that malignant transformation is frequently accompanied by antigenic changes on the cell surface. This observation has led to numerous efforts by research investigators to identify and characterize cell surface markers associated with tumor cells to gain a more basic understanding of neoplastic transformation and to advance the development of immunological approaches for diagnosis and therapy of cancer (28).

It is the purpose of this article to describe the biochemical and functional characterization of two such tumor cell surface markers that are synthesized by human melanoma cells and to delineate their potential for the diagnosis and therapy of malignant melanoma. The first of these is a non-cartilage, chondroitin sulfate-rich proteoglycan that presents an effective target for a monoclonal antibody (Mab 9.2.27) for the eradication of large, established human melanoma tumors in nude mice. The second is a disialoganglioside, i.e. GD_3 that is 9-0-acetylated at its terminal sialic acid residue and thereby becomes a uniquely specific melanoma antigen.

Biochemical Profile of a Melanoma-Associated Chondroitin Sulfate Proteoglycan Antigen

Pulse-chase studies and extensive immunochemical analyses indicated that human melanoma cells synthesize a non-cartilagenous type proteoglycan composed of a core protein of M_r 2.5 x 10^5 containing both N- and O-linked oligosaccharides, as well as O-glycosidically-linked chondroitin sulfate chains (4,5). This proteoglycan appears to be functionally relevant in cell-cell interactions important for anchorage-independent growth and cytoplasmic spreading of melanoma cells onto solid substrata (14). Two monoclonal antibodies, 9.2.27 and 155.8, have been described as recognizing distinct determinants on the core protein in absence and presence of attached chondroitin sulfate chains (12,13). By using Mab 9.2.27 in extensive pulse-chase analyses, it was shown that the biosynthesis of the melanoma type proteoglycan proceeds through a M_r 2.4 x 10^5 component having N-linked, high mannose oligosaccharides whose M_r decreases to 2.35 x 10^5 following digestion with endo-β-N-

169

acetylglucosaminidase H (Endo H). Almost immediately following the processing of high mannose oligosaccharides to the complex type and addition of O-linked oligosaccharides, forming a core glycoprotein of M_r 2.5 x 10^5, chondroitin 4- and/or 6-sulfate chains are initiated and elongated as is described for cartilage proteoglycans (5). The overall structural organization of this chondroitin sulfate rich, melanoma-associated proteoglycan was found to be quite similar to that of cartilage type proteoglycans (16,17). Although the core protein structure of proteoglycans may vary according to the tissue of origin, all proteoglycans share their extensive post-translational modifications that most likely occur by similar mechanisms. Thus, N-asparagine-linked "high mannose" type oligosaccharides are apparently added to the core protein chain co-translationally within the rough endoplasmic reticulum. These chains are then trimmed and terminally glycosylated with sialic acid to the "complex" form in Golgi-related vesicles. In the Golgi complex, O-linked glycosylation occurs practically simultaneously with initiation and elongation of glycosaminoglycan chains (11). The maturation of the completely glycosylated proteoglycan is followed by its rapid transport to the cell surface and exocytosis into the extracellular space (11,16,17).

In a separate study to be described in detail elsewhere (15), we obtained experimental evidence supportive for a hypothesis that acid compartments involved in certain Golgi-related functions make it possible for human melanoma cells to regulate proteoglycan biosynthesis by an efficient low-pH mechanism affecting fusion and thus interaction of vesicular compartments in the Golgi apparatus. Such low-pH mechanisms appear to be responsible for the delivery of mature core glycoprotein molecules to the site of glycosaminoglycan synthesis in Golgi-related vesicles. Finally, we observed that the addition of chondroitin sulfate side chains is not required for expression of the core protein on the surface of human melanoma cells and such core proteins, as well as intact proteglycans, once transported to cell surface are exocytosed by an apparent enzymatic cleavage to an extracellular form whose core protein has a molecular weight of 1.75 x 10^5 (15).

Eradication of Established Human Melanoma Tumors by Antibody-Directed Effector Cells with NK Activity

In previous work we observed that the growth of human melanoma tumors in nude mice could be partially suppressed by the simultaneous injection of Mab 9.2.27 specific for melanoma cells and splenocytes of BALB/c mice at the time of tumor cell inoculation (35). It was assumed that this antibody-dependent suppression of tumor growth was caused by a cell-mediated mechanism. The effector cells involved were believed to be NK cells since such cells express ADCC activity.

We present here highlights of a study described in detail elsewhere (36) that examines this hypothesis. To this end, BALB/c nu/nu mice were rendered NK-deficient by injection with anti-asialo GM_1 antiserum, and 24 hours later groups of treated and untreated mice were inoculated subcutaneously with either 2.5×10^6 or 5×10^6 M21 tumor cells. All animals that received 5×10^6 melanoma cells showed tumor growth after 20 days. The extent of this tumor growth was approximately the same as that observed on untreated animals, i.e. 220 m^3 versus 190 mm^3. However, a far more pronounced tumor growth was observed in all five animals injected with 2.5×10^6 melanoma cells, whereas only 1/5 mice in the untreated group exhibited tumor growth. Since we found in control experiments that injection of anti-asialo GM_1 efficiently eliminates NK activity, the data strongly suggest an important role for NK cells in the suppression of human melanoma tumor growth in nude mice.

Experiments were designed to determine whether simultaneous injection of Mab 9.2.27 and cell populations with NK activity can cause the eradication of established melanoma tumors (mean volume 90 mm^3) in nude mice. To this end, BALB/c nude mice bearing 2-week old melanoma tumors received a single intravenous injection as follows: 400 μg 9.2.27 IgG (Group 2); mononuclear BALB/c splenocytes (2×10^7) (Group 3); 2×10^7 mononuclear splenocytes and 400 μg 9.2.27 IgG (Group 4). A group of tumor-bearing control mice received no injection (Group 1). We observed that 7/10 animals in Group 4 were tumor-free four weeks after injection. All other animals treated with either antibody or splenocytes alone exhibited large tumors with the exception of one animal in Group 3 that received only splenocytes. Interestingly enough, mice that received only Mab 9.2.27 (Group 2) showed a mean tumor volume ($1285 + 151$ mm^3) that was almost the same as that of control animals (Group 1) ($1359 + 167$ mm^3) whereas tumors of mice that received only effector cells (Group 3) were 50% smaller ($605 + 120$ mm^3). Most interesting, the mean tumor volume of mice that received 9.2.27 IgG together with effector cells was less than 10% of that of control tumors, i.e. $127 + 16$ mm^3 versus $1359 + 167$ mm^3.

Additional experiments were done to determine whether the observed tumor eradication was attributable to T cells present in the normal BALB/c splenocytes that are otherwise lacking in nude mice. Mature T-cells are apparently not involved in this phenomenon, since we observed that a combination of 9.2.27 IgG and mononuclear splenocytes from BALB/c nude mice was equally effective in eradicating established melanoma tumors as mononuclear splenocytes from normal BALB/c mice. Furthermore, mononuclear splenocytes obtained from melanoma tumor-bearing BALB/c nude mice also were almost equally effective as effector cells obtained from either normal or nude mice of BALB/c origin.

Several observations strongly suggested that the effector cells involved in melanoma tumor destruction are cells with NK activity. First, splenocytes obtained from NK-deficient beige were incapable of inducing tumor regression. Specifically,

C57BL/6 nude mice with established human melanoma tumors were injected with 9.2.27 IgG, either together with splenocytes from normal C57BL/6 mice or with splenocytes from NK-deficient C57BL/6 mice that carried the homozygous beige mutation. None of ten mice that received normal C57BL/6 splenocytes and 9.2.27 IgG showed any tumor growth 4 weeks after injection. In contrast, 8/9 mice that received splenocytes from C57BL/6 bg/bg mice showed large tumors. Since beige mice have low NK activity (30,31), these data taken together, indicate that NK cells play a key role in the eradication of established human melanoma tumors in the nude mouse model system.

To further strengthen this conclusion, C57BL/6 nude mice with established human melanoma tumors were also injected with the cloned NK cell line B61B10. In this case, a single dose of only 2×10^6 cells, i.e a dose only one-tenth that of the splenocytes used in our other experiments, resulted in a pronounced suppression of tumor size ($>70\%$) in those mice that received 9.2.27 IgG plus NK cells. Complete tumor elimination was not accomplished, possibly because of the very large tumor size at the start of the experiment (mean volume = 185 mm^3) or due to a lack of effective migration of the cloned NK cells to the subcutaneous tumor site.

Because it is well known that NK cells perform antibody-dependent cell mediated cytolysis (ADCC) in vitro (2,25,32), we determined whether Mab 9.2.27 and effector cells with NK activity can lyse M21 human melanoma cells. For this purpose, BALB/c mononuclear splenocytes, mixed with M21 melanoma cells were assayed for cytolytic activity in ^{51}Cr release assays, either in the absence or presence of Mab 9.2.27. Effector cells lysed NK-sensitive YAC-1 target cells and caused 25% cytolysis of melanoma cells in the absence of Mab 9.2.27 as compared to 38% in the presence of this antibody. Removal of NK cells by treatment of splenocytes with anti-asialo GM$_1$ caused marked reduction of cytotoxicity, both in the absence and presence of Mab 9.2.27. Effector cells treated in this manner also failed to lyse YAC-1 target cells, indicating that NK activity was eliminated by this treatment. Other antibodies specific for NK cells, i.e., anti-Qa5 and anti-NK1.1 (19,26,41) essentially abolished any cytolytic effect of the effector splenocytes on M21 melanoma cells and YAC-1 target cells. C57BL/6 effector cells were found equally effective as BALB/c effector cells in mediating cytotoxicity against M21 melanoma cells. Treatment of the C57BL/6 effector cells with anti-Qa5 and anti-NK1.1, but not with anti-Lyt 6.2, completely abolished their cytolytic activity against YAC-1 and M21 cells, regardless of the presence of Mab 9.2.27. Finally, C57BL/6 bg/bg effector cells that have greatly reduced NK activity could not mediate any efficient cytotoxicity in the ^{51}Cr release assay.

Taken together, our results strongly suggest that NK cells are responsible for the antibody-dependent and antibody-independent cytolysis of human melanoma cells. Our in vivo data lead us to conclude that the cells chiefly responsible for tumor elimination are most likely NK cells. First, NK cells are present in splenocytes of T cell-deficient nude mice. Second, cloned cells with NK activity are also able to suppress growth of established human melanoma tumors in nude mice. Our conclusion is further strengthened by the fact that splenocytes were ineffective in suppressing tumor growth when obtained either from NK-deficient beige mice or from BALB/c mice treated with anti-asialo GM_1 antiserum, a treatment that is known to eliminate cells with NK activity. Since it is well established that murine NK cells are heterogeneous with differences in cell surface markers and in responsiveness to regulatory influences by interferon and IL2 (19,20,24), it is quite likely that the cells responsible for tumor regression are also heterogeneous. Our finding that cloned NK cells were less effective than normal spleen cells points to this possibility, especially since cloned NK cells were found much more effective in rejection of bone marrow allografts and protection from radiation induced leukemia (44). Our observation that injection of Mab 9.2.27 by itself into tumor-bearing nude mice that have NK cells is insufficient to cause tumor rejection is also interesting from a clinical point of view, especially if one considers eventual application of our regimen for the treatment of melanoma patients. We favor the explanation that antibody and effector cells have to be injected simultaneously so that the antibody can bind to the effectors, most likely via Fc receptors, and thereby "arm" them. It is likely that this antibody effector cell interaction will target the effector cells to the tumor in a more effective way. It may therefore not be too surprising that in some clinical studies (29,38), the injection of relatively large amounts of monoclonal antibodies "per se" resulted at best in only a partial regression of the tumor. Finally, our demonstration of the involvement of cells with NK activity in antibody-mediated tumor rejection does not at all preclude the participation of other cell types, e.g. neutrophils and macrophages which we also observed in preliminary experiments to be attracted to the tumor site, particularly at later stages of tumor destruction. It is also most likely that the sequence of events in antibody-mediated tumor destruction may vary in different tumor systems. In this regard, we observed resistance of lung cancer cells to NK lysis in vitro (data not shown) and several recent reports have demonstrated that macrophages effectively mediate antibody-dependent cytotoxicity against colorectal tumor cells (1,40).

Although our nude mouse model with human melanoma tumors may be regarded as somewhat artificial and is certainly not optimally suited to predict the outcome of clinical studies, we conclude that the results from our experiments outlined here at least suggest simultaneous injection of effector cells with a monoclonal antibody like 9.2.27 specifically directed to a melanoma cell surface antigen, may ultimately prove more effective than antibody alone for tumor elimination, particularly in melanoma patients that are deficient in NK and other effector functions. It is, of course, quite obvious that this contention remains to be proven by the results of clinical phase I trials.

Human Melanoma Cells Create a Unique Antigenic Determinant by O-Acetylation of Disialoganglioside GD$_3$

Monoclonal antibodies to a variety of human tumor-associated antigens have facilitated the characterization of molecular differences between tumors and normal cells and thereby considerably advanced an understanding of the functional role of some of these antigens. Most information gained initially involved mainly protein or glycoprotein antigens since these can be readily characterized by indirect immunoprecipitation from tumor cell lysates. More recently, technological advances also made it possible to use monoclonal antibodies (Mabs) for the characterization of a number of complex carbohydrate antigens on tumor cell surface-associated glycolipids (3,10,22,27,45). Monoclonal antibodies to melanoma-associated sialic acid containing glycolipids, i.e. gangliosides GD$_2$ (6) and GD$_3$ (27,45) have also been described. Gangliosides represent interesting molecules that may become most useful to mark differentiation events and thus provide markers for tumor metastasis. In this regard, the sialic acid of ganglioside have a considerable diversity, largely created by different types of O-substitutions, usually O-acetyl esters at the 4, 7, 8 and 9 positions of the parent molecule, neuraminic acid (34).

We outline here some of the highlights of studies described in detail elsewhere (7,8) delineating a highly unique and specific antigenic determinant on human melanonma cells that is comprised by the alkali-labile O-acetylated product of the neuroectoderm-associated disialoganglioside GD$_3$.

As shown in our initial studies, this antigen is highly restricted to human melanoma and is specifically recognized by Mab D1.1 (7), an antibody that was originally described by Levine et al. (21) to recognize a fetal rat neuroectoderm-associated ganglioside. The first clue that Mab D1.1 recognized an O-acetylated ganglioside came from our initial studies that indicated base treatment of this melanoma-associated ganglioside to cause a decrease in its migration on thin layer chromatography (TLC) (7). The purified, alkali-labile ganglioside migrated on TLC between the monosialylated ganglioside standards, GM$_1$ and GM$_2$. As shown in Fig. 1, increasing periods of alkali treatment first partially and then completely converted this ganglioside to a new doublet, migrating in the same position as GD$_3$. This observation suggested a structural relationship of this yet undefined ganglioside with GD$_3$, and the single downward shift in migration on TLC implied the removal of a single, base-labile O-acyl group.

We elected to use biochemical and immunochemical techniques rather than direct-probe mass spectrometry to confirm the structure of this ganglioside since it is relatively unstable and comprises at best only 5% of total melanoma ganglioside. In determining the antigenic characteristics of the de-O-acetylated GD$_3$, we used in addition to Mab D1.1, two other monoclonal antibodies, i.e. Mab R24 (27) and Mab 3.6 (9) that recognize only native GD$_3$ and fail to cross-react with any other

TLC MIGRATION OF D1.1 GANGLIOSIDE
AFTER BASE-TREATMENT

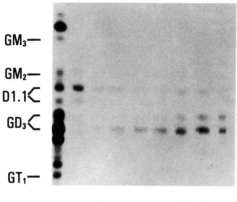

A B C D E F G H I

Figure 1: Effect of alkali-induced de-0-acetylation on the TLC
migration of the ganglioside recognized by Mab D1.1
    Lane A: ³H-labeled gangliosides isolated from
biosynthetically labeled Melur melanoma cells were separated by
thin layer chromatography and exposed to x-ray film as
previously described (7). The positions of Resorcinol
visualized standards are depicted to the left. Lane B: The
purified ganglioside recognized by Mab D1.1. Lanes C-I:
Ganglioside recognized by Mab D1.1 previously exposed to 2.5 N
ammonium hydroxide at 37°C for increasing 10-minute intervals.

gangliosides. We found that base-induced de-0-acetylation of
purified melanoma ganglioside completely destroyed their
reactivity with Mab D1.1 while causing at the same time a
reciprocal increase in the reactivity of Mab R24.

    We gained direct evidence that Mab D1.1 recognizes an
alkali-labile, acetylated form of GD_3 by parallel TLC analysis
of both total melanoma ganglioside and the purified ganglioside
recognized by Mab D1.1, either with or without prior base
treatment followed by direct immunostaining with monoclonal
antibodies. Base treatment, i.e. overnight incubation at room
temperature in an airtight chamber saturated with ammonia, had
three effects: first, it caused loss of reactivity with Mab
D1.1; second, it resulted in a decrease of mobility on TLC,
causing comigration with purified GD_3; and third, the base-
treated purified ganglioside now reacted exclusively with Mabs
R24 and MB3.6 that are specific for non-acetylated GD_3. We also
obtained further corroboration that base treatment of total
melanoma gangliosides causes de-0-acetylation of 0-acetylated
gangliosides with a subsequent decrease in mobility resulting in

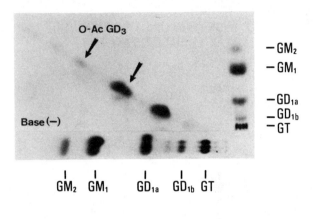

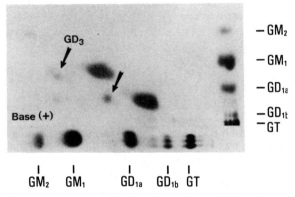

Figure 2: Two-dimensional TLC for identification of alkali-labile gangliosides

Purified gangliosides from M21 melanoma cells were subjected to two-dimensional TLC without intermediate base hydrolysis (top panel) and with base hydrolysis (bottom panel). Gangliosides were visualized with Resorcinol reagent. The first dimension was run from right to left. The designated arrows refer to O-acetylated GD_3 (7,8) and the unmarked arrows indicate the position of putative O-acetylated GD_2.

comigration with their parent gangliosides. Figure 2 (top panel) depicts the two-dimensional TLC profile of total melanoma ganglioside without alkali treatment. The arrows indicate the position of O-acetylated GD_3 and of a putative O-acetylated GD_2 which under these conditions cannot be distinguished as it is covered, in part, by GD_3. Base treatment produces de-O-acetylation and the resultant decrease in mobility that now clearly indicates the two de-O-acetylated ganglioside to comigrate with their parent gangliosides, GD_3 and GD_2, respectively. Coincidentally, these data provided our first evidence for the presence of O-acetylated GD_2 in a human melanoma cell extract (Figure 2, bottom panel).

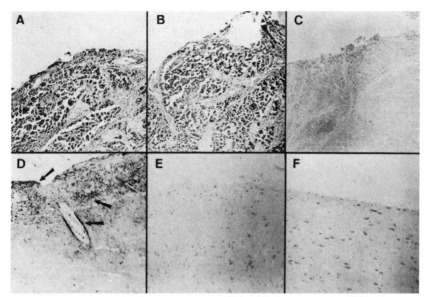

Figure 3:   Immunological reactivity of human melanoma and brain tissues with Mabs D1.1 and R24
Paraffin-embedded formalin-fixed human melanoma (A-C) or adult brain (D-F) were sectioned and stained by the immunoperoxidase anti-peroxidase technique as previously described (7). Monoclonal antibodies R24 (A,D), D1.1 (B,E) or the non-melanoma binding negative control Mab KS1/4 (C,F) recognizing a lung adenocarcinoma antigen (7) were used as primary antibodies. Arrows correspond to various areas of the brain tissue reactive with Mab R24.

Direct evidence was obtained indicating that the O-acetyl group of acetylated GD_3 was located on the 9-position of its terminal sialic acid residue. To this end, we performed periodate oxidation on gangliosides isolated from melanoma cells under conditions that were such that oxidation would occur only between the exocyclic (7,-8,-9) hydroxyl positions of terminal, unsubstituted sialic acid residues (23,42). In this regard, it was previously reported that an acetyl group in the 9-position sterically hinders this oxidation whereas substitutions on the 7- or 4- positions do not (39,43). Substitutions at the 8-position occurs very rarely because of rapid migration to the 9-position (33,34). We found that controlled periodate oxidation of total melanoma gangliosides completely eliminated their antigenic reactivity with Mabs R24 and MB3.6 that specifically recognize non-acetylated GD_3 as well as reactivity with Mab 126 that reacts specifically with GD_2 (37). However, antigenic reactivity with Mab D1.1 remained unchanged even at the highest periodate concentration employed (4 mM), strongly suggesting that the O-acetyl group is indeed located at the 9-position of the terminal sialic acid of GD_3. We could also confirm this finding by chemical means, using the mild acetylating agent N-acetyl-imidazole that is known to selectively O-acetylate the 9-position of the methyl ester/methyl glycoside of sialic acid under appropriate conditions of molar excess (18). The compound created by this procedure now migrated in the appropriate position on TLC between GM_1 and GM_2 and also specifically reacted with Mab D1.1.

We have shown previously that Mab D1.1 is highly restricted in its reactivity with human melanoma tissues and failed to react with a wide variety of normal adult tissues, fetal tissues, and tissues of other malignancies when tested by the frozen section immunoperoxidase assay (7). In contrast, it is well known that GD_3 is associated with various tissues of the neuroectoderm (27). As illustrated by Fig. 3, the GD_3 defined by Mab R24 is indeed present in tissues of human melanoma and adult brain, whereas the 9-O-acetylated GD_3, defined by Mab D1.1, appears only in melanoma tissues. Consequently, we postulated that the putative O-acetyl transferase responsible for O-acetylating the terminal sialic of GD_3 may be selectively expressed in human melanoma cells, possibly as a consequence of neoplastic transformation. We have now confirmed the existence of such an enzyme in human melanoma cells by de-O-acetylating melanoma cell-derived gangliosides, incubating them with lysates of melanoma cells and assaying for the synthesis of the antigen specifically recognized by Mab D1.1. Reactivity with this antibody was indeed generated in this manner as a function of protein concentration and time. Preheating the melanoma cell extract at 80°C for 20 minutes completely abolished this reactivity. Interestingly enough, presence of the putative acetyl transferase not only generated antigenic activity with Mab D1.1 but reciprocally decreased reactivity with Mab R24 that exclusively recognizes non-acetylated GD_3. Reactivity with Mab D1.1 could not be generated by gangliosides extracted from cells lacking GD_3. These data strongly suggest the existence of a melanoma-associated acetyl transferase capable of generating the antigenic epitope that is specifically recognized by Mab D1.1

SUMMARY

The biosynthesis of a melanoma-associated chondroitin sulfate proteoglycan is regulated by an efficient low-pH mechanism that is responsible for delivery of mature core glycoprotein molecules to the site of glycosaminoglycan synthesis in Golgi-related vesicles. This chondroitin sulfate proteoglycan antigen, expressed on the surface of human melanoma cells, presents an effective target for the eradication of established human melanoma tumors in nude mice by a specific monoclonal antibody that directs effector cells with NK activity to the tumor site. Finally, disialoganglioside GD_3 acetylated in the 9-position of its terminal sialic acid proved to be a unique and highly specific marker for human melanoma cells and has the potential to become an effective indicator of tumor cell metastasis.

ACKNOWLEDGEMENT

Work reported here was supported in part by U. S. Public Health Service Grant CA 28420. The authors with to thank Ms. Bonnie Pratt Filiault for preparation of the manuscript.

REFERENCES

1. Adams, D.O., Hall, T., Steplewski, Z., and Koprowski, H. (1984): Proc. Natl. Acad. Sci., in press.

2. Bradley, T.P. and Bonavida, B. (1982): J. Immunol. 130:2260.

3. Brockhaus, M., Magnani, J.L., Blaszczk, M., Steplewski, Z., Koprowski, H., Karlsson, K-H., Larson, G., and Ginsburg, V. (1981): J. Biol. Chem. 256:13223-13225.

4. Bumol, T. F. and Reisfeld, R.A. (1982): Proc. Natl. Acad. Sci. USA 79:1245-1249.

5. Bumol, T.F. Walker, L. E., and Reisfeld, R.A. (1984): J. Biol. Chem. in press.

6. Cahan, L.D., Irie, R.F., Sing, R., Cassidenti, A., and Paulson, J.C. (1982): Proc. Natl. Acad. Sci. USA 79:7629-7633.

7. Cheresh, D.A., Varki, A.P., Varki, N.M., Stallcup, W.B., Levine, J., and Reisfeld, R.A. (1984): J. Biol. Chem. in press.

8. Cheresh, D.A., Reisfeld, R.A., and Varki, A.P. (1984): Science, in press.

9. Cheresh, D.A., Harper, J.R., Schulz, G., and Reisfeld, R.A. (1984): Proc. Natl. Acad. Sci. USA, in press.

10. Hakomori, S., Patterson, C.M., Nudelman, E., and Sekiguchi, K. (1983): J. Biol. Chem.258: 11819-11822.

11. Hardingham, T. (1981): Biochem. Soc. Trans. 9:489-497.

12. Harper, J.R., Bumol, T.F., and Reisfeld, R.A. (1983): Hybridoma, 423-432.

13. Harper, J.R., Bumol, T.F., and Reisfeld, R.A. (1983): J. Immunol. 132: 2096-2104.

14. Harper, J.R., Bumol, T.F, and Reisfeld, R.A. (1983): J. Natl. Cancer Inst. 71:259-263.

15. Harper, J.R., Quaranta, V., and Reisfeld, R.A. (1984): J. Biol. Chem., in press.

16. Hascall, V.C. and Hascall, G.K. (1981): In: Cell Biology of Extracellular Matrix, edited by E. D. Hay, pp. 39-60, Plenum Press, New York.

17. Hascall, V.C. and Kimura J.H. (1982): Methods in Enzymol. 82:769-799.

18. Haverkamp, J., Schauer, R., Wember, M., Kamerling, P., and Vliegenthart, J.F.G. (1975) Hoppe Seyler's Z. Physiol. Chem. 356:1575-1581.

19. Koo, G.C., Jacobsen, J.B., Hammerling, G.J., and Hammerling, U. (1980): J. Immunol. 125: 1003-1006.

20. Lattime, E.C., Pecoraro, G.A., and Stuttman, O. (1981): J. Immunol. 126:2011-2014

21. Levine, J.M., Beasley, L., and Stallcup, W.B. (1984): J. Neurochem. 4:820-831.

22. Magnani, J.L., Nilson, B., Brockhaus, M., Zoph, F., Steplewski, Z., Koprowski, H., and Ginsburg, V. (1982): J. Biol. Chem. 257: 4365-4369.

23. McLean, R.L., Suttajit, M., Beidler, J., and Winzler, R. (1971): J. Biol. Chem. 246: 803-809.

24. Minato, N., Reo, L. and Bloom, B.R. (1981): J. Exp. Med. 154:750-762.

25. Ojo, E. and Wigzell, H. (1978): Scand. J. Immunol. 7: 297-306.

26. Pollak, S.B. and Hallenberg, L.A. (1982): Int. J. Cancer 29:203-207.

27. Pukel, C.S., Lloyd, K.P., Dippold, W.G., Oettgen, H.F., and Old, L.J. (1982): J. Exp. Med. 155:1133-1137.

28. Reisfeld, R.A. (1984): In: Cancer Markers III, edited by R. A. Reisfeld and S. Sell. Humana Press, Inc., Clifton, New Jersey, in press.

29. Ritz, S. and Schlossman, S.F. (1982): Blood 59:1-11.

30. Roder, J.C. (1979): J. Immunol. 123:2168-2174.

31. Roder, J.C., Lohmann-Matthes, M.L., Domzig, W., and Wiszell, H.J. (1979): J. Immunol. 123:2174-2181.

32. Santoni, A., Herberman, R.B., and Holden, H.T. (1979): J. Natl. Canc. Inst. 62:109-116.

33. Schauer, R. (1982): In: Sialic Acids: Chemistry, Metabolism and Function, edited by R. Schauer, Springer Verlag, New York.

34. Schauer, R. (1982): Adv. Carbohyd. Chem. Biochem. 40:131-234.

35. Schulz, G., Bumol, T.F., and Reisfeld, R.A. (1983): Proc. Natl. Acad. Sci., USA 80:5407-5411.

36. Schulz, G., Staffileno, L.K., Reisfeld, R.A., and Dennert, G. (1984): J. Exptl. Med., in press.

37. Schulz, G., Cheresh, D.A., Varki, N.M., Yu, A., Staffileno, L.K., and Reisfeld, R.A. (1984): Cancer Res., in press.

38. Sears, H.F., Mattis, J., Herlyn, D., Hayry, P., Atkinson, B., Ernst, C., Steplewski, Z., and Koprowski, H (1982): The Lancett ii: 762-765.

39. Shukla, A.K., and Schauer, R. (1982): Hoppe-Seyler's Z. Physiol. Chem. 363:255-261.

40. Steplewski, Z., Lubeck, M.D., and Koprowski, H., (1983): Science 221:865-866.

41. Stuttman, O. and Cuttita, M.J. (1981): Nature 290:254-256.

42. Van Lenten, L. and Ashwell, G. (1971): J. Biol. Chem. 246:1889-1894.

43. Varki, A. P. and Kornfeld, S. (1980): J. Exp. Med. 152:532-544.

44. Warner, J.F. and Dennert, G. (1982): Nature 300:31-34.

45. Yeh, M-Y., Hellström, I., Abe, K., Hakomori, S., and Hellström, K.E. (1982): Int. J. Cancer 29:269-275.

Molecular Biology of Tumor Cells, edited by
B. Wahren et al. Raven Press, New York © 1985.

Human Leukemia Viruses: The HTLV "Family" and Their Role in Human Malignancies and Immune Deficiency Disease

R. C. Gallo, F. Wong-Staal, P. D. Markham, M. Popovic, and
M. G. Sarngadharan

Laboratory of Tumor Cell Biology, Developmental Therapeutics Program, Division of Cancer Treatment, National Cancer Institute, Bethesda, Maryland 20205

Since the first isolation of a human retrovirus (leukemia virus) from cultured human leukemia T-cells (56,58), there have been numerous isolates of this and related viruses from many laboratories in different parts of the world (see ref. 20 for review). All of the known human retroviruses belong to one virus family collectively called human T-cell leukemia (lymphotropic) virus or HTLV because of their striking capacity for infection of human T-cells, especially the OKT4/leu3+(T4) subset. We can now distinguish three major HTLV subgroups, i.e., HTLV-I, HTLV-II, and HTLV-III. HTLV-I was the first to be isolated and is the cause of a particular form of adult T-cell leukemia (ATL) (20). More than 100 isolates of HTLV-I have been obtained. At least one variant (HTLV-Ib) has been isolated from an African T cell leukemia patient (26). Viruses closely related to HTLV-I have also been isolated from Old World monkeys (52). We call these primate T-cell leukemia/lymphoma virus (PTLV). HTLV-II has been only rarely found. HTLV-III is etiologically linked to the acquired immune deficiency syndrome (AIDS) (19,61,71,75). Already there are close to 100 isolates of HTLV-III. Thus, we now regard "HTLV" as a generic name for an enlarging family of retroviruses which have in common the following features: 1) T-cell tropism, especially with the OKT4/leu 3+(T4) phenotype; 2) a major core protein of about 24,000 daltons; 3) a 100,000 dalton reverse transcriptase, favoring Mg^{++} for its catalytic activity; 4) some cross reactive antigens; 5) the presence of a nucleotide sequence at the 3' end of the viral genome potentially coding for a novel protein

called pX; 6) the capacity to exert a cytopathic effect on some
of the infected T-cells and to induce formation of giant multi-
nucleated cells; 7) sequence homology of some region of the
genome under low stringency conditions; and 8) a probable
African origin.

This family of viruses currently presents to us an unusual
opportunity to study aspects of cell growth relevant to human
disease. In vitro infections of fresh primary human blood or
bone marrow-derived T4 cells with HTLV-I, the subtype linked to
T-cell leukemia, leads to the immortalized growth of some cells
(46,60,69) and these take on properties very similar to the
primary HTLV-I positive leukemic cells. Conversely, infection
of fresh human T4 cells with HTLV-III, the virus linked to AIDS,
often leads to in vitro death of these cells (19,61).

BACKGROUND

Temin's provirus hypothesis (87) and its subsequent verification has helped to clarify the scheme for the cycle of infection by retroviruses. Following penetration into the infected
cell viral RNA is transcribed into DNA which is then integrated
into the DNA of the host cell as the provirus. In some instances some or all of the viral DNA persist in an episomal or
unintegrated state. Infection by a retrovirus can have a spec-
trum of effects on the cell. There may be no change, no apparent change which may nonetheless contribute to a several-step
process leading to neoplasia, or immediate effects such as
neoplastic transformation. Infection with some retroviruses
can also lead to cytopathic changes culminating in cell degener-
ation.

We distinguish retroviruses by several biological and
biochemical criteria. One major subdivision is according to
their manner of transmission. Endogenous retroviruses are
transmitted in the germline as "normal" genetic elements from
parent to progeny. There is as yet no substantial evidence that
these rather ubiquitous viruses cause naturally occurring
diseases. A human endogenous retrovirus has not been isolated.
Exogenous retroviruses infect somatic cells and their genomes
are found only in the infected cells and their progeny. These
are usually the kind of retroviruses which cause disease.
Therefore, those retroviruses that induce neoplasia may be present only in tumor cells or in a very restricted number of
normal cells. The exogenous retroviruses may be further subdi-
vided according to their RNA genome and biological activities.

Acute vs Chronic Retroviruses. The acute leukemia viruses
or sarcoma viruses have acquired cellular derived onc genes (32),
usually at the expense of viral sequences. They are replication
defective. Each cell infected by these viruses is transformed

because of the direct oncogenic property of the protein encoded
by the v-onc gene (polyclonal transformation). Such viruses
when accompanied by a helper virus will cause cancer rapidly.
However, these viruses are rare in nature and are more often
generated in the laboratory. The chronic leukemia viruses in
contrast are relatively common. They are causes of naturally
occurring leukemia in chickens, mice, cats, cows, and gibbon
apes. Chronic leukemia viruses are replication competent. They
contain the full complement of genes for replication: the gag
gene coding for internal structural proteins, the pol gene coding for the reverse transcriptase, and the env gene coding for
the viral envelope. They do not contain cellular derived onc
genes. They take a long time to produce a malignancy which
invariably is monoclonal, and in general they do not transform
cells in vitro. How these viruses cause neoplastic disease is
a subject of great current interest. In some systems the mechanism probably involves specific integration events with the
enhancement of expression of specific cellular genes mediated
by regulatory sequences usually found in the viral long terminal
repeated sequences (LTR). For example, this seems to be an
early event in the induction of leukemia in chickens by avian
leukosis virus.

We initially classified HTLV as a chronic leukemia virus,
but it actually forms a new category of retroviruses which also
includes BLV and PTLV. These viruses might be thought of as a
hybrid between the acute and chronic leukemia viruses. They
have all the features of a chronic leukemia virus, notably they
contain the three genes for replication, produce monoclonal
tumors after a long latency period, and do not contain a cellular derived onc gene. However, HTLV-I and HTLV-II, do transform
(immortalize) fresh primary human T-cells in vitro efficiently,
and contain a sequence of about 1.6 Kb at the 3' end of the
viral genome (Fig. 1) (77). Although this sequence (pX) is
apparently not cell-derived, there are indications that its
product is involved in the first stages of HTLV-induced neoplasia (see Section VII).

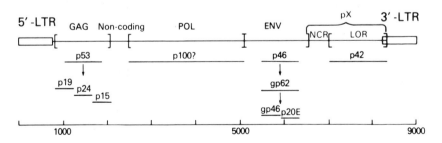

Fig. 1.   Genetic structure of the genomes of HTLV-I and HTLV-II.

ISOLATION OF HTLV

A T-Cell Growth Factor (TCGF) or Interleukin-2 (IL-2)

We had speculated that if a retrovirus is associated with any human leukemia, it would be present at very low levels and might not be fully expressed unless the cells were grown in culture. Successful isolation of virus would, therefore, depend on the ability to grow specific cells of interest. The eventual isolation of HTLV was possible because of the earlier discovery of TCGF which allowed the relatively long-term in vitro growth of human T-lymphocytes (53,66). It was first observed that TCGF does not bind to or induce proliferation of normal human T-cells unless they are first activated by lectins or antigens which induced the synthesis of TCGF receptors. In general, most T-cells from normal people do not bear significant TCGF receptors without activation. In contrast, when partially purified TCGF was used to study the proliferation of neoplastic T-cells from patients with different forms of T-cell malignancies, it was soon apparent that cells of many patients responded directly to TCGF (22,57), i.e., these cells were already activated. To date, all T-cell malignancies known to be positive for HTLV have been TCGF receptor (or TAC)-positive (43). Not only do the HTLV positive neoplastic T-cells have TCGF receptors, but they also contain these receptors in increased numbers compared to normal T-cells activated by lectins (24) (see Figure 2).

TCGF RECEPTORS IN MAN

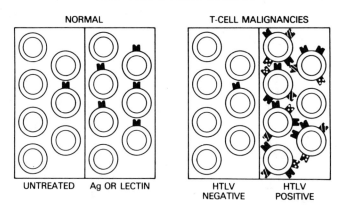

FIG. 2.   Schematic Illustration of Different Levels of Receptors for T-cell Growth Factor on the Surface of the Indicated Source of Cells

Isolation of HTLV-I

Procedures used for isolation of HTLV-I were basically a modification of those developed in this laboratory for culturing of human T lymphocytes in the presence of TCGF (57). Fresh peripheral blood or bone marrow cells of patients were banded on Ficoll-Hypaque, treated for 48-72 hours with PHA-P and then grown in complete growth media supplemented with fetal calf serum and TCGF. These cell cultures were monitored at regular intervals for distinct morphological changes and for expression of virus detected initially by the release of viral reverse transcriptase activity into supernatant fluids and by electron microscopic observation. Specific immunological and nucleic acid reagents were later prepared which greatly facilitated detection and characterization of viral proteins and nucleic acids.

HTLV-I was first detected in cultured T-cells from two adult Black U.S. patients with aggressive forms of T-cell malignancy. These were initially diagnosed as aggressive variants of mycosis fungoides and Sézary syndrome (56,58). Later it was appreciated that these were the same disease as the adult T-cell leukemia-lymphoma (ATL) described in Japan and the Caribbean (85,86,88). HTLV-I was observed to have a typical type-C retrovirus morphology and was seen budding from the cell membranes. (Figure 3). The size of HTLV-I virus varied from 900 to 1400Å.

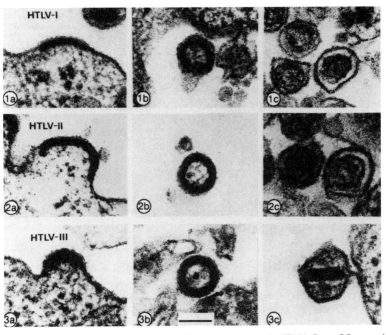

FIG. 3. Transmission Electron Micrograph of HTLV-I, -II, and -III Infected Cells With Budding Virus (a), and Complete Viral Particles (b,c).

The initial HTLV viruses were called HTLV type I, and the isolates are distinguished from each other by the initials of the
patients.

Since the first isolations of HTLV-I in the United States,
many additional isolates have been obtained in this laboratory
from patients in the U.S., the Caribbean, Japan, Africa, South
America, and Israel (20,60), independently by investigators in
Japan (51,93), in the U.S. (31), in Holland (90), and in England
(7). These isolates have chiefly been obtained from T-cells of
patients with ATL and in some cases from their relatives (70).

Following identification of HTLV-I-positive leukemic cells
after in vitro cultivation, these cells were lethally irradiated,
or treated with mitomycin C, and co-cultivated with various
sources of normal human T-cells to further transmit the virus
and to study their biological properties. Cord blood and bone
marrow mononuclear cells are excellent sources of sensitive
target cells. Using immunological cross reactivities of the
viral proteins, sequence homology by molecular hybridization,
cleavage sites of several restriction endonucleases, and more
recently by nucleotide sequence analyses, we determine that
these isolates belong to a group of very closely related viruses
of the same subgroup HTLV-I.

Isolation of HTLV-II

In collaboration with UCLA investigators we isolated a new
retrovirus from a patient with hairy cell leukemia (38). This
cell line also has T-cell properties even though hairy cell
leukemias are believed to be B-cell leukemias (74). This retrovirus is related to, but substantially different from HTLV-I
(38) and is called HTLV-II$_{MO}$. Recently, a second isolate of
HTLV-II was obtained in our laboratory from an intravenous drug
user.

Other variants having minor differences from HTLV-I in
their genome have also been recognized (26). Retroviruses
closely related to HTLV-I have also been isolated from at least
2 species of Old World nonhuman primates (52). We call these
primate T-cell leukemia virus (PTLV). Molecular analysis of
isolates of PTLV retroviruses revealed that these viruses are
closely related to but distinct from HTLV-I (25).

Isolation of HTLV-III

Retroviruses classified as HTLV-I and HTLV-II have occasionally been isolated from tissues obtained from AIDS and pre-
AIDS patients (18, and Popovic et al., unpublished). In contrast to these observations retroviruses belonging to a distinct
new subgroup of HTLV have been isolated at a very high frequency
from AIDS and pre-AIDS patients and from donors at high risk

for AIDS (19,61). These viruses, named HTLV-III, have several features in common with HTLV-I and HTLV-II, namely a preferred tropism for OKT4/leu3+ lymphocytes, a Mg^{2+}-dependent high molecular weight reverse transcriptase, similar size and content of structural proteins, some immunological cross-reactivity of both their major core proteins and envelope, presence of the pX sequence and limited nucleic acid homology. The first HTLV-III isolates were obtained in this laboratory in November 1982, but because of the difficulty in growing the infected T cells adequate characterization was difficult. Eventually, permissive subclones of an established T-cell line were obtained which could be infected by HTLV-III and yielded large amounts of virus (61). This development facilitated the preparation of immunological and nucleic acid reagents for detailed characterization and comparison of these viruses allowing us to link HTLV-III to the etiology of AIDS. In addition, this development opened the way to large-scale blood bank assays for serum antibodies to HTLV-III.

Peripheral blood, bone marrow, and serum from AIDS and pre-AIDS patients and other donors were collected, processed and tested for the presence of virus or the presence of antibody to viral proteins. The isolation of virus from fresh patient material, e.g., peripheral blood or bone marrow lymphocytes was accomplished using techniques similar to those used for the isolation of HTLV-I and HTLV-II. Procedures used for the detection of virus included: 1) monitoring of supernatant fluids for viral reverse transcriptase activity; 2) transmission of virus to fresh normal human T lymphocytes, e.g., umbilical cord blood, adult peripheral blood, or bone marrow leukocytes; 3) electron microscopic observation of fixed, sectioned cells; and 4) testing for antigen expression by indirect immunofluorescence or radioimmunoprecipitation procedures using serum from antibody positive donors or hyperimmune sera prepared using purified virus.

HTLV-III has been isolated from a large number of the AIDS and pre-AIDS patients and from some clinically normal carriers (Table 1). For example, HTLV-III was isolated from ~50% of AIDS and ~80% of patients with pre-AIDS syndromes. HTLV-III was not found in 125 samples from normal heterosexual donors. This incidence of virus isolation from the AIDS samples is clearly an underestimate of the true frequency since many more patients have been exposed to the virus as indicated by the high percentage seropositive for antibody to viral protein (71,75 and discussed below). Using freshly obtained specimens, and by testing repeated samples from the same donors, the incidence of HTLV-III isolation approaches 100% (our personal observation). In later sections we will summarize some serological and other results which combined with the above data on virus isolations strongly indicate that HTLV-III is the cause of AIDS.

TABLE 1. Summary of HTLV-III isolates.

Patients and Donors	Diagnosis	Number of HTLV-III Isolates[a]
Homosexual	AIDS	33
Males	Pre-AIDS	20
	Clinically Normal	13
Non-Homosexual		
Intravenous Drug Users	Pre-AIDS	2
Hemophiliacs and	AIDS	4
Other Transfusion	Pre-AIDS	1
Recipients		
Juveniles	AIDS	3
	Pre-AIDS	1
Mothers of	AIDS	1
Juvenile AIDS	Pre-AIDS	1
	Clinically Normal	2
Promiscuous Males	AIDS	2
	Pre-AIDS	6
Spouses of AIDS,	Pre-AIDS	1
Pre-AIDS Patients	Clinically Normal	2
Random Donors	Clinically Normal	0

[a]The incidence of virus isolation varied depending on condition of cells, health of donor, etc. For AIDS the overall incidence number of successful virus isolation/number of patients tested was ~50% and ~80% for pre-AIDS patients.

BIOLOGICAL EFFECTS OF HTLV

Transformation of Fresh Human T Lymphocytes by HTLV-I

Extensive studies have shown that HTLV-I from various sources can transform human T lymphocytes (51,46,60,69). The procedures used for these studies were similar to those used to initiate fresh leukemic T cells in cell culture. HTLV-I was transmitted to fresh human T-cells by cocultivation with leth-ally irradiated HTLV-positive leukemic cells from cell lines grown in vitro or as extracellular virus. Infected, replicating cells were observed within 3-6 weeks after exposure to HTLV-I and these cells eventually grew to populate the culture. These transformed cells usually did not need added TCGF, although the initial steps of transformation were usually facilitated by its inclusion. The most sensitive target cells for these studies were umbilical cord blood and adult bone marrow leukocytes. Fresh adult peripheral blood leukocytes were not easily infected by HTLV-I. Despite repeated attempts to transmit HTLV-I to these cells, successful infection has been a very rare event. HTLV-I transformed cells had a population doubling time between 40-60 hours, and reached a cell saturation level of ~2 x 10⁶ cell/ml.

Properties of transformed cells.

Like leukemic T cells, a percentage of the HTLV-I-infected T lymphocyte cells contained lobulated nuclei and some became polynucleated. These transformed cells expressed T-lymphocyte markers, including receptors for sheep erythrocytes and reactivity with T-lymphocyte-specific monoclonal antibodies. Histochemically, these cells stained positively with an atypical globular-granular staining pattern, for nonspecific esterase and acid phosphatase and lack other cytochemicals, e.g., myeloperoxidase, chloroacetate esterase, and Sudan Black staining. They did not contain B-lymphocyte markers, e.g., surface immunoglobulin, Epstein-Barr virus nucleic acids or antigens. Like leukemic T lymphocytes, the HTLV-I-transformed cord blood T lymphocytes were usually OKT4/leu 3a+ (helper T-cell phenotype). Unlike cord blood T-cells, transformed bone marrow T-lymphocytes could also express surface markers usually found in other T-cell subsets (47), i.e., either OKT4/leu 3a+ (helper/ inducer phenotype), OKT8/leu 2a+ (cytotoxic/ suppressor T-cell phenotype), or those showing neither marker. However, there appears to be no consistent correlation between cell phenotype and functional T-cell subclass in the in vitro HTLV-I transformed cells. They usually are either functionally inactive or possess cytotoxic activity.

Differences between HTLV-I-transformed T-lymphocytes and were also observed. For example, the density per cell of receptors for TCGF and HLA-DR markers were about 50-fold greater in HTLV-infected cells than in mitogen-stimulated normal human cord blood T-cells (24). HTLV-transformed T lymphocytes also expressed elevated levels of receptors for transferrin, as expected for rapidly dividing cells. Other surface markers detected on HTLV-I-infected T-cells include HLA-A and -B locus antigens that were not present on the EBV-transformed B-cells or fresh peripheral blood lymphocytes from the same patient (44). It is not clear whether these antigens are induced cellular gene products or actually related to expression of infecting viral antigens. Considering possible mechanisms of transformation, and a possibility of their being involved in a differing susceptibility to infection, these observations may be significant.

Cellular and Immunological Regulatory Potential of HTLV-I and II Infected T Lymphocytes

Several T lymphocyte functions are apparently mediated by the release of soluble, biologically active factors termed lymphokines. T lymphocyte cultures, established either from

the peripheral blood of HTLV-I-positive patients with T-cell
malignancies or from human umbilical cord blood or bone marrow
T-cells transformed in vitro by HTLV-I, were found to constitutively produce one or more of a number of lymphokines including:
macrophage migration enhancing factor; leukocyte migration inhi-
bitory factor; migration enhancing factor; macrophage activating
factor; differentiation inducing activity; colony stimulating
factor; eosinophil growth and maturation activity; fibroblast
activating factor; and gamma interferon (68). In addition to
these activities, preliminary tests suggested that biological
activities related B cell growth factor and platelet-derived
growth factor may also be released in some instances. Some
T-lymphocytes established in cell cultures from leukemic donors
were also shown to produce low levels of TCGF (22,41).

Earlier observations suggested that infection by HTLV-I or
HTLV-II can modulate T lymphocyte immune functions. For example, Essex and coworkers found that patients in an infectious
diseases ward in a HTLV-I endemic region in Japan had almost
three times the prevalence of antibodies to HTLV-I than the
general population in the area (11). Similar observations were
made by others in patients from the Caribbean (6,9) and Africa
(15). These results suggest that natural exposure to the virus
may induce immunosuppression and therefore increase the susceptibility of the population to various opportunistic infections
or neoplastic transformation.

It was recently observed (50) that a T-cell line derived
from a HTLV-I infected ATL patient with a prolonged survival,
possessed specific cytotoxic activity to neoplastic T-cells
expressing HTLV-I, provided that the target tumor cells also
expressed at least one HLA antigen (HLA-A1) in common with the
effector cells (50). However, a clone (K7) derived from this
parental line appeared to have lost its normal immune functions.
When exposed to tumor cells expressing HTLV-I antigens, this
clonal population ceased to proliferate and eventually died.
This aberrant T-cell clone was found to have 1 copy of HTLV-I
provirus per cell (M. Clarke, unpublished results).

Loss of immune functions was also demonstrated after in
vitro infection of helper T-cells and cytotoxic T-cells with
HTLV-I and HTLV-II (59). Before infection, a cloned human
helper T-cell line proliferated and provided help to B-cells
only in the presence of both a specific soluble antigen (key
hole limpet hemocyamin) and histocompatible antigen-presenting
cells (APC). Following infection with either HTLV-I or HTLV-II,
these cells responded with increased proliferation to stimulation of polyclonal immunoglobulin production by B-cells regardless of the histocompatibility of the APC or the presence of
the soluble antigen. Similarly, HTLV-I infection of a cytotoxic
T-cell clone led to a diminution or loss of their cytotoxic
function (59). These data suggested that HTLV-I infection of
T-cells might induce immune deficiency and cause polyclonal
B-cell activation. These data further suggested to us that a

T-lymphotropic retrovirus, possibly belonging to the family of
HTLV, might be involved in the acquired immunodeficiency syndrome.

BIOLOGICAL PROPERTIES OF HTLV-III
    In contrast to HTLV-I or HTLV-II transmission of HTLV-III
to fresh human lymphocytes was most effective with cell-free
virus preparations. These could be used to infect not only cord
blood and bone marrow lymphocytes, but also normal adult peripheral blood lymphocytes. Like HTLV-I and -II the primary targets of HTLV-III are T-cells with a helper phenotype OKT4/leu 3+.
The usual consequence of infection by HTLV-III was a burst of
virus production, usually within 1-2 weeks following infection.
During this period of time a pronounced cytopathic effect on
the infected cells was also observed. As shown in Figure 4 one
effect is the formation of polynucleatid giant cells. Following
infection, the viable cell number decreased over the first
2-3 weeks. The cells most affected were those with the OKT4/
leu 3+ phenotype which rapidly died after infection. There is
also some evidence that cells other than those with the OKT4/
leu 3+ phenotypes may serve as a reservoir of virus in natural
disease and that then cells can be infected by HTLV-III at low
levels, e.g., monocytic cells and B-lymphocytes (our personal
observation). As has been described previously (61) certain
established human leukemic T-cell lines could also be produc-
tively infected by HTLV-III.

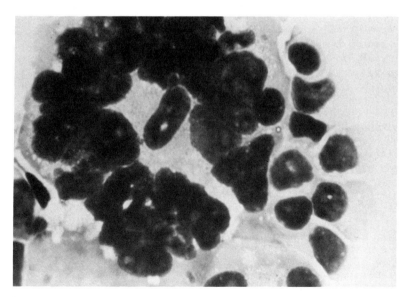

Fig. 4.   Cytopathic effect of HTLV-III on fresh human T lymphocytes.

As noted above, these cell lines are a valuable source of virus
in the preparation of reagents critical in the identification
and characterization of HTLV-III. Additional observations of a
retrovirus belonging to the HTLV-III group, were independently
made by other investigators. For example, a virus designated
lymphadenopathy virus (LAV) was first detected in cultured
lymphocytes from a patient with lymphadenopathy by Barré-
Sinoussi et al. (3). Additional isolations were found by the
same group from patients with AIDS but now called IDAV (89) and
later again as LAV (14). Preliminary comparison between these
HTLV-III and LAV demonstrated that they are closely related.

DISEASES CAUSED BY, OR ASSOCIATED WITH HTLV-INFECTION

HTLV-I Infection - Adult T-Cell Leukemia

A classification of human neoplastic lymphocytes into T
and B cells based on their distinctive cell surface markers
revealed that in general B-cell neoplasias are more common in
adults than T-cell malignancies such as Sézary syndrome, mycosis
fungoides, and acute lymphocytic leukemia of T-cell origin.
However, a slight elevation in the incidence of the T-cell
malignancies was observed in Japan (85,86,88). Although these
cases had some features of the classic Sézary syndrome and the
classic chronic lymphocytic leukemia of the T-cell type (T-CLL),
they were distinct. These T cell malignancies had the following
characteristics: Onset in adulthood and frequent dermal
involvement such as erythroderma and itching, and sometimes
cutaneous nodules. Histological examination of the skin lesions
often showed cutaneous and subcutaneous infiltration of numerous
abnormal cells, but unlike in Sézary syndrome and mycosis fungoides no epidermal infiltration like Pautrier microabsesses were
usually seen. Lymphadenopathy and hepatosplenomegaly were seen
in many cases. No mediastinal mass was observed and there was
no thymoma or thymic involvement. Frequently these patients
had unexplained hypercalcemia. Most importantly, the leukemic
cells had T-cell properties and they possessed distinctive
morphological features. The cells were pleomorphic and frequently had lobulated or indented nuclei. On clinical and pathological grounds, the disease represented a distinct syndrome
and was called adult T-cell leukemia (ATL) (28,85,86,88).
The original cases of ATL were identified in Kyoto, but
all of the patients came from one of two southernmost islands
of Japan, Kyushu or Shikoku. Since then it has been shown that
this disease clustered in these islands. The etiological significance of this geographic clustering became apparent subsequently, when it was shown that ATL is caused by HTLV-I infection (6,7,33,34,37,63,93).
Other geographic clusters of ATL have been identified in
the Caribbean basin, central and South America, and in some
parts of Africa. A low level of incidence of ATL is also seen

in the Southeastern United States, Israel, Italy, and in locations of African and Caribbean immigrants.

HTLV-III Infection - Acquired Immunodeficiency Syndrome

Acquired immunodeficiency syndrome (AIDS) has been recognized since 1981 as a unique clinical syndrome manifested by
opportunistic infections or neoplasms complicating an underlying
defect in the cellular immune system (13,23,40,48,80,83). The
major deficiency is a quantitative depletion of the helper
T-cell population. As a consequence, most AIDS patients present
with signs and symptoms secondary to opportunistic infections,
e.g., fever, pulmonary infiltrates, disseminated cryptococcal
disease, mental status changes associated with multiple CNS mass
lesions, etc. A definition of AIDS was based on the development
of opportunistic infections (40,83). This definition has limited usefulness for early diagnosis because it was primarily
designed to identify AIDS after the development of opportunistic
infections resulting from T-cell deficiency and was not based
on detailed clinical and epidemiological manifestations evident
in the early phases of the disease. Two common clinical characteristics of patients who develop AIDS are chronic extrainguinal
lymphadenopathy and subtle clinical manifestations of T-cell
deficiency due to an absolute depletion of T-cells (13).
Patients with generalized lymphadenopathy and helper T-cell
depletion, when followed, have developed AIDS (49). These
frequently observed manifestations of T-cell deficiency are
called lymphadenopathy syndrome, AIDS-related complex (ARC), or
pre-AIDS. Certain populations are at an increased risk for
AIDS. These include promiscuous homosexual males, intravenous
drug abusers, hemophiliacs, recent Haitian immigrants, heterosexual contacts of the above groups, newborns of high-risk
mothers, persons receiving blood transfusions, and most recently
promiscuous heterosexuals.

Some epidemiological studies indicate that transmission of
HTLV-III in semen may be one critical common route of infection
(21). Other body fluids such as saliva may also be involved as
a medium for infective transfer of the virus. In fact, virus
has been isolated from the saliva of 4 of 10 pre-AIDS patients
and 4 of 6 asymptomatic homosexual men at high risk for AIDS
(J.E. Groopman et al., submitted) and from lymphocytes found in
patient semen (D. Zagury et al., and M. Hirsch et al., submitted). Transfusion of infected blood probably rates the highest
in the efficiency of virus-transmission and thus the highest
risk factor for the acquisition of infection. Such infection
also happens frequently among intravenous drug users through
contaminated needles. AIDS in children of virus-infected
mothers probably occurs through infection by transplacental
maternal-fetal blood exchange.

EPIDEMIOLOGY

Epidemiology of HTLV-I

Seropeidemiology of HTLV-I.

Sera of patients with a variety of malignancies and control sera were screened for antibodies to HTLV-I proteins. The methods employed for these studies in our laboratory were: (a) solid phase immunoassay using disrupted viral particles; (b) radioimmune precipitation assays using pure HTLV-I p24, p19, and p15; and (c) indirect immunofluoresence against virus infected cells under live or fixed cell conditions (36,62-65). In some systems (e.g., (a) and (c)) positive results are further verified for specificity using appropriate controls. An example of results from such studies are shown on Table 2 and can be summarized as follows. Sera of patients with ATL are almost always positive for antibodies to HTLV-I. Normal individuals and patients with non-T-cell leukemias and lymphomas lack antibodies to HTLV-I as do patients with T-cell malignancies that are not the typical HTLV-I type. In the ATL-endemic geographic areas, prevalence of antibody positive asymptomatic carriers is significantly higher than in non-endemic areas. For instance, in Japan the range of antibody-positive normal subjects range from 0% in Hokkaido district in the north to as high as 16% in Nagasaki area and 15% in Kagoshima area in the Kyushu district in the southwest (64). The prevalence of antibody-positive cases parallels remarkably well the clustering pattern of ATL (63,64). A second well-documented endemic area for HTLV-I associated malignancies is the Caribbean basin. In one study, about 70% of all the adult non-Hodgkin's lymphoid malignancies studied in Jamaica over a one year period contained serum antibodies to HTLV-I (4-6). Antibodies to HTLV-I was also observed in sera from nearly 100% of the ATL patients among black Caribbean immigrants in England (6,7). Studies of healthy people from the Caribbean indicate that a range of 1% to about 12% are positive for antibodies to HTLV-I.

Antibody positive adult T-cell malignancies with clinical features similar to typical ATL have been found sporadically in the United States and Israel (17) and in a few limited surveys such cases have also been identified in Central and South America, Africa, and southern Italy. Since several regions are endemic in Africa, we anticipate that clusters of ATL patients will be identified there in additional studies. For instance, antibody prevalence of 2-10% have been found among normal populations from Capetown South Africa, Nigeria, Egypt, Tunisia, and Ghana (73).

In contrast to ATL where there is a clear etiological association between HTLV-I and the disease, the occasional antibody positive patients with non-T-cell leukemias or lymphomas or childhood leukemias may be victims of HTLV infection as a "passenger virus", probably by blood transfusions. However, in some HTLV-I endemic areas, antibody positive ATL and B-cell CLL have

TABLE 2.   Prevalence of natural antibodies to HTLV-I in sera
           of patients with mature T cell malignancies
                   and their healthy relatives

	Antibodies to HTLV-I
	No. positive/
	No. tested (%)
Healthy relatives of U.S. patients with HTLV-associated malignancy	5/35 (14)
Unrelated healthy donors, Washington, D.C.	1/185 (<1)
Unrelated healthy donors, Georgia	4/538 (<1)
Caribbean ATL patients	11/11 (100)
Healthy relatives of Caribbean patients	4/20 (20)
Random healthy donors, Caribbean	12/337 (4)
Japanese ATL patients	45/52 (87)
Healthy relatives of ATL patients	20/43 (47)
Random healthy donors, nonendemic area, Japan	9/600 (2)
Random healthy donors, endemic area, Japan	50/419 (12)

been found in the absence of blood transfusions and at a rate
of incidence greater than observed in the normal population.
It is possible that in these cases infection of normal T-cells
by HTLV leads to impaired T-cell function leading to an
increased risk of leukemias or lymphomas by other causes or
HTLV-I infected T-cells may stimulate proliferation of cells of
different lineages resulting in leukemias in which the leukemic
cell is not the infected cell.
    Seroepidemiological studies indicate that transmission of
HTLV-I may require close or intimate contact because: (i) The
single most antibody-prevalent group other than ATL patients
are family members of ATL patients.   In fact, in areas where
ATL is not endemic, they form the only significant group of
antibody positive people (65).   Within the families the data
suggest that transmission occurs from male to female and female
to child (84).   (ii) Antibodies to HTLV-I have been demonstrated
in people receiving transfusions of HTLV-positive blood such as
hemophiliacs (12,72,73) and the virus has been isolated from
intravenous drug users (unpublished data of M. Popovic and
R. Gallo).   One possible major source of transmission of HTLV-I
is the infected cell.   Modes of transmission might occur by sex
through lymphocytes in semen, by insect vectors, by blood transfusions, by contaminated needles during illicit drug use, by in
vitro maternal-fetus exchange, and possibly through mother's
milk.

Molecular epidemiology of HTLV-I

Availability of molecularly cloned DNA probes specific for the LTR and other regions of the HTLV-I genome enabled their use in screening cellular DNA of cultured cells as well as uncultured fresh tumors of patients with ATL and other malignancies for proviral sequences. These studies using Southern blot hybridization procedures primarily carried out by two groups (92,93) reached the same conclusions. (a) Fresh cells from all patients with typical ATL contain one or a few copies of HTLV provirus. (b) The provirus was complete in most instances but a few examples of proviral DNA consisting only of envelope and LTR were found. (c) Tumor cells from other types of malignancies involving immature T-cells, B-cells or myeloid cells in general lack HTLV-I sequences. (d) The results of the molecular hybridization survey and of the serum antibody surveys correlate very closely; however, in a few instances the neoplastic T-cells from patients negative for serum antibodies were positive for HTLV-I proviral sequences. (e) The site of integration of the HTLV-I provirus in different patients was different, i.e., no two patients had the same cellular sequences flanking the integrated provirus. (f) The infected cells are oligoclonal or monoclonal. This implies that the HTLV-I infection in each case preceded the neoplastic transformation. (g) The proviruses from all HTLV-I-associated malignancies worldwide (Japan, South America, the Caribbean, the United States, etc.) are essentially identical.

Seroepidemiology of HTLV-III

Sera of a large number of patients with AIDS, those with signs and symptoms often preceeding AIDS, homosexual males, hemophiliacs, and normal control subjects were analyzed for antibodies to HTLV-III. The techniques used included: (a) an enzyme-linked immunosorbent assay (ELISA); (b) a Western blot analysis, and (c) radioimmunoprecipitation of purified HTLV-III p24. In the ELISA system detergent-salt-disrupted HTLV-III was bound to microtiter plate wells and reacted with the test sera. Immune reactivity was detected using an enzyme labeled second antibody to human immunoglobulins. Western blot assays were performed by electrophoretically separating the viral antigens on a SDS-polyacrylamide gel and transferring the protein bands to a nitrocellulose sheet Longitudinal strips of the nitrocellulose sheet contaning the representative profile of viral protein bands were used to screen the sera for reactive antibodies (Fig. 5). Routinely, sera were initially screened by the ELISA system. Those that were negative in ELISA were rescreened by the Western blot. Sera were considered antibody positive if they reacted positive in the ELISA or if they reacted positive in the Western blot even if they were initially negative in the ELISA (67,71).

In a coded sample study, this system of screening scored
100% of all AIDS patients sera positive and none of the control
sera that included those from normal individuals and those with
non-AIDs related illnesses (67).   In addition to the nearly
total correlation between HTLV-III antibodies and AIDS, the
results also indicate that patients with lymphadenopathy sydrome
[AIDS-related complex (ARC)], have a high prevalence of antibodies to HTLV-III.   Others with antibodies to HTLV-III include
promiscuous homosexual men and intravenous drug users.   In
contrast, a large number of controls were negative for HTLV-III
antibodies.   Among individuals with no traditional risk factors
for AIDS, antibodies to HTLV-III were detected among recipients
of blood transfusions or blood products recipient of a kidney
transplant from a donor who was antibody positive and among
female sexual partners of men with HTLV-III infection.   Examples
of such studies carried out in our laboratory are shown in
Table 3.

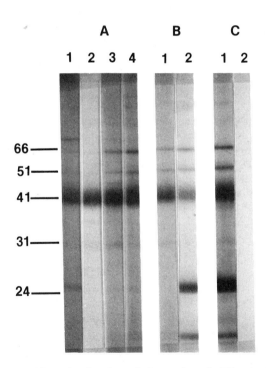

FIG. 5.   Western Blot Analysis of Sera for Antibody to HTLV-III
Structural Protein.   Proteins from disrupted HTLV-III were fractionated by electrophoresis on 12% polyacrylamide slab gels,
transferred to nitrocellulose sheets, and evaluated with sera
as described (67).   Panel A, serum from 4 AIDS patients, Panel B,
serum from 2 pre-AIDS patients, Panel C, sera from one sera-
positive (1) and one sero-negative (2) homosexual male.

TABLE 3.　Antibodies to HTLV III in sera of patients
with AIDS and AIDS related complex

Patients/Donors	Number / Number Positive / Tested (%)
Patients with AIDS	288/297 (97)
Patients with AIDS Related Complex	327/360 (91)
Asymptomatic Homosexual Men	96/235 (41)
High Risk Blood Donors	9/9
Renal Transplant Recipient from High Risk Donor	1/1
Controls	
Random Normal Donors	0/238
Black Women from Baltimore (1962 Collection)	0/100
Healthy Japanese from HTLV-I Endemic Regions	0/123
Patients with Leukemias and Other Malignancies from HTLV-I Endemic Areas	0/34
Healthy Surinamese (Methodone-Treatment Group)	0/54
Schizophrenics	0/30
Hodgkins Patients and Siblings	0/160
Renal Transplant Recipients	0/24
Other Immunosuppressed Cases	0/34
Miscellaneous Patients[a]	0/82

[a]These include heavily transfused patients and those with:
Hepatitis B virus infection, primary stage Syphilis, Rheumatoid
arthritis, Systemic lupus erythematosus, Acute mononucleosis,
Lymphatic leukemias, B- and T-cell lymphomas, Alopacia areata,
Idiopathic splenomegaly.

MOLECULAR BIOLOGY

The Genomes of HTLV-I and HTLV-II

The complete nucleotide sequence of one isolate of HTLV-I
has been determined (77). Figure 1 depicts the structure and
deduced coding regions of this genome. Many unusual features
are notable. First of all, the provirus is flanked by unusually
long Long Terminal Repeat (LTR) sequences as compared to those
of other retroviruses. The gag gene codes for three viron core
proteins, p19, p24 and p15 instead of four proteins usually
encoded by the gag gene of other retroviruses. By alignment of
the predicted, and sometimes actual, amino acid sequence of
these proteins to other mammalian retrovirus gag proteins, it
was concluded that a phosphoprotein (p10-p12) is lacking in
HTLV-I (reviewed in 29). A long non-coding sequence separating
the gag and pol genes of HTLV-I has distant homology to
sequences coding for the carboxyl terminal gag protein (p19) in

RSV or those at the beginning of the pol gene of MuLV possibly coding for a similar protein product. Therefore, HTLV-I lacks two structural proteins compared to these two retroviruses. Whether these deficiencies would attenuate the replication of HTLV-I remains to be determined.

In addition to open reading frames potentially coding for the gag, pol, and env precursor proteins, there is a region of about 1.6 kilobase between the carboxyl terminus of the env gene and 3' LTR that contains four open reading frames. This region, initially referred to as the pX region, is not closely homologous to cellular sequences of vertebrate cells, and therefore, is not a typical retroviral oncogene. Deletions in the first open reading frame (pX-1) found in a variant, HTLV-Ib, obtained from an African ATL patient (Hahn et al., in press) did not affect the transforming capacity of this virus (L. Ratner et al., in preparation). A better definition of the pX region was obtained by comparison to an analogous region in HTLV-II (see below), which indicated that only the 3' kb pX sequences may be functional.

HTLV-II has a very similar genomic organization as HTLV-I. The LTR resembles that of HTLV-I in the unusual lengths of R and U5 sequences and the lack of a Proudfoot-Brownlee consensus sequence upstream of the polyadenylation site (35,77,79,81). However, the actual sequences of the two LTRs differ markedly. Homologies are limited to short stretches at the 5' and 3' ends of the LTR, probably reflecting functional conservation for virus integration and transcription, and a 21 bp repeat sequence which is repeated imperfectly three times in HTLV-I and four times in HTLV-II (81). Although this repeat is not homologous to consensus transcriptional enhancer sequences (39), its presence as a tandomly repeated sequence in U3 upstream of the RNA initiation site suggests that it serves as a core enhancer sequence. Its different arrangement in HTLV-I and HTLV-II may determine differences in the disease potential of these two viruses, by analogy to some murine retroviruses in which rearrangement of enhancer sequences may affect their leukemogenicity (10,42).

Except for the LTRs, homology throughout the HTLV-I and -II genomes can be observed under relatively nonstringent conditions. Under stringent conditions, however, only a 1 kb stretch of homology within the pX region is seen. Nucleotide sequence of the pX region of HTLV-II revealed two domains: a 0.6 kb sequence that is markedly divergent from HTLV-I pX, and a highly conserved 1.0 kb sequence which contains a single long open reading frame (LOR) in both (30). Since the LOR region does not initiate with an ATG codon, the encoded protein is likely to be a fusion protein of at least 38 kd in size. A 42 kd protein has been identified in all HTLV-I transformed cells, and preliminary amino acid sequence data suggest that at least part of this protein is encoded by the LOR region (Lee et al., in preparation).

Possible Mechanism of Transformation and Leukemogenesis by HTLV-I and HTLV-II

Cells infected by HTLV-I and HTLV-II in vitro are initially polyclonal with respect to provirus integration and go through a growth crisis within 4-6 weeks. Some cells then emerge as immortalized cells, often becoming independent of exogenous TCGF (Il-2) for growth, and these cells are predominantly clonal (C. Grandori et al., unpublished). However, the site of provirus integration is variable in different infection events. We have followed cells from the time of infection through the progression to monoclonality and found that virus or viral structural proteins (reverse transcriptase, core and envelope proteins) are often not expressed during this process of clonal selection of infected cells. It is not clear whether expression of the LOR product alone is essential. The lack of a unique integration site for the provirus and the highly conserved nature of the LOR sequences between the two transforming HTLVs suggest that the LOR product, which is not homologous to any structural protein of retroviruses, may be directly involved in cellular transformation. Recently, Sodroski et al. (81,82), observed that a bacterial gene (CAT) linked to the enhancer-promoter sequences of the HTLV-I and HTLV-II LTR can be transcriptionally activated in cells that are infected with HTLV-I or HTLV-II, including cells that are not expressing any other viral protein except the 42 kd presumed LOR product. Therefore, it is speculated that the LOR protein acts in a trans manner to activate the enhancer-promoter sequences of the viral LTR in transcription. It has been further speculated that the LOR protein would activate specific cellular genes via cellular enhancer-promoter elements. If these genes are involved in T-cell proliferation, the cells may be locked in a constantly proliferative state and are thus transformed. There are a number of cellular genes that are known to be activated by infection with HTLV-I and HTLV-II. These include the gene for TCGF receptor (91), and two genes that are linked to T-cell activation (2,45). It will be of interest to find out if the LOR protein activates the transciption of these genes.

Although HTLV-I transforms cells efficiently in vitro, it induces ATL in infected people only after a long latency period. Furthermore, fresh ATL cells usually exhibit clonal chromosomal abnormalities even though the in vitro transformed cells retain a normal karyotype (54). Therefore, a second event may be necessary for development of frank malignancy. Fresh ATL cells rarely express detectable levels of viral mRNA, including LOR sequences (16). Additionally, although each ATL sample is monoclonal, containing 1-3 copies of HTLV-I, there is no conserved integration site from sample-to-sample (76). Therefore, the virus does not seem to function either in a cis or trans manner in maintaining the leukemic state. It is possible that expression of LOR is necessary to set off a chain of events leading to development of the disease but is not necessary to maintain it.

Characterization of the HTLV-III Genome

We have exploited the high producer cell line H9/HTLV-III to obtain molecular clones of HTLV-III using three approaches: 1) cDNA clones were obtained from a recombinant plasmid library of double-stranded cDNA synthesized from purified virion RNA in the presence of oligo-dT primers (1 and unpublished data). These clones mostly represent 1-2 kb sequences from the 3' end of the viral genome. 2) Clones of unintegrated proviruses were obtained from a recombinant phage library derived from Hirt supernatent DNA of acutely infected H9 cells. Three clones were analyzed in detail and found to be comprised of one full length genome and two fragments that possibly constitute one complete genome (27). 3) Clones of integrated proviruses with flanking cellular sequences were obtained from a genomic DNA library of H9/ HTLV-III cells (G. Shaw et al., submitted). H9/ HTLV-III was established by infection of H9 cells with pooled culture supernatents of short term cultured lymphocytes of several AIDS patients, and our analysis of the derived molecular clones indicated at least four highly related proviruses with some divergence in the restriction enzyme sites (Fig. 6). The widespread existence of HTLV-III variants was confirmed by screening DNA of other HTLV-III infected cells or of fresh tissues of AIDS patients by Southern hybridization. We have identified at least nine distinct HTLV proviruses out of 10 analyzed using four restriction enzymes. This extent of polymorphism was not found among different HTLV-I or HTLV-II isolates (26,27, 92) and may be due to the highly replicative nature of HTLV-III as opposed to the cryptic state of the HTLV-I and -II proviruses in vivo. It will be important to determine if the changes in HTLV-III cluster in any particular region of the virus genome and if they are significant enough to alter the immunological reactivities of the different virus isolates.

We also evaluated the homology between HTLV-III and other subgroups of HTLV (I, Ib and II) by Southern hybridization and heteroduplex mapping (1). The results showed short stretches of significant homology in the gag-pol region. Nucleotide sequence of the HTLV-III genome revealed extra coding sequence analogous to pX (unpublished data), which characterizes members of the HTLV family.

No hybridization was detected with the HTLV-III genome as probe to DNA of the uninfected HT, H9 and H4 cells as well as DNA of other normal human tissues, indicating that the virus is completely exogenous and does not carry a conserved cellular gene. Lymph node tissues and peripheral lymphocytes of AIDS patients were also examined. Infection with HTLV-III does not lead to a clonal cell expansion but, to the contrary, leads to death of the infected T-cell. Therefore, we expected that in the population of lymphocytes sampled from an AIDS patient, few would be infected. As anticipated, the results indicate that the infected cells are scarce. Only a few samples contain

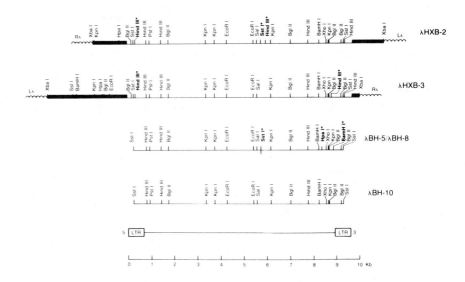

FIG. 6. Restriction endonuclease maps of four closely related
clones of HTLV-III. λHXB-2 and λHXB-3 represent full-length
integrated proviral forms of HTLV-III obtained from a lambda
phage library of H9/HTLV-III DNA. These clones contain the
complete provirus including two LTR regions (thin lines) plus
flanking cellular sequences (heavy lines). The lengths of the
LTRs are estimated. Clones λBH-10 and λBH-5/8 were derived from
the linear unintegrated replicative intermediate form of HTLV-
III in acutely infected H9 cells and have been reported elsewhere (1) Their restriction maps are shown here for comparison
with λHXB-2 and λHXG-3 and with Southern blots of genomic DNA
from other HTLV-III containing cells. It should be noted that
λBH-5/8 consists of two independent clones (λBH-5 and λBH-8)
which together comprise one HTLV-III genomic equivalent.
Differences in the restriction maps between these HTLV-III
clones are indicated by bold letters and asterisks using λBH-10
as a reference.

detectable levels of provirus which represent at best one
infected cell in a hundred. Lymphocytes from patients with
lymphadenopathy syndrome (LAS) were also tested. This is a
disorder exhibiting extensive lymphocyte proliferation, and
usually pre-dating the onset of frank AIDS. Very few specimens
revealed detectable proviral sequences. This result also rules
out HTLV-III as having a direct role in the proliferation of
lymphocytes in LAS patients. Our thinking is that LAS is secondary to other (secondary) infections and/or is due to indirect

effects of HTLV-III, i.e., a small number of infected T-cells promoting proliferation of other lymphocytes in early phases of the disease. Finally, Kaposi tumor tissues from AIDS patients also did not contain detectable levels of HTLV-III DNA, again ruling our a direct role of this virus for tumor induction.

Antigenic Properties of HTLV-I, II, III

SDS-polyacrylamide gel electrophoresis of sucrose-density banded HTLV-III indicated a protein profile similar to those of HTLV-I and HTLV-II with some minor differences (71,75). There were prominent Coomassie Blue stained bands at 40,000-46,000, 24,000 and 15,000-17,000 daltons. They presumably corresponded to the envelope glycoprotein and the major gag proteins of the virus. A comparison of the antigenic properties of HTLV-III with those of HTLV-I and HTLV-II was made using the Western blot analysis. Lysates of HTLV-I, HTLV-II and HTLV-III were subjected to polyacrylamide slab gel electrophoresis and the protein bands transferred to a nitrocellulose sheet. These blots were then reacted with rabbit antisera raised against HTLV-I, HTLV-II, and HTLV-III. The results demonstrated the following cross-reactivities in the p24 antigen between the viruses: While the strongest antibody reactions were with the homologous proteins, moderate reactivities were observed between: HTLV-I p24 and antibody to HTLV-II, and HTLV-III p24 and antibody to HTLV-II. Weak reactions were also seen between HTLV-I p24 and antibody to HTLV-III. The cross-reactivity between HTLV-II p24 and HTLV-III p24 appears to be a one-way reactivity because there appeared to be no significant reaction between the antibody to HTLV-III and HTLV-II p24.

Competition radioimmunoassays of HTLV-III p24 showed that HTLV-III is a unique retrovirus with a major core protein, p24, unrelated to most other retroviruses. The p24 of HTLV-III, however, does share a low but detectable level of antigenic cross-reactivity with HTLV-I and HTLV-II and not with other retroviruses. These cross-reactivities with HTLV-I and -II are seen more clearly in the Western blot analysis than in conventional competition radioimmunoassays. It is analogous to the detection of cross-reactivities between HTLV-I p24 and BLV p24 by the Western blot, although no such cross-reactivities could be demonstrated between the two viruses using competition radioimmunoassays (our personal observations). It is clear that HTLV-I and HTLV-II are more closely related to each other than HTLV-III is to either HTLV-I or HTLV-II. The properties of HTLV-III which place this virus in the HTLV family are summarized in Table 4.

TABLE 4. Relatedness of HTLV-III to HTLV-I and HTLV-II

Property	Subgroup of HTLV		
	I	II	III
1. General infectivity	Lym	Lym	Lym
2. Particular tropism	T4	T4	T4
3. RT size	~100K	~100K	~100K
4. RT divalent cation	Mg^{++}	Mg^{++}	Mg^{++}
5. Major core	p24	p24	p24
6. Common envelope epitope	+	+	+
			(Essex)
7. Common p24 epitope	+	+	+
8. Nucleic acid homology to I (stringent)		±	−
9. Nucleic acid homology to I (moderate stringency)		++	+
10. Homology to other retroviruses except PTLV	0	0	0
11. Genome contains a pX region	+	+	+
12. Produces giant multinucleated cells	+	+	+
13. African origin	Likely	?	Likely

SUMMARY AND FUTURE

HTLV is the generic name we gave to the first human retroviruses. To date there are more than 100 isolates since their
discovery in sporadic cases of adult T-cell malignancies in the
U.S. Isolation of HTLV has been made routine by the selection
of the proper patient and by the careful growth of the appropriate cell type with T-cell growth factor (TCGF), also known as
interleukin-2 (Il-2). The vast majority of isolates are very
closely related; we call them HTLV-I. HTLV-I is endemic (at
low rates) in some black populations of: the Caribbean, South
and Central America, southeast U.S., and especially Africa. It
is also endemic in some Indian populations in these regions and
Alaska and in Japanese from southern Japan. Transmission seems
to be only by intimate contact or by blood. Viruses closely
related to HTLV-I, but distinct from it, have been isolated from
Old World monkeys. This and other facts led us to propose that
the ancestral origin of HTLV is in Africa. Evidence indicates
that HTLV-I is the direct cause of an aggressive form of adult
T-cell leukemia and lymphoma, e.g.: (a) multiple animal models
of retrovirus induced T-cell leukemias/lymphomas; (b) consistent
epidemiology (case clusters where HTLV-I clusters); (c) reproducible identification of virus in this precise disease; (d) viral

sequences integrated in the DNA of the host tumor cell; (e) integration in many sites early after infection but in one site (monoclonality) of each cell of the tumor; (f) in vitro transformation of primary fresh human T-cells, converting these into immortalized cells with properties remarkably similar to HTLV-I positive primary T-cell malignancies, despite the fact that HTLV does not carry an onc gene as conventionally known. These cell lines are rich sources of many lymphokines and surprisingly become monoclonal a few months after infection.

The mechanisms involved in the in vitro immortalization and in vivo malignancy are not yet clear but apparently do not involve any visible consistent chromosomal change, consistent virus expression, or known onc gene. Current leads suggest involvement of: (1) the pX product (a region at the 3' end of all HTLV) in initiation of growth; (2) the TCGF receptors, since they are consistently present and in high numbers; (3) promiscuous response to Ia antigens acting as growth factors. Whichever the mechanism for growth induction by HTLV-I, its efficiency in causing malignancy may be because it has dual major effects on infected cells: (1) immortalization of some T-cells, and (2) interference with function and cytopathic changes in many others.

Recent data suggest that HTLV-I may also be indirectly involved in the origin of some B-cell malignancies, e.g., in Jamaica sera from 35% of patients with B-cell CLL have antibodies to HTLV-I, but the proviral sequences are present in the normal T-cells not the B-cell tumors.

We also discovered a second class of human T-lymphotropic retroviruses (HTLV-II). It shares many features with HTLV-I but has major genomic differences. This virus also can immortalize some T4 cells. It has been isolated only from one patient with hairy cell leukemia, and recently we isolated it again from a patient with AIDS. The role of HTLV-II, if any, in human disease is unknown.

Finally, we have obtained more than 100 isolates of HTLV-III. This retrovirus shares some antigenic cross reactivity and genomic homology with HTLV-I and II, is also highly T4 tropic, but has only the cytopathic not immortalizing effects. The common properties of HTLV-I, II and III are listed in Table 4. All isolates of HTLV-III have come from patients with AIDS or people at high risk for this disease. Sera from more than 95% of AIDS and pre-AIDS patients have antibodies specifically against this virus, whereas <1% of healthy heterosexuals are positive. These and some prospective studies indicate that HTLV-III is the cause of AIDS. Although usually cytopathic, HTLV-III can now be grown in large quantities in permanent cell lines. This offers the ability to screen large numbers of people for evidence of infection and also allows development of a vaccine to prevent infection.

The HTLV family offers unique opportunities to discover the mechanism and etiology of human disease. A schematic representation of its members is seen in Fig. 7. HTLV-I is an important cause of human leukemia/lymphoma in regions of the world such as southern Japan and the Caribbean. This virus provides us with the first in vitro model of leukemogenesis, whose mechanism has remained elusive. A new class of transforming genese has been elucidated, distinct from onc genes. These appear to be coded by the pX region of the genome. At this time, this family of viruses has been shown to be responsible for two human diseases, Adult T-cell leukemia/lymphoma and AIDS. These characterized viruses can now be used as nucleic acid or immunologic probes to explore other human diseases suspected of having a viral origin. Perhaps we will soon be uncovering other related members of this family and be able to provide a link to other disease etiologies.

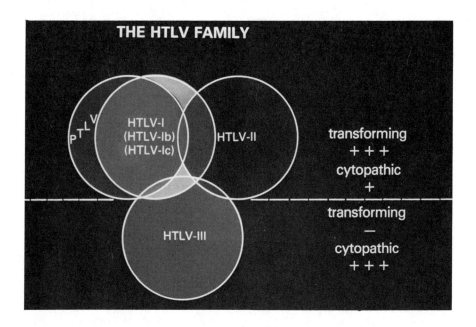

FIG. 7. Schematic representation of the relationship and biological properties of members of the HTLV family.

REFERENCES

1. Arya, S.K., Gallo, R.C., Hahn, B.H., Shaw, G.M., Popovic, M., Salahuddin, S.Z., and Wong-Staal, F. (1984): Science, in press.

2. Arya, S.K., Wong-Staal, F., Gallo, R.C. (1984): Molecular and Cell Biol., in press.
3. Barré-Sinoussi, F., Chermann, J.C., Rey, F., et al. (1983): Science, 220:868-871.
4. Blattner, W.A., Clark, J.W., Gibbs, W.N., Jaffe, E.S., Robert-Guroff, M., Saxinger, W.C., and Gallo, R.C. (1984): In: Human T-Cell Leukemia Viruses, pp. 267-274, edited by R.C. Gallo, M. Essex and L. Gross, Cold Spring Harbor Press, New York.
5. Blattner, W.A., Gibbs, W.N., Saxinger, C., et al. (1983): Lancet ii:61.
6. Blattner, W.A., Kalyanaraman, V.S., Robert-Guroff, M., Lister, T.A., Galton, D.A.G., Sarin, P.S., Crawford, M.H., Catovsky, D., Greaves, M. and Gallo, R.C. (1982): Int. J. Cancer, 30:257-264.
7. Catovsky, D., Greaves, M.F., Rose, M, Galton, D.A.G., Goolden, A.W.G., McCluskey, D.R., White, J.M., Lampert, I., Bourikas, G., Ireland, R., Brownell, A.I., Bridges, J.M., Blattner, W.A., and Gallo, R.C. (1982): Lancet i (#8273), 639-642.
8. Clapham, P., Nagy, K., and Weiss, R.A., (1984). Proc. Natl. Acad. Sci. USA. 81:2886-2888.
9. Clark, J.S., Hahn, B.H., Mann, D., et al. (1984): Submitted for publication.
10. DesGroseillers, L., Rossart, E., Jolieolur, P. (1983): Proc. Natl. Acad. Sci. USA, 80:4203-4207.
11. Essex, M.E., McLane, M.F., Tachibana, N., Francis, D.P. and Lee., T.-H. (1984): In: Human T-Cell Leukemia/Lymphoma Virus, edited by R.C. Gallo, M. Essex and L. Gross, Cold Spring Harbor Laboratory, New York, pp. 355-362.
12. Evatt, B.L., Francis, D.P., McLane, M.F., et al. (1983): Lancet, 1:698-700.
13. Fauci, A.S., Macher, A.M., Longo, D.L., et al. (1984): Ann. Int. Med., 100:92-106.
14. Feorino, P.M., Kalyanaraman, V.S., Haverkos, H.W., et al. (1984): Science, 225:69-72.
15. Fleming, A., Yamamoto, N., Bhusnarmath, S., et al. (1983): Lancet ii:334.
16. Franchini, G., Wong-Staal, F., Gallo, R.C. (1984): Proc. Natl. Acad. Sci. USA, in press.
17. Gallo, R.C., Kalyanaraman, V.S., Sarngadharan, M.G., et al. (1983): Cancer Res., 43:3892-3899.
18. Gallo, R.C., Sarin, P.S., Gelmann, E.P., Robert-Guroff, M., Richardson, E., Kalyanaraman, V.S., Mann, D.L., Sidhu, G., Stahl, R.E., Zolla-Pazner, S., Leibowitch, J., and Popovic, M. (1983c): Science, 220:865-867.
19. Gallo, R.C., Salahuddin, S.Z., Popovic, M., Shearer, G.M., Kaplan, M., Haynes, B.F., Palker, T.J., Redfield, R., Oleske, J., Safai, B., White, F., Foster, P., Markham, P.D. (1984): Science, 224:500-503.

20. Gallo, R.C. (1984): In: Cancer Surveys, pp.113-159, edited by L.M. Franks, L.M. Wyke, and R.A. Weiss, Oxford University Press, Oxford.

21. Goedert, J.J., Sarngadharan, M.G., Bigger, R.J., Weiss, S.H., Grossman, R.J., Greene, M.H., Bodner, A., Mann, D.L., Strong, D.M., Gallo, R.C., and Blattner, W.A. (1984): Lancet, in press.

22. Gootenberg, J.E., Ruscetti, F.W., Mier, J.W., Gazdar, A.F., and Gallo, R.C. (1981): J. Exp. Med., 154:1403-1418.

23. Gottlieb, M.S., Schrodd, R., Schanker, H.M., et al. (1981): N. Engl. J. Med., 305: 1425-1431.

24. Greene, W.C., and Robb, R.J. (1984): Receptors for T-cell growth factor: structure, function, and expression on normal and neoplastic cells. In: Contemporary Topics in Molecular Immunology. Edited by S. Gillis, Plenum Press, New York, in press.

25. Guo, H.-G., Wong-Staal, F., and Gallo, R.C. (1984): Science, 223:1195-1197.

26. Hahn, B.H., Shaw, G.M., Popovic, M., LoMonico, A., and Gallo, R.C. (1984): Int. J. Cancer, in press.

27. Hahn, B.H., Shaw G.M., Arya, S.K., Popovic, M., Gallo, R.C., and Wong-Staal, F. (1984): Nature, in press.

28. Hanaoka, M. (1981): Acta Haem. Japanese, 44:1420-1430.

29. Haseltine, W.A., Sodroski, J.G., and Patarca, R. (1984): Current Topics in Microbiol., in press.

30. Haseltine, W.A., Sodroski, J., Patarca, R., Briggs, D., Perkins, D., and Wong-Staal, F. (1984): Science, 225: 419-421.

31. Haynes, B.F., Miller, S.W., Palker, T.J., Moore, J.O., Dunn, P.H., Bolognesi, D.P., and Metzgar, R.S. (1983): Proc. Natl. Acad. Sci. USA, 80:2054-2058.

32. Hayward, W.S., Neel, B.G., and Astrin, S.M. (1981): Nature, 290:475-480.

33. Hinuma, Y., Komoda, H., Chosa, T., Kondo, T., Kohakura, M., Takenaka, T., Kikuchi, M., Ichimura, M., Yunoki, K., Sato, I., Matsuo, R., Takiuichi, Y., Uchino, H., and Hanaoka, M. (1982): International Journal of Cancer, 29:631-635.

34. Hinuma, Y., Nagata, K., Misoka, M., Nakai, M., Matsumoto, T., Kinoshita, K.I., Shirakawa, S., and Miyoshi, I. (1981): Proc.Nat. Acad.Sci.USA, 78:6476-6480.

35. Josephs, S.F., Wong-Staal, F., Manzari, V., Gallo, R.C., Sodroski, J.G., Trus, M.D., Perkins, D., Patarca, R., Haseltine, W.A. (1984): Virology, in press.

36. Kalyanaraman, V.S., Sarngadharan, M.G., Bunn, P.A., Minna, J.D., and Gallo, R.C. (1981a): Nature, 294:271-273.

37. Kalyanaraman, V.S., Sarngadharan, M.G., Nakao, Y., Ito, Y., Aoki, T., and Gallo, R.C. (1982a): Proc. Natl. Acad. Sci., USA, 79:1653-1657.

38. Kalyanaraman, V.S., Sarngadharan, M.G., Robert-Guroff, M., et al. (1982): Science, 218:571-573.

39. Khoury, G., and Gruss, P. (1983): Cell 33:313-314.
40. Lane, H.C., Masur, H., Edgar, L.C., Whalen, G., Rook, A.H., Fauci, A.S. (1983): N. Engl. J. Med., 309:453-458.
41. Le, J., Vilcék, J., Sadlik, J.R., Cheung, M.K., Balazs, I., Sarngadharan, M.G., and Prensky, W. (1983): J. Immun., 130:1231-1235.
42. Lenz, J., and Haseltine, W.A. (1983): J. Virol. 47:317-323.
43. Leonard, W.J., Depper, J.M., Uchiyama, T., Smith, K.A., Waldman, T.A., and Greene, W.C. (1982): Nature (London) 300:267-269.
44. Mann, D.L., Popovic, M., Sarin, P.S., Murray, C., Reitz, M.S., Strong, D.M., Haynes, B.F., Gallo, R.C., and Blattner, W.A. (1983): Nature, 305:58-60.
45. Manzari, U., Gallo, R.C., Franchini, G., Westin, E., Popovic, M., and Wong-Staal, R. (1983): Proc. Natl. Acad. Sci. USA, 80:11-15.
46. Markham, P.D., Salahuddin, S.Z., Kalyanaraman, V.S., Popovic, M., Sarin, P.S., and Gallo, R.C. (1983): Int. J. Cancer, 31:413-420.
47. Markham, P.D., Salahuddin, S.Z., Macchi, B., Robert-Guroff, M., and Gallo, R.C. (1984): Int. J. Cancer, 33:13-17.
48. Masur, H., Michelis, M.A., Greene, J.B., et al. (1981): N. Engl. J. Med., 305:1431-1438.
49. Metroka, C.E., Cunningham-Rundles, S., Pollack, M.S., et al. (1983): Ann. Int. Med., 99:585-591.
50. Mitsuya, H., Matis, L.A., Megson, M., Bunn, P.A., Murray, C., Mann, D.L., Gallo, R.C., and Broder, S. (1983): J. Exp. Med., 158:994-999.
51. Miyoshi, I., Kubonishi, I., Yoshimoto, S., Akagi, T., Ohtsuki, Y., Shiraishi, Y., Nagato, K., and Hinuma Y. (1981a): Nature, 294:770-771.
52. Miyoshi, I., Yoshimoto, S., Fujishita, M., Taguchi, H., Kubonishi, I., Niiya, K., and Minezawa, M. (1982): Lancet, ii, 658-659.
53. Morgan, D.A., Ruscetti, F.W., and Gallo, R.C. (1976): Science, 193:1007-1008.
54. Nagy, K., Clapham, P., Cheingsong-Povov, R., and Weiss, R.A. (1983) Int. J. Cancer, 32:321-326
55. Nowel, P.O., Finan, J.B., Clark, J., Sarin, P.S., and Gallo, R.C. (1984): J. Natl. Cancer Inst., in press.
56. Poiesz, B.J., Ruscetti, F.W., Gazdar, A.F., Bunn, P.A., Minna, J.D., and Gallo, R.C. (1980a): Proc. Natl. Acad. Sci. USA, 77:7415-7419.
57. Poiesz, B.J., Ruscetti, F.W., Mier, J.W., Woods, A.M., and Gallo, R.C. (1980b): Proc. Natl. Acad. Sci. USA, 77:6815-6819.
58. Poiesz, B.J., Ruscetti, F.W., Reitz, M.S., Kalyanaraman, V.S., and Gallo, R.C. (1981): Nature, 294:268-271.

59. Popovic, M., Flomberg, N., Volkman, D.J., Mann, D., Fauci, A.S., Dupont, B., and Gallo, R.C. (1984): Science, in press.

60. Popovic, M., Sarin, P.S., Robert-Guroff, M., Kalyanaraman, V.S., Mann, D., Minowada, J., and Gallo, R.C. (1983): Science, 219:856-859.

61. Popovic, M., Sarngadharan, M.G., Reed, E., and Gallo, R.C. (1984): Science, 224:497-500.

62. Posner, L.E., Robert-Guroff, M., Kalyanaraman, V.S., Poiesz, B.J., Ruscetti, F.W., Fossieck, B., Bunn, P.A., Jr., Minna, J.D., and Gallo, R.C. (1981): J. Exp. Med., 154:333-346.

63. Robert-Guroff, M., Nakao, Y., Notake, K., Ito, Y., Sliski, A., and Gallo, R.C. (1982): Science, 215:975-978.

64. Robert-Guroff, N. and Gallo, R.C. (1983a): Blut, 47:1-12.

65. Robert-Guroff, M., Kalyanaraman, V.S., Blattner, W.A., Popovic, M., Sarngadharan, M.G., Maeda, M., Blayney, D., Catovsky, D., Bunn, P.A., Shibata, A., Nakao, Y., Ito, Y., Aoki, T., and Gallo, R.C. (1983b): J. Exp. Med., 157:248-258.

66. Ruscetti, F.W., Morgan, D.A., and Gallo, R.C. (1977): J. Immunol., 119:131-138.

67. Safai, B., Sarngadharan, M.G., Groopman, J.E., et al. (1984): Lancet, 1:1438-1440.

68. Salahuddin, S.Z., Markham, P.D., Lindner, S.G., Gootenberg, J., Popovic, M., Hemmi, H., Sarin, P.S., and Gallo, R.C. (1984): Science 223:703-706.

69. Salahuddin, S.Z., Markham, P.D., Wong-Staal, F., Franchini, G., Kalyanaraman, V.S. and Gallo, R.C. (1983): Virology, 129:51-64.

70. Sarin, P.S., Aoki, T., Shibata, A., Ohnishi, Y., Aoyagi, Y., Miyakoshi, H., Emura, I., Kalyanaraman, V.S., Robert-Guroff, M., Popovic, M., Sarngadharan, M., Nowell, P.C. and Gallo, R.C. (1983): Proc. Natl. Acad. Sci. USA, 80:2370-2374.

71. Sarngadharan, M.G., Popovic, M., Bruch, L., Schüpbach, J., Gallo, R.C. (1984): Science, 224: 506-508.

72. Saxinger, W.A. and Gallo, R.C. (1982): Lancet, i (#8280), 1074.

73. Saxinger, W., Blattner, W.A., Lavine, P.H., et al. (1984): Science, in press.

74. Saxon, A., Stevens, R.H. and Golde, D.W. (1978): Ann. Int. Med., 88:323-326.

75. Schüpbach, J., Popovic, M., Gilden, R.V., Gonda, M., Sarngadharan, M.G. and Gallo, R.C. (1984): Science, 224: 607-610.

76. Seiki, M., Eddy, R., Shows, T.B., and Yoshida, M. (1984): Nature 309: 640-644.

77. Seiki, M., Hattori, S., Hirayama, Y. and Yoshida, M. (1983): Proc. Natl. Acad. Sci. USA, 80:3618-3622.

78. Shaw, G.M., Gonda, M.A., Flickinger, G.H., Hahn, B.H., Gallo, R.C., and Wong-Staal, F. (1984): Proc. Natl. Acad. Sci. USA 81:4544-4548.
79. Shimotohno, K., Golde, D.W., Miwa, M., Sugimura, T., and Chen, I.S.Y. (1984): Proc. Natl. Acad. Sci. USA, 81:1079-1083.
80. Siegel, F.P., Lopez, C., Hammer, G.S., et al. (1981): N. Engl. J. Med., 305:1439-1444.
81. Sodroski, J.G., Rosen, C.A. and Haseltine, W.A. (1984): Science, 225:381-385.
82. Sodroski, J., Trus, M., Perkins, D., Patarca, R., Wong-Staal, F., Gelmann, E., Gallo, R.C. and Haseltine, W.A. (1984): Proc. Natl. Acad. Sci. USA, in press.
83. Stahl, R.E., Friedman-Kien, A., Dubin, R., Marmor, M., Zolla-Pazner, S. (1982): Am. J. Med., 73:171-178.
84. Tajima, K., Tominaga, S., Suchi, T., Kawagoe, T., Komoda, H., Hinuma, Y., Oda, T., and Fujita, K. (1984): Gann., in press.
85. Takatsuki, K., Uchiyama, J., Sagawa, K. and Yodoi, J. (1977): In: Topics in Hematology, edited by S. Seno, F. Takaku, and S. Irino, pp. 73-77. Excerpta Medica, Amsterdan-Oxford.
86. Takatsuki, K., Uchiyama, T., Ueshima, Y. and Hattori, T. (1979): Jap. J. Clin. Oncol., 9:317-324.
87. Temin, H.M. (1964): Natl. Cancer Inst. Monograph 17:557-570.
88. Uchiyama, T., Yodoi, J., Sagawa, K., Takatsuki, K. and Uchino, H. (1977): Blood, 50:481-492.
89. Vilmer, E., Barré-Sinoussi, F., Rouzious, C., et al. (1984): Lancet, 1:753-757.
90. Vyth-Drees, F.A. and de Vries, J.E. (1983): Lancet, ii, 993.
91. Waldmann, T., Broder, S., Greene, W., Sarin, P.S., Saxinger, C., Blayney, D.W., Blattner, W.A., Goldman, C., Frost, K., Sharrow, S., Depper, J., Leonard, W., Uchiyama, T. and Gallo, R.C. (1983): Clin. Res., 31:5474-5480.
92. Wong-Staal, F., Hahn, B., Manzari, V., Colombini, S., Franchini, G., Gelmann, E.P. and Gallo, R.C. (1983): Nature, 302:626-628.
93. Yoshida, M., Miyoshi, I. and Hinuma, Y. (1982): Proc. Natl. Acad. Sci. USA, 79:2031-2035.

Molecular Biology of Tumor Cells, edited by
B. Wahren et al. Raven Press, New York © 1985.

Role of the Colony Stimulating Factors in the Emergence and Suppression of Myeloid Leukemia Populations

Donald Metcalf and Nicos A. Nicola

Cancer Research Unit, The Walter and Eliza Hall Institute of Medical Research, Royal Melbourne Hospital, Victoria, Australia

ABSTRACT

The glycoprotein colony stimulating factors (CSF's) regulate the proliferation and differentiation of granulocyte-macrophage populations. Primary myeloid leukemia cells remain dependent on extrinsic CSF for all cell proliferation although leukemia cells may exhibit intrinsic abnormalities in the ratio of CSF-stimulated self-replicative versus differentiative divisions. One CSF, G-CSF, has the pronounced capacity to induce differentiation in mouse myeloid leukemia cells and to suppress completely leukemia stem cell self-generation. Myeloid leukemia does not appear to be the consequence of unregulated CSF production by the leukemia cells themselves but the CSF's are likely to be mandatory for the proliferation and emergence of myeloid leukemia clones. Conversely, because of its differentiation-inducing action, G-CSF may prove to be a highly effective agent in the therapy of myeloid leukemia.

Extensive information now exists regarding the molecular control of the proliferation and differentiation of granulocyte-macrophage (GM) populations, particularly in the mouse. In vitro studies have indicated that a group of highly specific glycoproteins - the colony stimulating factors (CSF's) - interact to regulate the production and at least some aspects of the differentiation of granulocytes and macrophages (28). With the characterization and purification of these CSF's, specific questions can be raised concerning the role played by these CSF's in the transformation of normal granulocyte-macrophage (GM) cells to myeloid leukemia cells and in the emergence and progressive proliferation of myeloid leukemia clones and, conversely, whether the CSF's exhibit any ability to suppress myeloid leukemia populations. Indeed the GM population possibly represents the best available system at present in which to determine whether any of the current speculations regarding the origin and nature of cancer cells can be substantiated.

The CSF's and Their Actions on Normal GM Populations

Granulocytes and monocyte-macrophages are formed by the proliferative activity of specific progenitor cells identifiable by their capacity to generate colonies (clones) of progeny cells in semisolid cultures and known as the granulocyte-macrophage colony-forming cells (GM-CFC). In the mouse, the majority of GM-CFC are bipotential and are able to form both granulocytic and macrophage progeny although smaller subsets of monopotential progenitors exist that have a capacity to form only granulocytes or macrophages. GM-CFC are themselves the progeny of a self-generating population of multipotential hemopoietic stem cells. Most evidence indicates that normal GM-CFC are not capable of a significant level of self-generation but are a transit population of cells irreversibly committed to the GM pathway of differentiation that are expended in the generation of maturing granulocytes and macrophages. GM-CFC have a variable proliferative potential but each can generate from 200 - 20,000 progeny in vitro.

GM-CFC have the morphology of undifferentiated blast cells and form mature progeny by a sequential series of divisions accompanied by morphologically-recognizable differentiation. In the granulocyte pathway, the sequence is CFC $\rightarrow$ promyelocytes$\rightarrow$myelocyte $\rightarrow$ metamyelocyte $\rightarrow$ polymorph and in the monocyte pathway the sequence is CFC $\rightarrow$ promonocyte $\rightarrow$ monocyte $\rightarrow$ macrophage. Metamyelocytes and polymorphs are post-mitotic end cells incapable of further cell divisions. A substantial fraction of monocytes and macrophages retains the potential capacity for further extensive cell proliferation although in normal health this is not necessarily invoked, in which case they behave as end cells like polymorphs.

Analysis of the proliferation of mouse GM cells in vitro has led to the identification of four glycoproteins - the granulocyte-macrophage colony stimulating factors (CSF's) - that control the proliferation of GM-CFC and their differentiating progeny (28).

In humans, two comparable CSF's have been identified (34). Table 1 presents a summary of current information regarding the mouse CSF's. GM-CSF (MW 23,000) is able to stimulate the formation of both granulocytic and macrophage progeny (3). M-CSF (CSF-1) (MW 70,000) is a dimer of two apparently identical polypeptide subunits of MW 14,500 that stimulates the formation almost exclusively of macrophage cells (40,41). G-CSF (MW 25,000) in low or medium concentrations is an exclusive proliferative stimulus for granulocyte formation (35). Multi-CSF (also known as Interleukin 3, IL-3) (MW 23 - 28,000) has proliferative effects on a broad range of stem and progenitor cells but in the GM pathway functions in a manner similar to GM-CSF (18,28).

Prototype members of each of the four CSF's have been purified to homogeneity and partial or complete amino acid sequence data have been obtained. cDNA's for GM-CSF and Multi-CSF (the latter under the names mast cell growth factor or IL-3) have been cloned

TABLE 1

The major granulocyte-macrophage colony stimulating factors in the mouse

Name	M.W.	Purified from	Sequence	cDNA cloned	Antibody	Radio-labeled
M-CSF (CSF-1)	70,000 (Dimer)	L-cell C.M.	±		+	+
GM-CSF	23,000 (Monomer)	Lung C.M.	Full	+		+
G-CSF (MGI-2)	25,000 (Monomer)	Lung C.M.	±	+		+
Multi-CSF	23,000 (Monomer)	WEHI-38 C.M. and	Full	+	+	+
(IL-3, PSF, Mast		T-lymphocyte C.M				
cell growth factor)						

Alternative names used for the CSF's in some laboratories are shown in parenthesis.

C.M. = conditioned medium

PSF = persistent cell factor

and the full amino acid structure determined (10,9,45).

The CSF's are active at very low concentrations, the concentration required for 50 % of maximal stimulation of colony formation ranging from 10^{-11} - 10^{-13} M. The CSF's exhibit four major properties.

(a) They are required continuously for survival in vitro of GM precursor cells (30)

(b) They are required continuously to stimulate every cell division in the GM pathway. Withdrawal of CSF prevents most GM cells from completing cell cycles in progress at the time of withdrawal. Both the length of the cell cycle and the final number of progeny produced by GM-CFC are determined by the concentration of CSF used (23).

(c) Where GM-CFC are bipotential, the appropriate CSF is able to commit such cells to the restricted formation of cells of one or other of the two available differentiation pathways, e.g. M-CSF commits cells irreversibly to macrophage formation, while high concentration of GM-CSF commit cells irreversibly to granulcyte formation (29). The commitment process is relatively slow, requiring 1 - 2 cell divisions in the presence of the committing CSF, is irreversible and is notably asymmetrical (28).

(d) The CSF's are able to stimulate the level of expression of a variety of functions of mature granulocyte (G) and monocyte (M) cells. These range from adherence, phagocytosis and cytotoxicity to the synthesis of specific products as prostaglandin E (PGE) or plasminogen-activating factor (19,20,28).

This combination of functional effects probably requires actions at multiple locations in the responding cells. For example, irreversible commitment would seem to require events at the gene level, whereas the rapid action of CSF's in stimulating adherence or phagocytosis by mature cells could well be mediated at or near the membrane.

Binding studies for G-CSF and GM-CSF on normal GM progenitors and their maturing progeny indicate that receptor numbers are relatively low (average number 300 to 700 per cell) although from autoradiographic studies there is an almost tenfold range in receptor numbers expressed at any one time by cells of a particular class (Nicola, N.A., Metcalf, D., Walker, F. and Burgess, A.W., unpublished data). Receptor numbers for M-CSF appear to be considerably higher (1,000 - 70,000) (40). At least for G-CSF, half-maximal proliferative effects are achieved with 10 % occupancy of receptors i.e. approximately 30 - 70 receptors bound per cell. From studies using ^{125}I G-CSF, loss of membrane receptors is not the basis for the postmitotic state of polymorphs since receptor numbers actually increase progressively from the myelocyte to polymorph stage (Metcalf, D. and Nicola, N.A., unpublished data).

Two comments need to be made regarding the uniqueness of the role of CSF's in ther functional actions. There are no agents other than the CSF's that are able to induce proliferation in GM cells. All agents appearing to stimulate proliferation in these populations do so via CSF. On the other hand, the CSF's are certainly not the only agents able to influence the functional activity of mature GM cells.

The CSF's represent a control system with a surprising degree of apparent overlap and redundancy. Thus G-CSF, GM-CSF and Multi-CSF can all stimulate the formation of granulocytes and M-CSF, GM-CSF and Multi-CSF the formation of macrophages (Fig. 1).

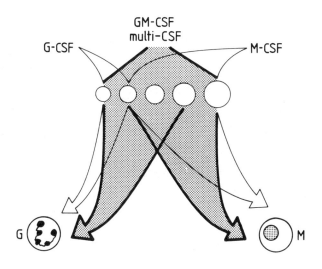

Figure 1: Schematic diagram of the manner in which the four mouse granulocyte-macrophage colony stimulating factors interact on a heterogeneous population of progenitor cells to control granulocyte and monocyte-macrophage formation.

Despite considerable heterogeneity in GM progenitor populations and some evidence that subsets of progenitors may respond preferentially to one or other CSF, it has also been observed using reciprocal clone transfers that GM-CSF and Multi-CSF can both stimulate the proliferation of the same clone to generate what appear to be identical GM progeny (28). This latter situation is intriguing for two reasons. (a) The amino acid sequences for GM-CSF and Multi-CSF share no homology and the two molecules differ radically in predicted secondary structure (10) yet both can exhibit the same functional activity on the same target cells. (b) Binding data indicate that many GM progenitor cells simultaneously express unique receptors for more than one CSF. Despite this, a significant fraction (30 - 40 %) of receptors appears to bind more than one type of CSF e.g. both GM-CSF and Multi-CSF or both GM-CSF and G-CSF.

It can be questioned how a receptor can discern some similarity between GM-CSF and Multi-CSF where there is no similarity in primary or secondary structure of the two polypeptides. Furthermore, the carbohydrate portion of the molecules is known not to be necessary for in vitro activity and therefore is presumably not mandatory for recognition of the CSF by the receptor. It is also curious that different regulator molecules and/or receptors should be able to initiate a series of cellular events with much in common.

In part, the answer to these apparent paradoxes may lie in the capacity of the CSF's to exert multiple effects on responding GM populations. While GM cells generated in response to GM-CSF stimulation may resemble in general those generated in response to stimulation by Multi-CSF, there may nevertheless be subtle differences between these populations either in terms of clonal derivation or the exact functions exhibited by the cells.

2D gel analyses using purified GM progenitor cells or mature polymorphs have shown that the CSF's initiate changes in the synthesis rates of a number of nuclear and cytoplasmic proteins (42, Stanley, I.J., Nicola, N.A. and Burgess, A.W., unpublished data) but it has not been possible yet to determine which are the earliest proteins affected. In view of the suggested association between the actions of specific growth regulators and onc genes, it is of considerable interest that GM-CSF has been shown to induce major phosphorylation changes in the proteins of GM progenitor cells, one of the most obvious being to increase, for a 5 - 15 hour period, phosphorylation of a P21 that appears to be the Kirsten/Harvey ras gene product (Stanley, I.J., Nicola, N.A. and Burgess, A.W., unpublished data). This raises the possibility that the CSF's and onc genes may activate a final common pathway of cellular events, an arrangement fitting well with current speculations concerning possible interactions between these two agents. In this context, a computer search has failed to identify homologies between the cDNA's of GM-CSF or Multi-CSF and known onc genes, although possible homologies between CSF receptors and onc gene products are not yet able to be investigated.

The multiple actions of the CSF's on responding GM cells create an unusual situation in which there is the potentiality for antagonistic end results. The CSF's stimulate, and are essential for, all cell divisions yet at the same time have at least the potentiality to suppress cell divisions by differentiation commitment and stimulation of mature cell functional activity. Which element of these two actions is dominant in any one situation may well be determined by the genetic programming of the target cell and, particularly in the case of leukemia cells where there may be an abnormal linkage between programming for cell proliferation and differentiation, these antagonistic effects of the CSF's can result in quite complex end results (22,26).

Control by CSF's of Cell Division in Myeloid Leukemia Cells

The most important question concerning the proliferation of myeloid leukemia cells is whether, as is true for normal GM cells, all cell divisions remain dependent on stimulation by exogenous CSF. The answer is best established for cells from patients with chronic myeloid leukemia (CML) and acute myeloid leukemia (AML). Data from many hundreds of patients have indicated that the proliferation of leukemia cells from all patients with myeloid leukemia remain absolutely dependent in vitro on stimulation by added CSF (28). There are no reported exceptions to this statement. In early studies some apparently spontaneous proliferation was reported in cultures of human myeloid leukemia cells but analysis subsequently showed that this low level of background proliferation is due to the synthesis of CSF by cells in the cultures. When leukemic CFC are purified, such cells are incapable of any cell division in unstimulated cultures (12,32).

Fewer data are available for primary myeloid leukemias in the mouse because of the rarity of this disease but from the limited data available the same situation appears to exist as with human myeloid leukemia cells (16).

Measurement of the quantitative responsiveness of human myeloid leukemia cells to stimualtion by CSF has indicated that their responsiveness is very close to that of normal cells with CSF concentrations required for half-maximal stimulation being essentially identical. Human CSF's have yet to be purified and radiolabeled and no binding studies have yet been possible to determine receptor numbers for human CSF's on human leukemia cells. However, initial studies have indicated that mouse G-CSF is a relatively efficient stimulus for the proliferation of human promyelocytes and myelocytes and receptor numbers for mouse G-CSF on human acute myeloid leukemia blast cells and promyelocytes appear similar to those on corresponding normal human cells (Metcalf, D., Begley, G. and Nicola, N.A., unpublished data).

These findings eliminate the simplest version of the autocrine hypothesis that would propose that leukemia cells produce their own growth factors (CSF's) and thereby exhibit the capacity for autonomous proliferation in unstimulated cultures. While apparently autonomous proliferation is exhibited in vitro by cells of long-established mouse and human leukemia cell lines, e.g. M1, WEHI-3B, HL60, this property was acquired at some stage in the tissue culture history of these cell lines and is not the characteristic of myeloid leukemia cells taken directly from a patient or animal with primary leukemia.

There is no question that some leukemia cells can synthesize CSF. In interpreting the significance of these observations, it needs to be kept in mind that the CSF's are synthesized by a wide range of normal cell types and indeed possibly by all cell types and that CSF synthesis is increased by exposure to microorganisms and their products, such as endotoxin (28).

There have so far been no reports that primary leukemia stem cells or normal progenitor cells can synthesize CSF but these cells have yet to be tested at high enough concentrations to establish this point. What has been established is (a) that leukemia-derived monocytes in AML or CML can produce CSF but not in larger amounts than are produced by normal monocytes, and (b) that many leukemic continuous cell lines can synthesize one or other form of CSF (37). Table 2 lists some examples of data recently obtained in this laboratory on this latter point. There are four comments worth making about data of this type. Firstly, some leukemia cell lines only produce detectable CSF after stimulation by endotoxin, a normal inducing agent for CSF synthesis (28). Secondly, the amounts of CSF produced by leukemia cell lines, although high, are no higher than those produced by normal peritoneal macrophages. Thirdly, as shown by the two examples in the Table, CSF production by tumor cells is not unique to leukemia cells since a wide variety of tumors of non-hemopoietic origin can produce large amounts of CSF. Fourthly the molecular nature of the CSF's produced by leukemia cells is not abnormal, and chemical characterization of some of these has indicated them to be probably identical with the CSF's produced by normal cells (Nicola, N.A. and Metcalf, D., unpublished data).

While the ability of at least some leukemia cells to produce CSF again raises the possibility of autocrine stimulation of growth, it must be re-emphasized that primary leukemia cells are absolutely dependent on exogenous CSF for proliferation. This appears to eliminate the possibility that CSF/receptor binding occurs in the cytoplasm of the leukemia cells at the site of synthesis of these molecules and renders the cells autonomous. If leukemia cells produce CSF it would appear to be inactive within the cell and to need to be secreted and bind to membrane receptors before being able to stimulate the cell producing it. Once the necessity of this step is accepted, it becomes difficult to imagine the first leukemia cell being able to synthesize sufficient CSF to build up any sort of effective concentration in the body fluids moving past the cell. Furthermore, the total amount of CSF able to be produced by a small emerging leukemia clone would be quite trivial in comparison with the CSF produced by all normal tissues in the body and could not reasonably be expected to produce a perceptible increase in proliferative stimuli impinging on the leukemia cells.

What is a more likely possibility is that onc gene-induced changes in a leukemia stem cell may have altered the cell's response to the cytoplasmic signals generated by CSF-receptor binding and internalization of the CSF-receptor complex. While the cell proliferates as do normal GM progenitors in response to these signals, the proportion of self-generative divisions resulting may well be excessively high in leukemia cells, resulting in a progressive expansion of the population of cells remaining capable of further divisions - the essential feature of a cancer population.

TABLE 2

Production of CSF's by monocyte-macrophage tumor cell lines

Cells	Type	Primer	CSF Units produced per 10^6 cells		
			GM-CSF	G-CSF	Other
WEHI-38	Myelomonocytic leukemia	-	0	0	Multi-CSF 1,500 M-CSF 200
J774	Monocytic leukemia	-	80	80	0
		Endotoxin	160	160	0
RAW 264	Monocyte-macrophage leukemia	-	0	160	0
		Endotoxin	0	4,000	0
WR 19	Monocyte-macrophage leukemia	-	0	400	0
		Endotoxin	0	8,000	0
R 309	Monocyte-macrophage leukemia	-	0	400	0
		Endotoxin	0	8,000	0
WEHI-274	Monocyte-macrophage leukemia	-	7,000	0	0
		Endotoxin	8,000	0	0
WEHI-265	Monocyte-macrophage leukemia	-	0	0	0
		Endotoxin	0	4,000	0
Peritoneal macrophages	Normal	Endotoxin	70	300	0
LB3 T lymphocyte line	Normal	Con A	60,000	10,000	Multi-CSF 70,000
Krebs II ascites cells	Carcinoma	-	600	600	0
		Endotoxin	4,000	5,000	0
RIII cell line	Breast cancer	-	0	3,000	Some M-CSF

Table 2: 1 x 10 cells/ml were incubated for 4 days then the medium harvested and assayed. Endotoxin 200 ng/ml or concanavalin A 5 μg/ml were used as priming stimuli. GM-CSF assayed on 75,000 C57BL marrow cells and 300 FDC-Pl cells. G-CSF assayed on 300 WEHI-3B D^+ cells. Multi-CSG assayed on 300 32D cells. M-CSF assayed on 75,000 C57BL marrow cells. 50 units of CSF is concentration stimulating half-maximal colony formation or colony differentiation in the various assays.

Induction by G-CSF of Differentiation
and Stem Cell Suppression in Leukemia Cells

Most of the work on the induction of differentiation in mye-loid leukemia cells has been carried out using two mouse myeloid leukemia cell lines, the M1 and WEHI-3B that no longer exhibit de-pendency on extrinsic CSF for proliferation (17,28,38).

Analysis in this laboratory of the WEHI-3B model using puri-fied preparations of the CSF's has indicated that M-CSF and Multi-CSF have no obvious differentiation-inducing effects (25) and while GM-CSF has some capacity to induce mainly monocytic diffe-rentiation, the action is relatively weak (22). In contrast, G-CSF has a powerful capacity to induce differentiation in WEHI-3B co-lony cells at concentrations similar to those required for stimu-lation of normal GM colony formation (half-maximal effects at 3 X X 10^{-12} M concentrations) (31,35). At high G-CSF concentra-tions both granulocytic and monocytic differentiation results and with low concentrations only monocytic differentiation (31).

Although the differentiating granulocytes and monocytes pro-duced by mouse and human leukemia cells are recognizable morpholo-gically and exhibit some of the functions and membrane markers of corresponding normal cells (17,38), they are almost certainly not entirely normal since they exhibit abnormalities in nuclear and cytoplasmic shape and somewhat abnormal patterns of reactivity to monoclonal antisera (7). They are however clear examples of diffe-rentiation to post-mitotic cells and therefore represent cells removed from the proliferating pool of leukemia cells by enforced differentiation.

A wide variety of chemical agents has been documented to be able to induce comparable differentiation in mouse and human mye-loid leukemia cell lines and in at least some primary leukemia populations (17,38). In some cases, the actions of these agents may be indirect and involve the induction of G-CSF synthesis by the leukemia cells but in other instances this is not the likely mechanism (28).

While the induction of differentiation is a spectacular pheno-menon, induced differentiation alone will not result in suppres-sion of a leukemia population unless stem cell self-generation is also suppressed. In the case of some chemical agents, e.g. the ac-tion of butyrate on human HL60 cells, the induced monocytic diffe-rentiation appears to be virtually complete and to be associated with the loss of all clonogenic cells (1) but little evidence has been published on this question for most of the agents used(8,13).

Stem cell self-generation in the WEHI-3B model is easily moni-tored because of the capacity of the stem cells to generate colo-nies in semisolid cultures. In untreated WEHI-3B colonies, appro-ximately 90 % of the colony cells are stem cells able to generate further colonies which in turn contain comparable numbers of stem cells. When G-CSF is added to such cultures there is a notable suppression of stem cell self-generation within developing colo-nies and if colonies are recloned for two to six cycles in the

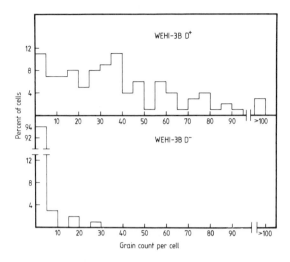

Figure 2: Autodiographic analysis of the binding of ^{125}I G-CSF to differentiation responsive WEHI-3B D$^+$ leukemic cells compared with that of differentiation-unresponsive WEHI-3B D$^-$ cells. Note that the vast majority of unresponsive cells fail to bind detectable amounts of G-CSF.

presence of G-CSF, complete suppression of all clonogenic cells can be achieved (24). Not only does G-CSF treatment reduce clonogenic cell levels as analyzed in vitro but it also reduces the leukemogenicity of such cells when transplanted to syngeneic recipients (25) and can even result in suppression of established transplanted myeloid leukemias (21).

Analysis of the action of G-CSF on WEHI-38 cells has shown that two types of suppression occur: (a) affected cells may remain clonogenic but form spontaneous differentiating colonies containing reduced numbers of clongenic cells, or (b) affected cells become non-clonogenic, usually undergoing one or at most two, further cell divisions with the production of differentiated progeny that then die (26). These two types of suppression may represent a sequence or may merely reflect the heterogeneity of clonogenic cells and their variable responsiveness to suppression.

The effects of G-CSF are irreversible but require the presence of G-CSF's throughout 1 - 2 full cell divisions and suppression is commonly an asymmetrical event affecting only one member of the daughter cell pair (26). These characteristics of G-CSF action closely resemble the action of the CSF's in enforcing differentiation commitment in normal GM progenitors. The process possibly involves modification of daughter chromatids during chromosome duplication, the suppressed daughter cell receiving one or more chromosomes modified by methylation or some other irreversible change in the genes controlling self-generation or the expression of differentiation commitment.

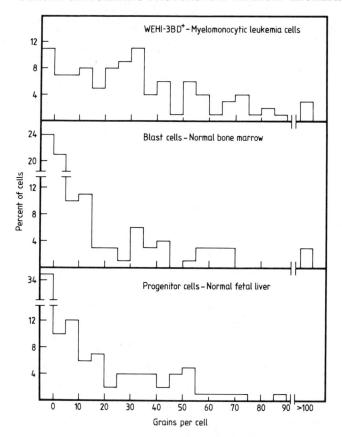

Figure 3: Autoradiographic analysis of the binding of ^{125}I G-SCF to WEHI-3B D$^+$ myelomonocyticleukemia cells in comparison with binding of ^{125}I G-CSF by corresponding blast cells in normal adult mouse bone marrow and with progenitor cells from normal mouse fetal liver populations, purified by fluorescence-activated cell sorting. Note that within each population, the level of binding is variable but that, overall, the three populations bind similar amounts of G-CSF.

Subclones of both WEHI-3B and M1 cells can be derived that are unresponsive to differentiation induction by G-CSF. In the case of unresponsive (D$^-$) WEHI-3B cells, analysis has shown such cells do not express membrane receptors for G-CSF (Fig. 2) whereas the differentiation-responsive WEHI-3B (D$^+$) cells exhibit receptor numbers comparable with those of normal progenitor cells (Fig. 3) (33).

This may not be the only basis for unresponsiveness since cells on the leukemic J774 macrophage cell line exhibit normal numbers of G-CSF receptors yet appear refractory to differentiation induction by G-CSF (33).

Many chemical agents have been shown to induce responsiveness to G-CSF in (D⁻) cells and it will be of interest to determine whether such cells then express membrane receptors for G-CSF.

The ability or otherwise of CSF's to induce differentiation and thereby to suppress leukemic populations may hinge on the presence and nature of genetic rearrangements within the leukemic cell that are permissive for such G-CSF effects or render the cell refractory to induced differentiation. There are suggestions in the human myeloid leukemias of major differences in such genetic programming. Thus most AML cells when proliferating in vitro in the presence of CSF exhibit little evidence of normal differentiation and where differentiation occurs the cells are of bizarre morphology. On the other hand, studies using promyelocytic leukemic cells suggest that as a group, they are more readily inducible by chemical agents to exhibit differentiation than are other acute leukemias (2). In this context it is of interest that preliminary studies have indicated unusually strong binding of G-CSF to both normal and leukemic promyelocytes (Metcalf, D., Nicola, N.A. and Begley, G., unpublished data).

In the case of CML cells, a curious situation appears to exist. This clonal disease originates in the multipotential population ancestral to the GM progenitor cell stage and excessive self-generation by the stem cells of the clone results in an extreme increase in the numbers of all progenitor cells - GM, eosinophil (EO), erythroid burst forming unit (BFU-E) and Multi-CFC (15). While this suggests an intrinsic genetic derangement distorting the balance between self-generation and the differentiative divisions, this situation cannot be irreversible. Those progeny becoming GM progenitor cells form colonies in semisolid medium with very high cloning efficiency after stimulation by CSF. Furthermore, like normal GM colonies, these CML-derived colonies do not themselves contain clonogenic cells and the colony cells exhibit essentially normal differentiation to mature granulocyte and macrophage cells. If genetic derangements in the cell initiating the CML clone were involved in the original clonal expanison, such derangements appear to be reversible or correctable during CSF-stimulated clonal proliferation once the cells are committed to become GM progenitors.

What Role do the CSF's Play in the Emergence of Myeloid Leukemia?

Because primary myeloid leukemia cells are absolutely dependent on CSF for proliferation, CSF would appear to be mandatory for the emergence of a leukemia clone. An example of this role might be the failure of myeloid leukemia to develop in irradiated germfree mice (43). Such mice have extremely low serum CSF levels since the major stimulus for CSF synthesis is infections (28). Irradiated germfree mice exhibit elevated serum CSF levels if conventionalized (4) and this procedure also results in subsequent myeloid leukemia development (43), possibly because the abnormal GM cells are now stimulated to proliferate in vivo. This role of CSF might simply be a permissive one by stimulating the clonal proliferation of a cell with intrinsic abnormalities induced by some quite different mechanism. However an alternative view is that the CSF's might also be involved in the original transformation event. The evidence referred to earlier that CSF's induce phosphorylation of at least one onc gene translation product raises the possibility that CSF and onc genes could interact in producing the intrinsic changes needed.

Multi-CSF might play a role of particular importance in leukemogenesis. Addition of Multi-CSF to bottle cultures of bone marrow cells promotes the emergence of continuously proliferating hemopoietic cell lines which in many cases involves some type of immortalization, the cells involved becoming dependent thereafter on Multi-CSF for proliferative stimulation (36). A few such continuous cell lines exhibit an associated responsiveness to GM-CSF. Transplantation tests have suggested that these cell lines are not leukemic but the cells exhibit properties intermediate between normality and leukemia (Metcalf, D., unpublished data). The immortalization apparently induced by Multi-CSF could well provide a susceptible target cell population for subsequent onc gene tranformation to the leukemic state. It must be accepted however that the events in bottle cultures could be quite abnormal since there is little evidence to suggest that immortalized hemopoietic cells of this type exist in vivo. Even though the system could be quite artificial it is certainly intriguing that acquisition of leukemogenicity by such cells has been noted as having been accompanied by acquisition of the ability of the cells to secrete Multi-CSF constitutively (14,39).

For the reasons advanced above, primary myeloid leukemia probably cannot be viewed simply as a consequence of a GM cell acquiring the capacity to synthesize its own CSF in an uncontrollable or dysregulated manner. An even simpler hypothesis is to propose that no intrinsic changes exist in myeloid leukemia cells and CML might well be the most reasonable candidate for such a situation. In this propositon it could be argued that a chronic imbalance of CSF's and CSF inhibitors exist in the body favoring chronic overstimulation and consequent population enlargement. There are two major arguments against this proposal (a) CML and AML are clonal diseases arising from a single cell, not polyclonal as would be predicted from the overstimulation hypothesis, and (b) measurements of CSF levels in AML and CML, while not easy to interpret, have given no consistent evidence of excess CSF levels except perhaps in CML in acute transformation (28). The clonality of leukemia populations virtually demands an intrinsic heritable defect in the initiating cell, a conclusion strongly supported by the wealth of karyotypic data indicating a high frequency of non-random translocations.

If, as has been discussed above, at least one CSF has the capacity to suppress myeloid leukemia populations, does leukemia result from a failure of CSF suppression via induced differentiation? The answer is probably affirmative but again the reason for failure of suppression is more likely to be the consequence of an intrinsic abnormality in the affected cells rather than simply to an abnormally low G-CSF level in the patient. AML and CML patients appear able to produce elevated serum G-CSF levels in response to infections as effectively as do non-leukemic patients (27) although a relative inability of marrow stromal cells to produce CSF (of uncharacterized type) has been reported in some patients with established AML (11). It cannot be excluded at present that some patients developing AML may have a relatively ineffective G-CSF production system and that emerging leukemia cells, despite their intrinsic abnormality, would have been suppressed very effectively in persons with a more adequate G-CSF-producing cell population.

It is clear that the exact role of the CSF's in the emergence of myeloid leukemia is yet to be fully clarified. However, from the evidence so far available, autologous and unbalanced CSF production by the leukemia cells appears to be excluded as a realistic basis for myeloid leukemia development.

Unresolved Problems

Central to the current hypothesis of cancer development is the proposal that chromosomal translocations might result in activation of growth factor production or the synthesis of receptors for such factors (5,6,44). In the case of mouse myeloid leukemia, deletion of a portion of one chromosome 2 is the only reported consistent defect. It is not documented whether this material is translocated elsewhere. Of the four known CSF's, the chromosomal location of only one is known. The GM-CSF gene appears to be on chromosome 11 (10). The location of the other three CSF's genes needs to be established to determine whether any might be involved by the karyotypic abnormalities described for mouse myeloid leukemias.

It remains unclear in man which type of CSF is analogous with the anti-leukemic G-CSF of the mouse and whether this human CSF would be effective in suppressing human myeloid leukemia cells. At present, GM-CSF appears to be the best candidate for an analogue of mouse G-CSF. GM-CSF , like G-CSF, primarily stimulates granulocyte colony formation (34), is able to induce differentiation in both WEHI-3B and HL60 leukemic cells (27) and cross-competes for G-CSF binding sites on WEHI-3B cells (Nicola, N.A. and Metcalf, D. unpublished data). Conversely, mouse G-CSF binds strongly to receptors on human GM cells particularly promyelocytes and binds also to AML cells. This suggests the possibility of structural homology between mouse G-CSF and GM-CSF and that a probe based on mouse G-CSF might succeed in indentifying the gene for human GM-CSF.

Work on the mouse myeloid leukemia models has indicated that G-CSF or its human analogue should prove to be highly effective when used as a therapeutic agent to suppress myeloid leukemia. However, a major problem preventing exploitation of the CSF's in the treatment of myeloid leukemia is the minute amount available from separative protein chemistry on even the richest source materials. The CSF's have short serum half-lifes of at most a few hours and large amounts will be necessary for even the short-term use of CSF's in vivo. This problem is unlikely to be solved by conventional mass-production of CSF by cultured cell lines and almost certainly will require cloning of the CSF genes in high expression translation systems. Attempts to clone the human CSF genes are actively in progress and this logistical problem could be solved relatively quickly, provided the mouse cDNA probes are able to identify the analogous human genes.

Acknowledgements

This work was supported by the Carden Fellowship Fund of the Anti-Cancer Council of Victoria, The National Health and Medical Research Council, Canberra and The National Institutes of Health, Bethesda, Grant Nos. CA-22556 and CA-25972.

REFERENCES

1. Boyd, A.W. Metcalf, D. Leukemia Res. (In press)
2. Breitman, T.R., Collins, S.J. and Keene, B.R. (1981) Blood 57:1000-1004
3. Burgess, A.W., Camakaris, J. and Metcalf, D. (1977) J. Biol. Chem. 252:1998-2003
4. Chang, C.F. and Pollard, M. (1973) Proc. Soc. Exp. Biol. Med. 144:177-180
5. Doolittle, R.F., Hunkapillar, M.W., Hood, L.E., Devare, S.G., Robbins, K.C., Aronson, S.A. and Antoniades, H.N. (1983) Science 221:275-277
6. Downward, J., Yarden, Y., Mayes, E., Scrace, G., Totty, N., Stockwell, P., Ullrich, A., Schlessinger, J. and Waterfield, M.D. (1984) Nature 307:521-527
7. Ferrero, D., Pessano, S., Pagliardi, G.R. and Rovera, G. (1983) Blood 61:171-179
8. Fibach, E., Peled, T. and Rachmilewitz, E.A. (1982) J. Cell. Physiol. 113:152-158
9. Fung, M.C., Hapel, A.J., Ymer, S., Cohen, D.R., Johnson, R.N., Campbell, H.D. and Young, I.G. (1984) Nature 307:233-237
10. Gough, N.M., Gough, J., Metcalf, D., Kelso, A., Grail, D., Nicola, N.A., Burgess, A.W. and Dunn, A.R. Nature (In press)
11. Greenberg, B.R., Wilson, F.D. and Woo, L. (1981) Blood 58:557-564
12. Griffin, J.D., Beveridge, R.P. and Schlossman, S.F. (1982) Blood 60:30-37
13. Griffin, J.D., Munroe, D., Major, P. and Kufe, D. (1982) Exp. Hematol. 10:774-781
14. Hapel, A.J., Lee, J.C., Farrar, W.C. and Ihle, J.N. (1981) Cell 25:179-186
15. Hara, H., Kai, S., Fushimi, M., Taniwaki, S., Ifuku, H., Okamoto, T., Ohe, Y., Fujita, S., Noguchi, K., Kanamura, A., Nagai, K. and Inada, E. (1981) Exp. Hematol. 9:871-877
16. Heard, J.M., Fichelson, S., Choppin, J. and Varet, B. (1983) Int. J. Cancer 31:337-344
17. Hozumi, M. (1983) Adv. Cancer 38:121-169

18. Ihle, J.N., Keller, J., Henderson, L., Klein, F. and Palaszynski, E. (1982) J.Immunol., 129:2431-2436.

19. Kurland, J.I., Pelus, L.M., Ralph, P., Bockman, R.A. and Moore, M.A.S. (1979) Proc.Natl.Acad.Sci.(USA), 76:2326-2330.

20. Lopez, A.F., Nicola, N.A., Burgess, A.W., Metcalf, D., Battye, F.L., Sewell, W.A. and Vadas, M.A. (1983) J.Immunol., 131:2983-2988.

21. Lotem, J. and Sachs, L. (1981) Int.J.Cancer, 28:375-386.

22. Metcalf, D. (1979) Int.J.Cancer, 24:616-623.

23. Metcalf, D. (1980) Proc.Natl.Acad.Sci.(USA), 77:5327-5330.

24. Metcalf, D. (1980a) Int.J.Cancer, 25:225-233.

25. Metcalf, D. (1982) Natl.Cancer Instit. Monograph, 60:123-131.

26. Metcalf, D. (1982a) Int.J.Cancer, 30:203-210.

27. Metcalf, D. (1983) Leukemia Res., 7:117-132.

28. Metcalf, D. (1984) The Hemopoietic Colony Stimulating Factors. Elsevier Science Publishers B.V., Amsterdam (in press).

29. Metcalf, D. and Burgess, A.W. (1982) J.Cell.Physiol., 111:275-283.

30. Metcalf, D. and Merchav, S. (1982) J.Cell.Physiol., 112:411-418.

31. Metcalf, D. and Nicola, N.A. (1982) Int.J.Cancer, 30:773-780.

32. Metcalf, D., Johnson, G.R., Kolber, S. and Dresch, C. (1978) In "Advances in Comparative Leukemia Research 1977" Elsevier/North-Holland. Eds. Bentvelzen, P. et al, 307-310.

33. Nicola, N.A. and Metcalf, D. In press, Proc.Natl.Acad.Sci. (USA).

34. Nicola, N.A., Metcalf, D., Johnson, G.R. and Burgess, A.W. (1982) Blood, 54:614-627.

35. Nicola, N.A., Metcalf, D., Matsumoto, M. and Johnson, G.R. (1983) J.Biol.Chem., 258:9017-9023.

36. Palaszynski, E.W. and Ihle, J.W. (1984) J.Immunol., 132:1872-1878.

37. Ralph, P., Broxmeyer, H.E., Moore, M.A.S. and Nakoinz, I. (1978) Cancer Res., 38:1414-1419.

38. Sachs, L. (1982) J.Cell.Physiol. Suppl., 1:151-164.

39. Schrader, J.W. and Crapper, R.M. (1983) Proc.Natl.Acad. Sci. (USA), 80:6892-6896.

40. Stanley, E.R. and Guilbert, L.J. (1981) J.Immunol.Methods, 42:253-284.

41. Stanley, E.R. and Heard, P.M. (1977) J.Biol.Chem., 252:4305-4312.

42. Stanley, I.J. and Burgess, A.W. (1984) In press, J.Cell. Biochem.

43. Upton, A.C., Jenkins, V.K., Walburg, H.E., Tyndall, R.L., Conklin, J.W. and Wald, N. (1966) Natl.Cancer Instit. Monograph, 22:329-347.

44. Waterfield, M.D., Scarce, G.T., Whittle, N., Stroobant, P., Johnsson, A., Wasteson, A., Westermark, B., Heldin, C-H., Huang, J.S. and Deuel, T.F. (1983) Nature, 304:35-39.

45. Yokota, T., Lee, F., Rennick, D., Hall, C., Arai, N., Mosmann, T., Nabel, G., Cantor, H., and Arai, K. (1984) Proc.Natl. Acad.Sci. (USA), 81:1070-1074.

Molecular Biology of Tumor Cells, edited by
B. Wahren et al. Raven Press, New York © 1985.

Phorbol Ester (TPA)-Induced Differentiation of B-Type Chronic Lymphocytic Leukemia Cells

Kenneth Nilsson, Thomas Tötterman, Antero Danersund,
Klas Forsbeck, *Lars Hellman, and *Ulf Pettersson

*Department of Pathology, and *Department of Medical Genetics, University of Uppsala,
S-751 85 Uppsala, Sweden*

In the normal hemopoiesis development of mature cells from the
pluri- and unipotent stem cell compartments is regulated by specific growth and differentiation factors and involves both stepwise,
cell lineage specific phenotypic changes (differentiation) of the
cells and concomitant proliferation. The latter allows for the
necessary self renewal of the pluripotent stem cell pool, and for
the expansion of the progeny of the unipotent stem cells (20).
Differentiation and proliferation appear to be coupled processes.
The proliferative capacity is highest for the most immature cells
and will eventually come to an end when a cell of a given differentiation lineage has reached the stage of terminal differentiation (18). The proliferation arrest (block in the G1 phase of the
cell cycle) of the fully mature bone marrow cells is irreversible
for myeloid cells. In the case of lymphoid and perhaps also monocytic cells, however, the cell-cycle block is reversible. A second
round of differentiation and proliferation may be induced in these
cell types by specific signals (e.g. antigen) leading to the development of fully immunocompetent cells (i.e. plasma cells, T-cells
with specific helper or suppressor/killer function and macrophages,
respectively) (1). Lymphoid cells, B-cells in particular, appear
to have the option to mature without concomitant proliferation
when stimulated by "B-cell differentiation" factors, at least in
vitro (21).

Phenotypic studies of biopsy cells and established cell lines
of human and animal hemopoietic tumors have suggested that, with
few exceptions (e.g. chronic myeloid leukemia, myeloma), they
represent clonal expansions of a genetically defect cell arrested
at a particular stage along the differentiation lineage (1,11).
Until recently, this "uncoupling" of the two processes proliferation and maturation has been assumed to be irreversible. However,
following the lead of Sachs and collaborators studying the inducible differentiation in vitro in a mouse leukemia (28) it is
now clear that also in human leukemia/lymphoma differentiation may
be induced, and that the cellular changes toward the terminally

differentiated phenotype are associated with a proliferation arrest in the G1 phase of the cell cycle (14, 15). The differentiation, which has been best studied in the HL-60 promyelocytic leukemia (14, 23) and the U-937 histiocytic lymphoma (22, 23) cell lines, appears to be equivalent to that of normal cells as judged from analyses of the stepwise phenotypic changes and from studies on the DNA synthesis.

Attempts to induce differentiation in malignant human lymphoid cells have met with less success. In the case of B-cell lines increases in Ig production have been demonstrated but further analyses are required to elucidate if this should be regarded as an induced change in the genetic B-cell differentiation program and not merely as a modulation of the capacity to secrete Ig (23, 27). Some T-leukemic cell lines, on the other hand, have been found to undergo phenotypic changes, and have a decreased proliferative capacity, similar to those observed in normally differentiating T-cells. However, those studies were not extensive enough in the examination of differentiation markers and of the cell-cycle changes to justify the conclusion that terminal differentiation had been induced (23).

Due to the imperfection of the established B-lymphoid cell lines as tools for studies of various aspects of B-cell differentiation we have initiated studies of human chronic lymphocytic leukemia (CLL) cells of the B-lymphocytic type. CLL cells have several advantages over the established B-cell lines, the most important one being that cells of this leukemia are readily inducible to maturation toward lymphoblasts-plasmablasts by a phorbol ester, 12-0-tetradecanoyl-phorbol-13-acetate (TPA) (30).

In the following we will summarize our own results, and to some extent those of others, with the TPA-CLL system. The points will be made that this human clonal system of neoplastic B-cells appears to be useful not only for studies of the deranged genetic control mechanisms underlying the malignant behaviour of CLL in vivo but also as a model for studies of the terminal events in normal B-cell differentiation.

INDUCERS OF DIFFERENTIATION OF CLL CELLS

B-CLL is a heterogeneous leukemia both with respect to cellular phenotype and clinical behaviour. The characteristics of most tumors correspond to that of immature B-cells but some CLL clones are phenotypically similar to resting B-cells, and even far more to differentiated B-cells (patients having serum M-components) (9, 13, 25).

Attempts in the early 1970ties to induce proliferation and differentiation in CLL cells using conventional T- and B-cell mitogens were negative. However, Maino et al (19) found an increased secretion of a single isotype light Ig chain in some CLL populations cultured with phytohemagglutinin (PHA). Fu et al (5,6), using CLL cells from two patients with serum M-components, then

demonstrated that mitogen and allogeneic helper cells/factors
induced plasmacytoid differentiation. Later, Robèrt et al (16,
26) successfully induced non-Ig secretory CLL to proliferation
and Ig secretion using T-cell dependent (PHA, PPO, LPS, DxS) and
independent (EBV) B-cell mitogens. Work by Kishimoto largely confirmed and extended the observations of Fu et al and showed that
PWM and allogeneic T-cells induced Ig secretion, proliferation
and class-switch in a secretory CLL population (29). Recently,
these studies were further refined and it was claimed that three
signals were neccessary to induce Ig secretion in this particular
secretory CLL population, namely anti-Ig, Il-2 and TRF, in this
sequence (37).

In 1980 we made the observation that TPA is an efficient inducer of lymphoblastoid/plasmacytoid differentiation with an increase in cytoplasmic Ig but without significant proliferation
(30). This TPA effect has been confirmed by several other groups
(2, 10, 12, 24). Compared with other inducers, TPA was the most
effective (33). Successful differentiation was inducible in 60-
70 % of the tested CLL clones with an increase in Ig production
demonstrable in 80-90 % of the cells. In the case of mitogens,
the frequency of responding CLL populations as well as the fraction of cells aquiring a plasmablast morphology and capacity for
Ig secretion appears to be lower than with TPA.

Except for TPA we have found that anti-Ig M (F(ab')$_2$ fragments)
supernatants from JM (T-leukemic cell line) producing Il-2 and
U-937 (monoblastic cell line secreting Il-1) and the mitogens
Con-A and PHA induce differentiation although, as pointed out
previously, less regularly than TPA. Anti-IgD, anti-β_2-microglo-
bulin, retinoic acid, DMSO, choleratoxin have all been ineffective as inducers (33).

PHENOTYPIC CHANGES DURING TPA-INDUCED DIFFERENTIATION

Following treatment with 0.16 - 16x10^{-7}M TPA, responsive CLL
cells will undergo certain characteristic alterations of the
phenotype summarized in Table 1. Drastic changes of the morphology take place which, as demonstrated by studies at the ultra-
structural level, correspond to those found in populations of
normal B-cells undergoing maturation towards plasma cells, e.g.
development of rough endoplasmic reticulum, a prominent Golgi
apparatus, an increase in the number of mitochondria and changes
of the nuclear chromatin.

The cell surface changes are pronounced. Cells aggregate
rapidly (within a few hours) after TPA exposure and general
changes of the composition of surface glycoproteins and glycolipids have been demonstrated (30, 36). Glycocalyx alterations
(decrease in sialic acid) were also found (36). A reflection of
these surface changes appears to be an increased sensitivity for
natural killer cells (7, 8, 34, 36).

TABLE 1. Phenotypic changes in CLL cells following TPA treatment (1.6 x 10^{-7}M, 72 hours)

Characteristic	Reference
Morphology	
Development of a lymphoblastoid-plasmablastoid morphology	12, 30, 32
Cytochemistry	
Increase in B-glucuronidase activity	33
Cell surface	
Altered surface glycoprotein composition	a
Altered surface glycolipid composition	7, 8, 36
Increased stimulation capacity in MLR and AMLR	17, 24
Increased expression of HLA-DR antigens	12, a
Altered (increased or decreased) expression of B-cell differentiation antigens	10, a
Decreased amounts of sialic acid	36
Decreased expression of mouse erythrocyte- and Fcγ-receptors	32
Immunoglobulin (Ig) production	
Decrease in cell surface IgD and IgM	2, 4, 31, 32
Aquisition of capacity for Ig secretion	2, 4, 24

[a] Danersund, Forsbeck, Nilsson, Tötterman, unpublished observations and data to be published

Some specific surface changes have been defined by monoclonal antibodies against B-cell differentiation antigens (10) and by rosette assays for C3, Fcγ and mouse erythrocyte receptors (32). With no exception the alterations noted are those found during maturation of normal B-cells.

Studies on the most important functional hallmark of B-cell differentiation - Ig production - also agree that TPA-responsive CLL populations, when induced, will follow the same differentiation pathway as normal B-cells. The changes in Ig gene locus activity appear to equate that of normal cells in that surface Ig will be reduced in expression and that secretory Ig will be synthesized (2,4). Even class switch (IgM → IgG) has been observed although this may occur only in CLL clones being arrested at a more advanced stage of differentiation than the prototype non-secretory CLL.

To study the level(s) of control of Ig synthesis during the differentiation-associated change in Ig production (surface Ig expression → Ig secretion) we have performed a study on the bio-synthesis of μ-chains and of the levels of cell surface and secretory μ-chain mRNA (4).

As is clear from Table 2, even non-differentiated cells express a μm mRNA and also μs mRNA. The μs mRNA message is translated to cytoplasmic μ-chains. However, little, if any, of these cytoplasmic μ-chains appear to assemble to pentameric secretory IgM.

TABLE 2. Alterations in μ-chain production after TPA induced differentiation of CLL cells

	Control cells	TPA induced cells
μ_m mRNA	++	↓+
μ_m surface expression	+++	↓+
μ_s mRNA	++	↑+++
μ_s cytoplasm	+	↑++
IgM secretion	(+)	↑+++

Upon TPA, induced differentiation changes although only small, are found in μm mRNA and μs mRNA levels demonstrating that some transcriptional control takes place. However, the most important cellular mechanism involved to change the functional state from that of marginal Ig secretion to a high level Ig secretion appears to be an increase in translation and a change in post-translational modification of the Ig molecules, allowing the formation of secretory pentameric IgM and its efficient transport to the exterior of the cell.

MECHANISM(S) OF TPA INDUCED DIFFERENTIATION

As pointed out before, normal B-cell differentiation is regulated by lymphokines and monokines. We have therefore initiated studies aiming at understanding the role of accessory cells in the induction of differentiation of CLL cells. In early studies we noted that autologous and allogeneic T-cells, and to some extent also monocytes, played an important role in assisting the CLL cells to differentiation after TPA exposure (33). These studies have now been extended. Experiments have been performed along three lines. Firstly, in pilot experiments we have examined the effect of TPA on single CLL cells and shown that they will not respond by proliferation or morphological changes while blast transformation was evident when the cells were exposed to supernatants from TPA-treated conventional CLL cultures containing T-cells and monocytes. These experiments must, however, be regarded as technically imperfect as it cannot be excluded that single CLL cells, without physical contact with other cells, will not respond by differentiation to TPA.

We have therefore conducted a second series of experiments where T-cells and monocytes were selectively removed by E-rosetting followed by Percoll gradient centrifugation and further depletion of T-cells by the anti-T monoclonal antibodies OKT 3, OKT 4, OKT 8 and OKM 1 plus complement (3). Except for the depletion experiments, several enrichment experiments involving additions of purified T-cells to purified B-CLL cells were also performed. Taken together, these experiments suggest that the CLL cells are dependent on one or several small subsets (~ 1 %) of autologous T-cells expressing low-avidity E-receptors and the T 3, T 4 and T 8 antigens. Thus we favour a model where TPA-induced IgM secretion in biopsy B-CLL cells is regulated by minute numbers of autologous T-helper cells via lymphokines as illustrated in Fig. 1.

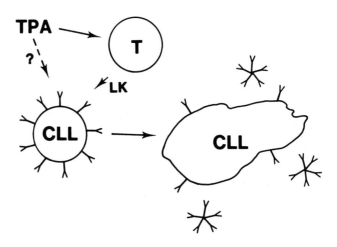

FIG. 1.   The hypothetical role for TPA, T-cells and lymphokines (LK) in the induction of differentiation of CLL cells by exposure to TPA.

It is likely that the low level of proliferation found in the TPA-stimulated CLL cultures to a large extent represents proliferation of T-cells as TPA is a well documented mitogen for T-cells and that the TPA activation of the T-cells leads to production of lymphokines. Such lymphokines should be of the B-cell differentiation (maturation) factor (BCDF) type rather than having growth factor properties (BCGF), since proliferation of CLL cells after TPA treatment is at best minimal.

CLINICAL STUDIES

The finding that TPA may induce in vitro differentiation in

CLL cells indirectly via the T-cells raised the question whether a similar modulation of the differentiation stage of the leukemic cells can take place in vivo during the course of the disease and if so would this alter the clinical behaviour of the tumor? In a comparative study (35) of the surface glycoprotein profiles of CLL clones from patients with active and inactive disease using galactose-oxidase tritiated sodium borohydride labelling we found that consistent differences in expression of some major surface glycoproteins indeed could be demonstrable between the two groups. As surface glycoprotein differences between lymphoid cells have been found to mainly reflect differences in the differentiation stage, one may assume that also in CLL this would be indicative of differences in maturation level.

A follow-up of the in vitro TPA response of the leukemic cells in a group of 16 CLL patients during the course of their disease demonstrated that TPA inducibility with few exceptions correlated with active disease (34). In patients whose disease activity fluctuated there was a parallel fluctuation in TPA inducibility. As we have demonstrated that TPA induction is dependent on one or two subsets of infrequent T-cells it is possible that the (in vitro) activity of these T-cells may vary during the course of the disease.

Taken together, these two studies thus suggest that the disease activity may be associated with the stage of differentiation of the leukemic B-cells and that this fluctuating level of differentiation may result from an interplay between T-cells and the CLL-cells. If so, CLL would be an example of a B-cell malignancy regulated to some extent by immune mechanisms in vivo.

CONCLUSIONS

1. CLL exemplifies a malignancy of B-cells usually arrested at a stage of differentiation corresponding to that of a cell slightly less mature than a peripheral resting B-cell.

2. The differentiation block in CLL cells is reversible since further differentiation is inducible in vitro by TPA and lymphokines.

3. The phenotypic changes during induced differentiation of CLL cells are those expected for non-neoplastic B-cells undergoing differentiation. No evidence for aberrant gene expression has been found.

4. The induced differentiation (maturation) occurs without little, if any, concomitant cell proliferation and is not completely terminal.

5. The control of surface and secretory μ-chain synthesis appears to be transcriptional, translational and post-translational.

6. The effect of TPA is mainly indirect via stimulation of T-cells producing CLL-directed differentiation factors.

7. It is conceivable that the CLL tumor cells in vivo are not autonomous but can be regulated with respect to differentiation stage (and perhaps also aggressiveness) by the patients' T-cell populations.

ACKNOWLEDGEMENTS

Work by the authors reported here was supported by grants from the Swedish Cancer Society.

REFERENCES

1. Biberfeld, P., and Nilsson, K. (1980): In: Malignant Lymphoproliferative Diseases, edited by J.G. van den Tweel, C.R. Taylor and F.T. Bosman, pp. 31-48. Leiden University Press, The Hague/Boston/London.

2. Cossman, J., Neckers, L.M., Braziel, R.M., Trepel, J.B., Korsmeyer, S.J., and Bakhshi, A. (1984): J.Clin.Invest., 73:587-592.

3. Danersund, A., Tötterman, T.H., Nilsson, K., Egle-Jansson, I., Kabelitz, D., and Sjöberg, O. Submitted.

4. Forsbeck, K.Ö., Danersund, A., Hellman, L., Tötterman, T.J., Pettersson, U., and Nilsson, K. Submitted.

5. Fu, S.M., Chiorazzi, N., Kunkel, H.G., Halper, J.P., and Harris, S.R. (1978): J. Exp. Med. 148:1570-1578.

6. Fu, S.M., Chiorazzi, N., and Kunkel, H.G. (1979): Immunol. Rev. 48:23-44.

7. Gidlund, M., Nilsson, K., Tötterman, T.H., and Wigzell, H. (1982): In: Modern Trends in Human Leukemia V, Vol. 28, edited by Neth et al, pp. 81-1 - 81-4. Springer-Verlag, Berlin-Heidelberg-New York.

8. Gidlund, M., Nose, M., Axberg, I., Wigzell, Tötterman, T., and Nilsson, K. (1982): In: NK Cells and other Natural Effector Cells, edited by R.B. Herberman, pp. 733-741. Academic Press, New York.

9. Gordon, J., Mellstedt, H., Åman, P., Biberfeld, P., Björkholm, M., and Klein, G. (1983): Blood, 62:910-917.

10. Gordon, J., Åman, P., Mellstedt, H., Biberfeld, P., and Klein, G. (1983): Leukemia Res. 7:133-138.

11. Greaves, M.F. (1979): In: Tumour Markers, edited by E. Boelsma and P. Rümke, pp. 201-211. Elsevier, Amsterdam.

12. Guy, K., Van Heyningen, V., Dewar, E., and Steel, C.M. (1983): Eur.J.Immunol. 13:156-159.

13. Hamblin, T., and Hough, D. (1977): Br. J. Haematol. 36: 359-365.

14. Huberman, E., and Callaham, M.F. (1979): Proc. Natl. Acad. Sci. USA 76:293-297.

15. Ivhed, I., Mattsson, P., and Nilsson, K. To be published.

16. Juliusson, G., Robèrt, K.-H., Hammarström, L., Smith, C.I.E., Biberfeld, G., and Gahrton, G. (1983): Scand. J. Immunol. 17:51-59.

17. Kabelitz, D., Tötterman, T.H., Nilsson, K., and Gidlund, M. Clin. Immunol. Immunopathol. In press.

18. Lajtha, L.G., Lord, B.I., Dexter, T.M., Wright, E.G., and Allen, T. (1978): In: Cell Differentiation and Neoplasia, edited by G.F. Saunders, p. 179. Raven Press, New York.

19. Maino, V.C., Kurnick, J.T., Kubo, R.T., and Grey, H.M. (1977): J. Immunol. 118:742-748.

20. Mak, T.W., and McCulloch, E.A. (editors) (1982): J. Cell Physiol. Suppl. 1.

21. Melchers, F., Andersson, J., Lernhardt, W., and Schreier, M.H. (1980): Eur. J. Immunol. 10:679-785.

22. Nilsson, K., Forsbeck, K., Gidlund, M., Sundström, C., Tötterman, T., Sällström, J., and Venge, P. (1981): In: Haematology and Blood Transfusion, vol. 26, edited by R. Neth, R.C. Gallo, T. Graf, K. Mannweiler, and K. Winkler, pp. 215-221. Springer-Verlag, Berlin-Heidelberg.

23. Nilsson, K., and Tötterman, T.H. (1984): Immunol. Clin. 3, 1-19.

24. Okamura, J., Letarte, M., Stein, L.D., Sigal, N.H., and Gelfand, E.W. (1982): J. Immunol. 128:2276-2280.

25. Preud'Homme, J.-L., Brouet, J.-C., and Seligmann, M. (1977): Immunol. Rev. 37:127-151.

26. Robèrt, K.-H. (1979): Immunol. Rev. 48:123-143.

27. Rosén, A., and Klein, G. (1983): Nature 306:189-190.

28. Sachs, L. (1980): Proc. Natl. Acad. Sci. USA 77:6152-6156.

29. Saiki, O., Kishimoto, T., Kuritani, T., Muraguchi, A., and Yuichi, Y. (1980): J. Immunol. 124:2609-2614.

30. Tötterman, T., Nilsson, K., and Sundström, C. (1980): Nature 288:176-178.

31. Tötterman, T.H., Nilsson, K., Claesson, L., Simonsson, B., and Åman, P. (1981): Human Lymphocyte Diff. 1:13-26.

32. Tötterman, T.H., Nilsson, K., Sundström, C., and Sällström,J. (1981): Human Lymphocyte Diff. 1:83-92.

33. Tötterman, T.H., Danersund, A., Nilsson, K., Gidlund, M., Kabelitz, D., and Wigzell, H. (1982): In: B and T Cell Tumors, Vol. 26, edited by E.S. Vitetta, pp. 419-423. Academic Press, New York.

34. Tötterman, T.H., Gidlund, M., Nilsson, K., and Wigzell, H. (1982): Br. J. Haematol. 52:563-571.

35. Tötterman, T.H., Forsbeck, K., Nilsson, K., Simonsson, B., Sundström, C., Sällström, J. (1983): Scand. J. Haematol. 30:79-88.

36. Yogeeswaran, G., Welsh, R.M., Gronberg, A., Kiessling, R., Patarroyo, M., Klein, G., Gidlund, M., Wigzell, H., and Nilsson, K. (1982): In: NK Cells and other Natural Effector Cells, edited by R.B. Herberman, pp. 765-770. Academic Press, New York.

37. Yoshizaki, K., Nakagawa, T., Kaieda, T., Muraguchi, A., Yamamura, Y., and Kishimoto, T. (1982): J. Immunol. 128: 1296-1301.

Molecular Biology of Tumor Cells, edited by
B. Wahren et al. Raven Press, New York © 1985.

Change in Expression of Oncogenes *(sis, ras, myc,* and *abl)* During *In Vitro* Differentiation of L6 Rat Myoblasts

Thomas Sejersen, *J. Pedro Wahrmann, †Janos Sümegi, and
Nils R. Ringertz

*Department of Medical Cell Genetics, Medical Nobel Institute, Karolinska Institutet, S-104 01
Stockholm, Sweden; *Institut de Pathologie Moléculaire, 75214 Paris, France; †Department of
Tumor Biology, Karolinska Institutet, S-104 01 Stockholm, Sweden*

The acutely oncogenic retroviruses contain sequences in their genomes that are responsible for neoplastic transformation in vivo and in vitro. These sequences, termed viral oncogenes, have their progenitors in the normal cellular genome (3). Although their precise role in normal cell metabolism is unknown, their high degree of evolutionary conservation suggests that these genes may be of key importance in the control of cell multiplication and differentiation. Studies of hematopoietic cells (4, 10, 25), a variety of normal tissues from chickens (10, 21) and mice (16) have demonstrated that the expression of proto-oncogenes show various degrees of specificity for tissue (4, 10, 21, 16), stage of histotypic differentiation (25) and stage of embryogenesis (4, 16). It is not clear, however, to what extent oncogene expression is related to cell proliferation as such, to the commitment of cells for specific developmental pathways (determination), and to expression of markers of histotypic differentiation. In order to answer these questions, further knowledge is required about the expression of proto-oncogenes in differentiating cell systems. The present investigation examines if proliferating and quiescent cells of a myogenic rat myoblast line (L6J1) and of a differentiation defective myoblast line (Ama 420) express the proto-oncogenes sis, ras, abl, src, fes, mos, myb, myc, and erb. For each of the cell-lines L6J1 and Ama 420, the expression of proto-oncogenes was correlated to the extent of DNA synthesis (^{3}H-TdR-incorporation) and to the degree of differentiation (creatine kinase assay).

The two subclones of the rat L6 myoblast line (26) selected for this study, L6J1 (19) and Ama 420 (6), can both be maintained as exponentially growing, mononucleate cells. As myoblasts of the line L6J1 attain high cell densities they stop DNA synthesis, fuse and form multinucleate myotubes. Synthesis of contractile proteins and enzymes typical of skeletal muscle occurs after fusion and can be used as quantitative markers of differentiation. (For a review of in vitro myogenesis see reference 17). The other subclone, Ama 420, is a differentiation defective derivative of L6 which is unable to form myotubes even at high cell densities and to undergo terminal differentiation.

Cells of the L6J1 line, plated and grown under the conditions specified in Figure 1, divide during the first three days in culture with a doubling time of about 24 hours. As the monolayer of cells becomes confluent, replication slows down. Fusion starts after 4-5 days in culture and continues until day 10 or 11, when more than 80% of all nuclei in the culture have been incorporated in the myotubes.

The Ama 420 mutant used in this study did not undergo fusion. Similar to the L6J1 cultures the mutant myoblasts first grew exponentially and then showed reduced rate of replication beginning on day 4. Occasionally short myotubes were observed in confluent cultures after 8-10 days. The extent of fusion, however, was much lower than in L6J1 cultures. Maximum proportion of nuclei in myotubes in these cultures was less than 2%. As can be seen in Figure 1, ^{3}H-TdR incorporation decreased in cultures of cells from both lines reaching a low level after 6-7 days.

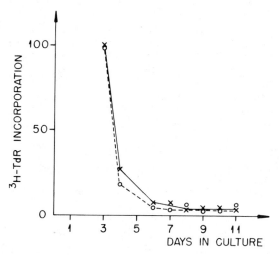

FIG. 1. ^{3}H-Thymidine incorporation into L6J1 and Ama 420 cells. L6J1 myoblasts (x——x) and Ama 420 myoblasts (o------o) were cultured in Dulbecco's modified Eagle's medium (DMEM) supplemented with 5% fetal calf serum (FCS) and antibiotics. At the times indicated, the cultures were incubated with 2 µCi/ml ^{3}H-thymidine for 22 h. Radioactivity was precipitated with 10% cold trichloroacetic acid on GF/C filters. After washing the filters, radioactivity was correlated to DNA-content. DNA-determinations were carried out as described (12). ^{3}H-TdR incorporation is expressed as percentage of the maximum value obtained for each cell-type.

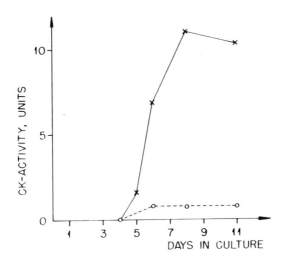

FIG. 2. Creatine kinase (CK) assay in L6J1, and Ama 420 cells. Cells were cultured as in figure 1. Enzyme activity in cell homogenates were measured at the times indicated, using a Merck test kit (CK NAC activated). NADPH was measured spectrophotometrically at 340 nm and CK-activity was expressed as μM NADPH/min/mg of DNA. p^5-Di(adenosin-5'-) pentaphosphate (300 μM) was included in the assay in order to inhibit myokinase (5). L6J1 (x———x), Ama 420 (o------o).

The extent of myogenic differentiation was measured by determining creatine kinase (CK) specific activity (see figure 2). A temporal relationship between the degree of morphological differentiation and CK specific activity has previously been reported by Shainberg et al., (20). The increase in CK-activity has been shown to be due to the synthesis of the MM form of the enzyme, i.e. the enzyme characteristic of skeletal muscle (14, 13). As can be seen in figure 2, no activity could be detected in cells of the L6J1 line until the fifth day of in vitro growth. The activity then increased sharply until day 8-11. Confluent cells of the myogenic, defective mutant Ama 420, which stopped dividing on day 6 in culture, showed only a very low specific activity.

Proliferating, undifferentiated myoblasts and non-cycling, differentiated myotubes of the cell line L6J1 were screened for expression of sequences homologous to nine oncogenes. Five of these: src, fes, mos, myb, and erb were not expressed in any of the samples applied to the dot blot analysis. Four others: sis, ras, myc, and abl, were found to be expressed differently during the in vitro differentiation of L6J1 myoblasts (see figure 3).

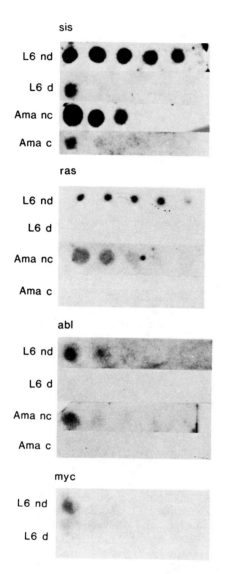

sis

L6 nd

L6 d

Ama nc

Ama c

ras

L6 nd

L6 d

Ama nc

Ama c

abl

L6 nd

L6 d

Ama nc

Ama c

myc

L6 nd

L6 d

FIG. 3. Poly(A)+RNA "dot blots" for semi-quantitative analysis of proto-oncogene like sequences in L6 and Ama 420 cells. Cells were cultured as in figure 1. They were harvested at day 2-3 (L6 nd, Ama nc) and at day 9-10 (L6 d, Ama c). Total RNA was extracted by hot phenol extraction (7) and selected for poly(A)+ RNA by chromatography on oligo(dT)-cellulose (2) twice, or occasionally once. Poly(A)+ RNA was dissolved in TE-buffer (10 mM Tris-Cl, 1mM EDTA, pH 7.6) and dotted onto freshly activated DBM (diazobenzyloxymethyl)-paper (1) as follows: Sis:L6 nd and Ama nc in a 1:2 dilution series, L6d and Ama c in a 1:4 dilution series. Ras: L6nd, L6d and Ama c in a 1:2 dilution series, Ama nc in a 1:4 dilution series. Abl: L6 nd, L6 d, Ama nc and Ama c in a 1:4 dilution series. Myc: L6 nd and L6d in a 1:4 dilution series. The most concentrated sample contained 2.0 (myc-hybridization) or 2.5 (all other hybridizations) μg of poly(A)+ RNA. The concentration was determined spectrophotometrically at 260 nm, where an optical density (OD) of 1 corresponds to 40 μg RNA/ml. The ratios between the readings at 260 nm and 280 nm were larger than or equal to 1.9. Dotted papers were prehybridized for 16-20 h at 42°C. Subsequently, the papers were hybridized for approximately 20 h at 42°C with 0.9-2.4 x 10^6 cpm of nick-translated probe per ml of hybridization buffer. Buffers for prehybridization and hybridization were essentially as described by Wahl et al (24). After hybridization, papers were washed for 4-8 h in 50% formamide, 50 mM sodium phosphate pH 7.0,5 x ssc (1 X SSC: 0.15 M NaCl, 15 mM sodium citrate). The papers were then exposed to X-ray films with intensifying screens at -70°C for 5-7 days. For rehybridization, papers were washed in 99% formamide at 56°C for 25 min.

The following cellular and viral oncogene probes were used: v-sis(pc14) cloned EcoR1-EcoR1 (600 bp; ref.9); c-ras^{Ki} (rat) (Hi-hi3), EcoR1-EcoR1 (1kb; ref.8); v-abl (pk5), Eco-R1-Eco-R1 (600 bp; ref. 22); c-myc (mouse) (pM c-myc 54), Pst1-Pst1 (2.2 kb; ref. 23).

Abbreviations: L6nd = proliferating, non-differentiated L6J1 myoblasts, L6d = quiescent, differentiated L6J1 myotubes. Ama nc = proliferating, non-confluent Ama 420 myoblasts, Ama c = quiescent, confluent Ama 420 myoblasts.

Sequences homologous to sis were seen in 2.5 μg of poly(A)+ RNA from differentiated L6J1 myotubes. However, the intensity of hybridization was much higher with undifferentiated L6J1 myoblasts, from which 0.16 μg of poly(A)+ RNA sufficed to give a well detectable hybridization. Hybridization with ras showed the greatest difference in expression pattern. Thus, 0.16 μg of poly(A)+ RNA from undifferentiated L6J1 myoblasts gave a visible hybridization signal with the ras probe, whereas 2.5 μg from differentiated L6J1 -myotubes could not be detected at all. Myc-related transcripts were readily detectable in 2.0 μg of poly(A) + RNA from undifferentiated L6J1 myoblasts. Hybridization with myc was also detectable in poly(A) + RNA from differentiated L6J1 myotubes. However, the intensity of the latter hybridization signal was 2-3 times lower than that obtained with RNA from undifferentiated L6J1 myoblasts. Abl-homologous sequences were barely, if at all, detectable in 2.5 μg of poly(A)+RNA from differentiated L6J1-myotubes, while 0.625 μg of poly(A)+RNA from proliferating, undifferentiated L6J1 myoblasts gave a visible hybridization signal with the abl probe. Preliminary data indicate that non-polyadenylated RNA from exponentially growing L6J1 myoblasts also contained sis and ras (Ki) transcripts (data not shown). Similar to the situation with the polyadenylated RNA fraction, the poly(A)-RNA from L6J1 myotubes did not contain detectable quantities of oncogene transcripts.

Also the differentiation defective, α-amanitin resistant L6J1 mutant (Ama 420), failed to express src, fes, mos, myb, or erb. The expression of myc-like sequences in Ama 420 has not yet been investigated with the probe (2nd and 3rd exon of mouse c-myc) used to detect myc-expression in L6J1 cells.

Sis-like sequences were found in non-confluent, proliferating Ama 420-myoblasts. Thus, 0.06 μg of poly(A)+ RNA from these cells gave a visible hybridization signal with the sis-probe. In confluent, non-cycling Ama 420-cells, 0.625 μg of poly(A)+ RNA was needed to detect sis-like sequences. Sequences homologous to ras were detected in 0.16 μg of poly(A)+ RNA from exponentially growing Ama 420 cells. No ras homologous sequences were detected in poly(A)+RNA from confluent Ama 420 myoblasts. Abl-like sequences were demonstrable in non-confluent, proliferating Ama 420-myoblasts from which 0.16 μg of poly(A)+ RNA gave a visible hybridization signal. In confluent Ama 420-cells, abl-like sequences were barely, if at all, detectable at the highest concentration of poly(A)+ RNA, corresponding to 2,5 μg.

In order to further explore the relationship between oncogene expression on the one hand, and differentiation and cell proliferation on the other, myogenic cell lines offer certain advantages in that the cultures pass through well defined stages of
differentiation. Though the in vitro model of myogenesis has not
yet been used in studies of oncogene expression some information
exists concerning oncogene expression in muscle. Thus expression
of some proto-oncogenes (myb, myc, erb, and yes) has previously
been reported in normal chicken muscle (4, 10, 21). It is also of
interest that transforming DNA segments from two human embryonal
rhabdomyosarcomas contain the c-ras (Ki) (18) and a transforming
gene (15), later found to be N-ras. However, in no case has a
correlation been established between the state of myogenic differentiation and expression of proto-oncogenes.

Our results show that some oncogenes (c-sis, c-ras (Ki), c-
myc, and c-abl) are expressed in exponentially growing myoblasts
and that expression decreases as the cells stop dividing. It is
noteworthy that a transient increase of c-ras (Ha) transcripts has
been observed in hepatocytes during rat liver regeneration (11).
It is interesting to note that proto-oncogene expression was reduced both in the differentiating L6J1 line and in the differentiation defective Ama 420 line. The reduced expression of at
least c-sis, c-ras (Ki), and c-abl does not correlate with myogenic differentiation as such but with reduced DNA replication. However, a decreased expression of one or more of these proto-oncogenes may be a necessary but, as such insufficient, prerequisite
for differentiation of L6 myoblasts.

SUMMARY

The expression of oncogenes during myogenesis was examined by
analyzing polyadenylated RNA from rat L6J1 myoblasts, L6J1 myotubes and differentiation defective Ama 420 myoblasts for nucleotide sequences complementary to cloned oncogenes. Using a dot
blot hybridization procedure, it was found that the proto-oncogenes sis, ras, and abl are expressed in exponentially growing
L6J1 and Ama 420 cells but not at all, or to a lesser degree in
L6J1 myotubes and confluent, stationary Ama 420 myoblasts. Also,
the expression of c-myc was found to be 2-3 times higher in exponentially growing L6J1 myoblasts than in L6J1 myotubes.

Acknowledgement

This investigation was supported by grants from the Swedish
Medical Research Council. J.P.W. was supported by a fellowship
from the NFR-CNRS exchange program. We thank Mrs. Ulla Krondahl
for technical assistance and Mrs. Vivi Jacobson for typing the manuscript. We are indebted to the following colleagues for providing us with cloned oncogenes: Drs. S.A. Aaronson (v-abl), M.A.
Baluda (v-myb), J.M. Bishop (v-src), R.W. Ellis (c-ras), R.C.
Gallo (c-fes), G.F. Van de Woude (c-mos), B. Vennström (v-erb), F.
Wong-Staal (v-sis), and K.B. Marcu (c-myc).

REFERENCES

1. Alwine, J.C., Kemp D.J., and Stark, G.R. (1977): Proc. Natl. Acad. Sci.U.S., 74:5350-5354.

2. Aviv, H., and Leder, P. (1972): Proc. Natl. Acad. Sci. U.S., 64:1408-1412.

3. Bishop, J.M. (1983): Ann. Rev. Biochem., 52:301-354.

4. Chen, C.H. (1980): J. Virol., 36:162-170.

5. Cohen, A., Buckingham, M., and Gros, F. (1978): Exptl.Cell Res.,115:201-206.

6. Crerar, M.M., Andrews, A.J., David, E.S., Somers, D.G., Mandel,J.-L, and Pearson, M.L. (1977): J. Mol. Biol., 112:317-329.

7. Edmonds, M., and Caramela, M.C. (1969): J. Biol. Chem.,244: 1314-1324.

8. Ellis, R.W., DeFeo, D., Shih, T.Y., Gonda, M.A., Young, H.A., Tsuchida, M., Lowy, D.R., and Scolnick, E.M. (1981): Nature (London), 292:506-511.

9. Gelman, E.P., Petri, E., Cetta, A., and Wong-Staal, F. (1982): J. Virol.,41:593-604.

10. Gonda, T.J., Sheiness, D.K., and Bishop, J.M. (1982): Mol. Cell. Biol., 2:617-624.

11. Goyette, M., Petropoulos, C.J., Shank, P.R., and Fausto, N. (1983):Science, 219:510-512.

12. Kapuscinski, J., and Skoczylas, B. (1977): Anal. Biochem. 83: 252-257.

13. Koniezcny, S.F., McKay, J., and Coleman, J. (1982): J. Dev. Biol., 91:11-26.

14. Luzzati, D., Loomis, W.F., Drugeon, G., and Wahrmann, J.P. (1973): In: Normal and pathological protein synthesis in higher organisms, edited by G. Schapira, J.C. Dreyfus, and J. Kruh, pp.475-483. Inserm Publ., Paris.

15. Marshall, S.J., Hall, A., and Weiss, R.A. (1982): Nature (London), 299:171-173.

16. Müller, R. (1982): In: Teratocarcinoma Stem Cells, vol. 10, edited by L.M. Silver, G.R. Martin, and S. Strickland, pp. 451-468. Cold Spring Harb.Conf. on Cell Proliferation.

17. Pearson, M.L., and Epstein, H.F. (1982): Muscle development. Molecular and cellular control. Cold Spring Harb. Lab., Cold Spring Harb., New York.

18. Pulciani, S., Santos, E., Lauver, A.V., Long, L.K., Aaronson, S.A., and Barbacid, M. (1982): Nature (London), 300:539-542.

19. Ringertz, N.R., Krondahl, U., and Coleman, J.R. (1978): Exptl. Cell Res., 113:233-246.

20. Shainberg, A., Yagil, G., and Yaffe, D. (1971): Dev. Biol. 25:1-29.

21. Shibuya, M., Hanafusa, H., and Balduzzi, P.C. (1982): J. Virol., 42:143-152.

22. Srinivasan, A., Reddy, E.P., and Aaronson, S.A. (1981). Proc. Natl. Acad. Sci. U.S., 78:2077-2081.

23. Stanton, L.W., Watt, R., and Marcu, K.B. (1983): Nature (London), 303:401-406.

24. Wahl, G.M., Stern, M., and Stark, G.R. (1979): Proc. Natl. Acad. Sci. U.S., 76:3683-3687.

25. Westin, E.H., Gallo, R.C., Arya, S.K., Eva, A., Souza, L.M., Baluda, M.A., Aaronson, S.A., and Wong-Staal, F. (1983): Proc. Natl. Acad. Sci. U.S., 79:2194-2198.

26. Yaffe, D. (1968): Proc. Natl. Acad. Sci. U.S., 61:477-483.

Molecular Biology of Tumor Cells, edited by
B. Wahren et al. Raven Press, New York © 1985.

Activation and Differentiation *In Vitro* of Human Lymphoma Cells: A New Method for the Cytological Evaluation of the Lymphoma Patient

Karl-Henrik Robèrt, Gunnar Juliusson, Gösta Gahrton, and
*Peter Biberfeld

*Division of Clinical Hematology and Oncology, Department of Medicine, Huddinge Hospital
and Karolinska Institute, S-141 86 Huddinge, Sweden; *Department of Pathology, Karolinska
Hospital, S-104 01 Stockholm, Sweden*

It is almost a truism that the functional properties of tumor cells play the most decisive role for the pathogenesis and prognosis in neoplasia. However, the main diagnostic considerations are still dependent on static judgements of the cancer cells, such as morphology, membrane markers, and the cellular biochemical composition. During the last few years, data have accumulated on in vitro activation of malignant lymphocytes as an additional method for the characterization of various types of B-cell lymphomas.

Activation of normal B lymphocytes

Lymphocytes provide unique possibilities for the study of regulation of cellular growth and differentiation due to their ability to become activated by antigens, and due to the existence of well defined markers for their metabolic activity and differentiation.

One of the major concepts of B-cell activation has been the one non-specific signal hypothesis[17]. It implies that the role of the surface membrane Ig (SmIg) is to concentrate specific antigens to the corresponding B-cell clones, after which a non-specific signal induces the activation process. This hypothesis evolved from the finding that high concentrations of thymus-independent antigens can activate a high proportion of B cells polyclonally. The responding cells, irrespective of their idiotypic specificity, share the same receptor for activation. The corresponding antigens, or rather epitopes of antigens, are referred to as polyclonal B cell activators PBA, and can be used to define functionally different B cell subsets.

A more complex model for the activation of B cells has been described lately. This includes the description of cellular interactions with other cell populations, and the detection of distinct growth and differentiation factors synthesized by accessory cells such as T-helper cells and macrophages (for review, see 12).

Activation of malignant B lymphocytes

When attending the question of malignant B-cell activation, one has to face certain problems inherent to the characteristics of malignant cell clones and their influence on other cells. The heterogeneity in primary malignant cell clones in comparison with malignant cell lines is of great importance in clonal activation. This heterogeneity has been shown for a number of variables studied, and can be observed with regard to variables that are associated with differentiation and metabolic or proliferative activity. Therefore one does not necesserily expect a hundred-percent response to activation in a primary malignant cell clone. Furthermore, since there, irrespective of the purification methods used, is a certain contamination of normal cells, reliable markers for monoclonality of the reponding cells are needed. These can be either chromosomal aberrations (that can be detected in many malignancies), light chains or idiotypes of malignant B-cell immunoglobulins.

Another crucial point for the activation of malignant B cells, would be that the receptors to different PBA:s are restricted to various B-cell subsets. Since the vast majority of lymphomas, including the B-lymphocytic leukemias, phenotypically correspond to different B cell subsets[1,15,16], a panel of PBA:s therefore has to be used in order to activate these cells[19].

Finally the clonal expansion in vivo eventually leads to the reduction of contaminating normal accessory cells, that secrete various lymphokines of importance for the activation procedure[21-22]. Therefore, for an optimal response in such assays, it may be important to add conditioned medium or to ensure a sufficient number of accessory cells in each culture.

Characterization of the responding cells

In contrast to previous opinions, it has been shown that malignant lymphocytes during optimal culture conditions, and considering the objectives pointed out above, have the ability to respond to activating substances, such as dextran sulphate (DxS), lipopolysaccharide from E.coli (LPS), anti-beta2-microglobulin (anti-beta2-m), purified protein derivate (PPD), conditioned media from phytohemagglutinin (PHA)-stimulated normal cell cultures, pokeweed mitogen (PWM), Epstein-Barr virus (EBV), and various phorbol esters (TPA)[5,18-22,28]. These responses have been characterized by proliferation and blast transformation of the malignant cells and furthermore by monoclonal immunoglobulin secretion. These effects generally show an interrelationship, i.e. the higher the DNA synthesis and proliferation, the more pronounced the blast transformation and secretion of immunoglobulins[20].

The present methods of activation leaves about 25% of the tested cell populations unactivated, i.e. a response is not always observed. Furthermore the magnitude of response varies between patients[8,14,23]. As expected, there is a heterogeneity of the response also within each clone, i.e. when successfully activated, only a proportion of the cells (20-80%) transform into blasts and only a few percent secrete antibodies[20,25].

Generally, more than one ligand can be used to activate each clone, probably indicating an intraclonal heterogeneity with regard to ligand reactivity. However, the optimal ligand(s) for activation is constant during the course of the disease and can thus be said to constitute a new marker system for various malignant subsets[23].

CLINICAL APPLICATIONS
Activation as a new marker system

In chronic lymphocytic leukemia cells, high responses to dextran sulphate and LPS are associated with a more aggressive course of the disease[14,23]. In our hands, the PBA-responding properties of the malignant cells give more prognostic information then conventional staging or classification systems such as those according to Rai or the Kiel-classification. The finding is similar to that observed by Tötterman et al[28], observing higher reponses to TPA in active phases of the diseases. These data imply, that cell clones that are easy to activate in vitro probably are more active also in vivo.

Chromosomal analysis

Chromosomal analysis in low-grade malignant B cell lymphomas, such as CLL, has previously revealed a normal karyotype in most cases[4,26]. In this group of malignancies the spontaneous mitotic index is very low. Thus, if the B-lymphocytic lymphoma cells are activated by T-cell mitogens there is, due to proliferation of normal cells, a high risk of misinterpretating the chromosomal data as being normal.

We have demonstrated that PBA:s can be used to induce metaphases in malignant lymphocytes, and also that most cases of low-grade malignant lymphomas have chromosomal abnormalities[6-7,14,24]. Most chromosomes can be involved in either structural or numerical aberrations, but some forms seem more common than others. The most common aberration is an extra chromosome 12, either alone or in combination with other aberrations. Extra chromosome 12 is present in nearly 50 percent of the properly evaluated cases (25% of the malignant clones cannot be activated, see above). Of particular interest is the association between +12 and unfavourable prognosis[14,24].

Of further interest is the finding, that patients with nonevaluable karyotypes (mainly due to a low frequency of metaphases) have the most favourable prognosis. This is in agreement with our previous finding cited above, that cell clones with a low response to PBA:s, such as DxS and LPS, have a more favourable prognosis[23]. Finally, cell clones with more than two aberrations run the most aggressive course of disease[14].

Interrelationships between lymphocytic malignancies

Chronic lymphocytic leukemia cells represent a resting stage of lymphocytes in various stages of differentiation. In these patients the disease mostly has a benign course with slow progression and a relatively low frequency of clinical complications[16]. The cytological picture is characterized by a pronounced homogeneity - all cells have a small nucleus without nucleoli and with a tiny border of cytoplasm. According to the Kiel classification[16], the "pure" CLL cases are devoid of antibody-secreting cells at plasmacytoid levels of differentiation. Malignant cell clones that include cells at this stage of differentiation are referred to as "immunocytomas" (IC). These cases may have monoclonal serum spikes, and are said to run a more active course of the disease in comparison with CLL. Furthermore, they often develop immune-associated complications, such as hemolytic anemia.

Another related B-cell malignancy is referred to as B-cell prolymphocytic leukemia (B-PLL). The cell picture is homogeneous with a blast-like appearance (nucleoli and a relatively high cytoplasm/nuclei ratio). This subgroup of low-grade malignant lymphomas is fairly distinguished also clinically from CLL and IC. It is a relatively aggressive disease that shows only a moderate response to various chemotherapy regimens. The spleen is often large, and the primary treatment of choice should be splenectomy[9,16].

B-PLL represents a relatively mature stage of B-lymphocyte differentiation with regard to immunological markers. Thus, these cells express strong SmIg and lack receptors for mouse red blood cells[3,11]. Furthermore, Catovsky et al[3] have demonstrated membrane reactivity with a new monoclonal antibody, FMC7, which is not expressed by ALL and CLL cells.

These phenotypic characteristics indicative of a relatively high degree of maturity, may seem contradictory to the immaturity implied by the blast-like appearance of these cells. However, after activation in vitro with LPS, CLL cells may display all characteristics typical for PLL[2,25]. Thus no such implicit contradiction exists. The blast-like appearance of PLL cells rather implies, that these cells represent a maturation arrest in a metabolically active stage, corresponding to that of physiologically activated and relatively mature B cells.

The type of phenotypical change in the activated CLL cells is influenced by the individual characteristics of the tested cells but also by the ligands used. The latter point is in agreement with findings in normal lymphocytes, where certain ligands are effective to induce differentiation and others proliferation[10]. In the experiment referred to above[25], LPS was used. This ligand is a potent inducer of blast transformation and proliferative activity in certain CLL cases. However, for the induction of monoclonal antibody secretion, other ligands, such as PWM and particularly Cowan staphylococci are usually more effective[13,23].

The latter has been used to induce differentiation as far as to a switch of immunoglobulin production from IgM to IgG in a fraction of the leukemic cell population[13]. Thus, before stimulation only my chains were detected on the surface of unstimulated cells, whereas after activation with Cowan, a few cells were able to secrete monoclonal gamma chains. It is not clear whether this reflects some sort of modulation of cells that had already undergone an in vivo immunoglobulin gene rearrangement to IgG secretion, or if it represents a real differentiation at the DNA level[13]. However, it is of great interest for the understanding of the pathogenesis in these diseases, since some cells in the immunocytomas show a spontaneous ability to differentiate to in vivo antibody secretion. In some cases, these cells secrete Ig gamma chains as demonstrated by the presence of monoclonal gamma chain spikes in serum.

In conclusion, it is possible to induce changes in CLL cells in vitro, that make these cells resemble other malignancies such as IC and PLL. The close relationship between these malignancies is demonstrated both by the mutual chromosomal aberations such as the +12 abnormality, and the possibility to transform the phenotypes of these cells to one another in vitro. The reason why the malignant lymphocytes in IC and PLL spontaneously achieve phenotypes characteristic of in vitro activated CLL cells is not clear. However, the difference between these malignancies on a cellular level seems to be on the level of metabolic activity in the cell rather than in differences in tumor initiation or different levels of differentiation blockage. A prognostic evaluation of a lymphoma clone should therefore take into consideration not only the level of differentiation, but also the level of cellular metabolic activity[25]. Most likely, the level of metabolic activity is also relatively more important for the clinical course, than "low" or "high" levels of differentiation per se. Thus, the higher level of differentiation in IC, PLL, and myeloma in comparison with CLL, is not necessarily in conflict with the generally more aggressive course of these diseases, since they mostly display a spontaneous high degree of metabolic activity.

SUMMARY

Activation of freshly sampled malignant lymphocytes provides a potential for the further understanding, and thereby for a clinically relevant evaluation of individual lymphoma patients. This method has been shown to give prognostic information both directly as a new marker system, but also indirectly through the evaluation of chromosomal abnormalities. Furthermore, it provides new perspectives for the analysis of tumor evolution. Of particular interest is the possibility to abrogate the maturation arrest in some clonally restricted cells.

Finally, the possibility to overcome the maturation arrest might even lead to therapeutical implications, since the differentiation blockage plays a fundamental role in the clonal expansion and pathogenesis in tumors.

REFERENCES

1. Aisenberg, A.C., Bloch, K.J. (1972): N Engl J Med 287: 272-6.
2. Caligaris-Cappio, F., Gobbi, M., Bergui, L., Compana, D., Chilosi, M., Foa, R., Malavasi, F., Janossy, G. International Society of Haematology, European and African Division. Seventh Meeting, Barcelona, Spain, September 4-6 1983. Abstract, p. 16.
3. Catovsky, D., Cherchi, M., Brooks, D., Bradley, J., Zola, H. (1981): Blood 58: 406-8.
4. Fleischman, E.W., Prigogina, E.L. (1977): Hum Genet 35: 269-79.
5. Fu, S.M., Chiorazzi, N., Kunkel, H.G., Halper, J.P., Harris, S.R. (1978): J Exp Med 148: 1570.
6. Gahrton, G., Robèrt, K-H., Bird, A.G., Zech, L. (1979): N Engl J Med 301: 438-9.
7. Gahrton, G., Robèrt, K-H., Friberg, K., Zech, L., Bird, A.G. (1980): Lancet 1: 146-7.
8. Gahrton, G., Robèrt, K-H., Friberg, K., Zech, L., Bird, A.G. (1980): Blood 56: 640-7.
9. Galton, D.A.G., Goldman, J.M., Wiltshaw, E., Catovsky, D., Henry, K., Goldenberg, G.J. (1974): Br J Med 27: 7.
10. Gronowicz, E., Coutinho, A. (1975): Transplant Rev 24: 3-40.
11. Gupta, S., Pawha, R., O'Reilly, R.J., Good, R.A., Siezal, F.P. (1976): Proc Natl Acad Sci 73: 919-22.

12. Howard, M., Paul, W. (1983): Ann Rev Immunol 1: 307-33.
13. Juliusson, G., Robèrt, K-H., Hammarström, L., Smith, C.I.E., Biberfeld, G., Gahrton, G. (1983): Scand J Immunol 17: 51-9.
14. Juliusson, G., Robèrt, K-H., Öst, Å., Friberg, K., Biberfeld, P., Nilsson, B., Zech, L., Gahrton, G. Prognostic information of cytogenic analysis in chronic B-lymphocytic leukemia and leukemic immunocytoma. Submitted for publication.
15. Korsmeyer, S.J., Arnold, A., Bakhshi, A., Ravetch, J.V., Siebenlist, U., Hieter, P.A., Sharrow, S.O., LeBien, T.W., Kersey, J.H., Poplack, D.G., Leder, P., Waldmann, T.A. (1983): J Clin Invest 71: 301-13.
16. Lennert, K., Mohri, N. (1978): pp. 111 ff. Springer-Verlag, Berlin-Heidelberg.
17. Möller, G., Coutinho, A., Persson, U. (1975): Scand J Immunol 4: 37-52.
18. Nowell, P., Shankey, T.V., Finan, J., Guerry, D., Besa, E. (1981): Blood 57: 444-51.
19. Robèrt, K-H., Möller, E., Gahrton, G., Eriksson, H., Nilsson, B. (1978): Clin Exp Immunol 33: 302-8.
20. Robèrt, K-H., Bird, A.G., Möller, E. (1979): Scand J Immunol 10: 447-52.
21. Robèrt, K-H., Nilsson, B. (1979): Scand J Immunol 10: 127-33.
22. Robèrt, K-H. (1979): Clin Exp Immunol 37: 517-22.
23. Robèrt, K-H. (1979): Immunological Rev 48: 123-43.
24. Robèrt, K-H., Gahrton, G., Zech, L. (1982): Scand J Haematol 82: 163-8.
25. Robèrt, K-H., Juliusson, G., Biberfeld P. (1983): Scand J Immunol 17: 397-401.
26. Rowley, J.D. (1978): In: Levy R, Kaplan HS, eds. Malignant Lymphoma. UICC Technical Report Series 37: 71.
27. Sadamori, N., Han, T., Minowada, J., Matsui, S., Sandberg, A.A. (1983): Cancer Res 43: 3287-91.
28. Tötterman, T.H., Nilsson, K., Claesson, L., Simonsson, B., Âman, P. (1981): Human Lymphocyte Differentiation 1: 13-26.

Molecular Biology of Tumor Cells, edited by
B. Wahren et al. Raven Press, New York © 1985.

Regulators of Growth, Differentiation, and the Reversion of Malignancy: Normal Hematopoiesis and Leukemia

Leo Sachs

Department of Genetics, Weizmann Institute of Science, Rehovot 76100, Israel

Abstract: Our development of systems for the in vitro cloning
and clonal differentiation of normal hematopoietic cells, made it
possible to identify the regulators of growth and differentiation
of these normal cells and the changes in normal controls that
produce leukemia. We have mainly used myeloid cells as a model
system. Experiments with normal hematopoietic precursors have
shown that normal cells require different proteins to induce
growth and differentiation. Differentiation-inducing protein, but
not growth-inducing protein, is a DNA-binding protein. We have
also shown that in normal myeloid precursors, growth-inducing protein induces both growth and production of differentiaion-indu-
cing protein, so this ensures the coupling between growth and differentiation that occurs in normal development. The origin of malignancy involves uncoupling of growth and differentiation. This
can be produced by changes from inducible to constitutive expression of specific genes which results in asynchrony in the co-ordination required for the normal developmental program. Normal myeloid precursors require an external source of growth-inducing protein for growth, and we have identified different types of leukemic cells. Some no longer require, and others constitutively produce their own growth-inducing protein. But addition of the normal
differentiation-inducing protein to these malignant celss still
induces their normal differentiation, and the mature cells are
then no longer malignant. Genetic changes which produce blocks in
the ability to be induced to differentiate by the normal inducer
occur in the evolution of leukemia. But even these cells can be
induced to differentiate by other compounds, including low doses
of compounds now being used in cancer therapy. This differentiation of leukemic cells has been obtained in vitro and in vivo,and
our in vivo results indicate that this may be a useful approach to
therapy. In some tumors, such as sarcomas, reversion from malignant to a non-malignant phenotype can be due to karyotypic changes
that suppress malignancy. In myeloid leukemia the cessation of
growth in mature cells by induction of differentiation by-passes
the genetic changes that produce the malignant phenotype. These
conclusions can also be applied to other types of normal and malignant cells.

The described cultures seem to offer a useful system for a quantitative kinetic approach to hematopoietic cell formation and for experimental studies on the mechanism and regulation of hematopoietic cell differentiation (25).

Reversibility of Malignant Cell Transformation

The change of normal into malignant cells involves a sequence of genetic changes including specific chromosome changes (See 2, 40,84,85). Evidence has, however, been obtained with various types of tumors, including sarcomas (85), myeloid leukemias (85,86,88) and teratocarcinomas (15,69), that malignant cells have not lost the genes that control normal growth and differentiation. This was first shown in sarcomas by the finding that it was possible to reverse the malignant to a non-malignant phenotype with a high frequency in cloned sarcoma cells (79-81,85). A comparison of sarcomas with myeloid leukemias then showed that reversion of the malignant phenotype can be achieved by two mechanisms. Chromosome studies on normal fibroblasts, sarcomas and revertants from sarcomas which have regained a non-malignant phenotype have indicated, that the difference between malignant and non-malignant cells is controlled by the balance between genes for expression (E) and suppression (S) of malignancy. When there is enough S to neutralize E, malignancy is suppressed; and when the amount of S is not sufficient to neutralize E, malignancy is expressed (Fig. 1; 30, 79,80, 85,105). Genes for expression of malignancy (E) are now called oncogenes (4,43), and these experiments indicate there are other genes, S genes, that can suppress the activities of oncogenes. In the mechanism found with sarcomas reversion was obtained by chromosome segregation, resulting in a change in gene dosage due to a change in the balance of specific chromosomes (Fig. 1; 80). This reversion of malignancy by chromosome segregation, with a return to the gene balance required for expression of the non-malignant phenotype, occurred without hybridization between different types of cells (30,79-81,85,105). The non-malignant cells were thus derived from the malignant ones by genetic segregation. Reversion of the malignant phenotype associated with chromosome changes has also been found after hybridization between different types of cells (41,82,104).

In addition to this reversion of malignancy by chromosome segregation, another mechanism of reversion has been found in myeloid leukemia. In this second mechanism, reversion to a non-malignant phenotype was also obtained in certain clones with a high frequency but, in contrast to sarcomas, this reversion was not associated with chromosome segregation. Phenotypic reversion of malignancy in these leukemic cells was obtained by induction of the normal sequence of cell differentiation by the physiological inducer of differentiation (85,86,88-90). In this reversion of the malignant phenotype, the cessation of growth in mature cells by induction of differentiation by-passes the genetic changes that produce the malignant phenotype. This second mechanism will now be discussed.

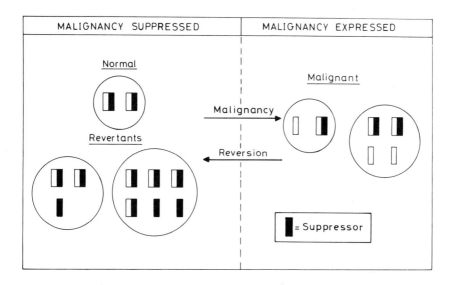

Fig. 1. Gene dosage and the expression and suppression of malignancy. From experiments with normal fibroblasts, sarcoma cells and their non-malignant revertants. Genes for □ expression and ■ suppression of malignancy (80).

Cloning and Clonal Differentiation of Normal Hematopoietic Cells in Culture

The cloning and clonal differentiation of normal hematopoietic cells in culture, made it possible to study the controls that regulate growth (multiplication) and differentiation of different hematopoietic cell types (See 85,86,88-90). We first showed (25, 77), as was then confirmed by others (5), that normal mouse myeloid precursor cells cultured with a feeder layer of other cell types can form clones of granulocytes and macrophages in culture. We also found that the formation of these clones is due to secretion, by cells of the feeder layer, of specific inducers that induce the formation of clones and the differentiation of cells in these clones to macrophages or granulocytes in mice (37,77,78), and in humans (74). After we first detected their presence in culture supernatants (37,78), these protein inducers have been referred to by a number of names and I shall use the name macrophage and granulocyte inducers (MGI; Table 1). These proteins can be produced and secreted by various normal and malignant cells in culture and in vivo (85). Their production can be induced by a variety of compounds (18,22,58,103) and some cells produce these proteins constitutively (1,37,44,50,93). MGI are a family of proteins that exist in a number of molecular forms that have different biologi-

Table 1: <u>In vitro</u> cloning and clonal differentiation of normal
hematopoietic cells

Cloning and differentiation in liquid medium (mast cells and gra-
nulocytes (25)
Cloning and differentiation in agar (macrophages) (77)
Inducer for cloning and differentiation secreted by cells (77)
Inducer in conditioned medium from cells (for macrophages and gra-
   nulocytes) (37,78)
Different inducer for macrophages and granulocyte clones (37)
Cloning and differentiation of macrophages and granulocytes in
   methyl-cellulose (37)
Confirmation of cloning and differentiation in agar (5)
Production of inducer for cloning by some leukemic cells (72)
Cloning and differentiation of human cells (74,76)
Protein inducer of differentiation that does not induce cloning
   (23)

Terminology used for proteins that induce cloning and differentiation of normal macrophages and granulocytes

Mashran gm (38)
Colony stimulating factor (CSF) (67)
Colony stimulating activity (CSA) (1)
Macrophage and granulocyte inducers (MGI) (44)
MGI-1 (=mashran gm, CSF, CSA) for cloning; MGI-2 (=D factor, DF)
   for differentiation (48,51,61,88)

cal activities. This cell culture approach has led to the cloning
and isolation of growth factors for all the different types of
hematopoietic cells including different types of lymphocytes.

Normal Growth-Inducing and Differentiation-Inducing Proteins

The family of MGI proteins include some proteins that induce
cell growth (multiplication) and others that induce differentiation. Those that induce growth, which are also required for normal
cell viability, we now call MGI-1. These include proteins that induce the formation of macrophage clones (MGI-IM) (37,51,93), granulocyte clones (MGI-IG) (37,51,70), or both types of clones (MGI-
IGM) (8,44,50). MGI-1 has previously been referred to as mashran
gm (38), colony stimulating factor (CSF) (67), colony stimulating
activity (CSA; 1) and MGI (44 ; Table 1). The existence of an
antibody that does not react with all forms of MGI-IM or MGI-IG
has shown, that there can be different antigenic sites on molecules that belong to the same form of MGI-1 (51,64). The other main
type of MGI, which we now call MGI-2 (48,51,88), induces the differentiation of myeloid precursor cells, either leukemic (20), or
normal (48,88), without inducing colony formation. This differentiation-inducing protein (20,23) has also been referred to as MGI
(20), D factor (63,106) and GM-DF (9). It has been suggested that
there are different forms of MGI-2 for differentiation to macrophages or granulocytes (48). The regulation of MGI-1 and MGI-2
appears to be under the control of different genes (18). Differen-

tiation-inducing protein MGI-2, but not the growth-inducing protein MGI-1, is a DNA-binding protein (102).

These macrophage and granulocyte inducers can be proteins or glycoproteins, depending on the cells in which they are produced, and the presence of carbohydrates does not appear to be necessary for their biological activity (50). Their molecular weights are mostly around 23,000 or multiples of this number (51,71,86), and MGI-2 activity is more sensitive to proteolytic enzymes and high temperature than MGI-1 activity (50). MGI-2 has a shorter half-life in serum than MGI-1 (60). The separability of the different forms of MGI seems to depend on the cells from which they are derived (51). Further studies should determine whether different forms of MGI are derived from a common precursor, and whether tumor cells with the appropriate gene re-arrangements and possibly even normal cells under certain conditions, may produce hybrid molecules of different forms of MGI including hybrid molecules with MGI-1 and MGI-2 activity (48).

Control of Growth and Differentiation in Leukemia

Normal myeloid precursor cells isolated from bone marrow (54) require an external source of MGI-1 for cell viability and growth. There are, however, myeloid leukemic cells that no longer require MGI-1 for viability and growth, so that these leukemic cells can then multiply in the absence of MGI-1 (86,88). This gives the leukemic cells a growth advantage over the normal cells when there is a limiting amount of MGI-1. Starting with a decreased requirement for MGI-1, this eventually leads to a complete loss of this requirement. Other myeloid leukemic cells constitutively produce their own MGI-1 (70,72) and these leukemic cells also have a growth advantage compared to normal cells that require an external source of MGI-1 (Fig. 2). A change in the requirement of MGI-1 for growth, either a partial or complete loss of this requirement, or the constitutive production of MGI-1, thus both give a growth advantage to leukemic cells.

The existence of myeloid leukemic cells that either no longer require MGI-1 for viability and growth or constitutively produce their own MGI-1, raises the question whether these leukemic cells can still be induced to differentiate to mature cells by the normal differentiation-inducing protein MGI-2. This question has been answered by showing that there are clones of myeloid leukemic cells that no longer require MGI-1 for growth, but can still be induced to differentiate normally to mature macrophages and granulocytes by MGI-2 (Fig. 3) via the normal sequence of gene expression (See 86,88-90). These mature cells are then no longer malignant in vivo (21,60,64). Among the many differentiation-associated properties induced in these cells by MGI-2 is the ability to respond by chemotaxis (Fig. 4) to a variety of chemoattractants (94). Injection of these myeloid leukemic cells into embryos has shown that after such injection the leukemic cells can participate in hematopoietic differentiation in apparently healthy adult animals (28, 101).

Type of myeloid cells	Requirement of MGI-1 for growth
Normal	External source
Leukemic	Decrease ⟶ no requirement or Constitutive production

Fig. 2. Differences in MGI-1 requirement for growth in normal and leukemic myeloid cells.

Injection of MGI-2 into animals, or in vivo induction of MGI-2 by a compound that induces the production of this differentiation-inducing protein, results in an inhibition of leukemia development in animals with such leukemic cells (Fig. 5) (60,64). There are also myeloid leukemic cells that constitutively produce their own MGI-1 and that can be induced to differentiate by MGI-2. Our results indicate that induction of normal differentiation in myeloid leukemic cells by MGI-2 can be an approach to therapy based on the induction of normal differentiation in malignant cells (20,57,60,

TABLE 2

Induction of Differentiation in Different MGI^+D^+
clones of Myeloid Leukemic Cells by Different Forms of MGI-2

Source of MGI-2	Induction of differentiation in:		
	Mouse Clone 11	Mouse Clone 7-M12	Human HL-60
Krebs tumor cells	+	+	−
Mouse endotoxin serum	+	−	−
Mouse macrophages	+	−	−
Mouse granulocytes	+	−	−
Mouse WEHI-3B cells	−	+	−
Human lymphocytes	+	−	+

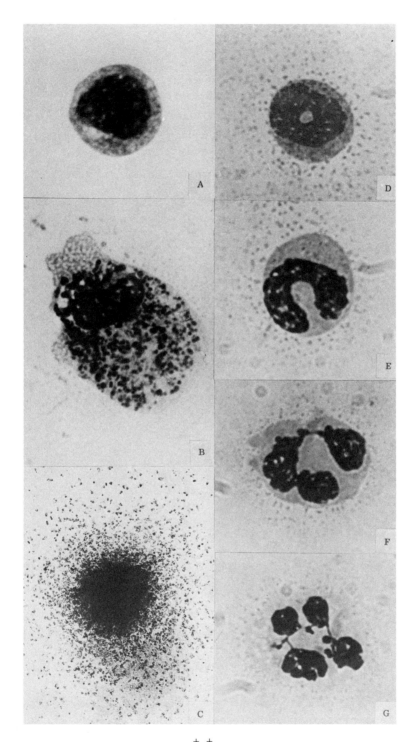

Fig. 3. Differentiation of MGI$^+$D$^+$ myeloid leukemic cells to mature macrophages and granulocytes by the normal myeloid differentiation-inducing protein MGI-2. (A) Leukemic cell; (B) macrophage; (C) colony of macrophages; (D-G) stages in differentiation to granulocytes (20).

63,64,74,85-87). There are various forms of MGI-2, which differ in their ability to induce differentiation in different clones of myeloid leukemic cells (57,58,63,64 and <u>Table 2</u>).

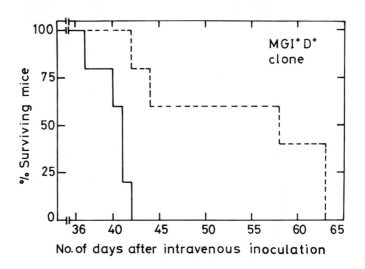

No. of days after intravenous inoculation

Fig. 5. Effect of treatment with MGI-2 on the survival of mice intravenously inoculated with MGI$^+$D$^+$ myeloid leukemic cells (60).

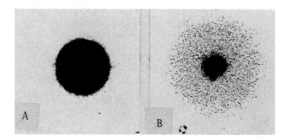

Fig. 4. Colony from (A) a MGI$^-$D$^-$clone and (B) from a MGI$^+$D$^+$clone cultured with MGI-2 (28). The differentiating cells in the MGI$^+$D$^+$clone migrate from the colony when the cells are induced to respond to chemotactic stimuli (94).

Leukemic clones that can be induced to differentiate to mature cells by MGI-2 have been found in different strains of mice (9,19,

20,35,36,55). They are referred to as MGI^+D^+ (MGI^+ to indicate that they can be induced to differentiate by MGI-2; D^+ for differentiation to mature cells). MGI^+D^+ leukemic cells have specific chromosome changes compared to normal cells (2,28). These chromosome changes thus seem to involve changes in genes other than those involved in the induction of normal differentiation. There are other clones of myeloid leukemic cells that can also grow without adding MGI-1 but that are either partly (MGI^+D^-) or almost completely (MGI^-D^-) blocked in their ability to be induced to differentiate by MGI-2 (Fig. 6) (19,31,33,36,51, 91,92). These differentiation-defective clones have specific chromosome changes compared to MGI^+D^+cells (2,28).

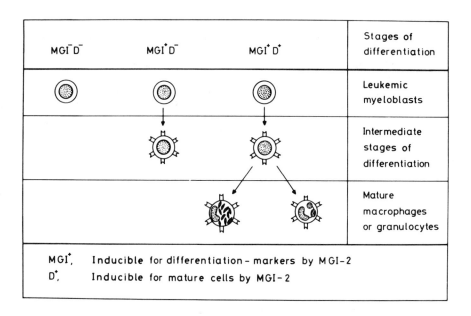

Fig. 6. Classification of different types of myeloid leukemic cell clones according to their ability to be induced to differentiate by MGI-2.

There are a variety of compounds, other than MGI-2, that can induce differentiation in MGI^+D^+ clones. Not all these compounds are active on the same MGI^+D^+ clone, and they do not all induce the same differentiation-associated properties. The inducers include certain steroids, lectins, polycyclic hydrocarbons, tumor promoters, lipopolysaccharide, x-irradiation and compounds used in cancer chemotherapy (59,86) (Table 3).

TABLE 3
Compounds used in cancer therapy that can induce differentiation
in clones of myeloid leukemic cells at low doses

Adriamycin, cytosine arabinoside, daunomycin, hydroxyurea, methotrexate, mitomycin C, prednisolone, X-irradiation

The existence of clonal differences in the ability of x-irradiation and cancer chemotherapeutic chemicals to induce differentiation, may help to explain differences in response to therapy in
different individuals (86). As a result of these experiments we
have suggested that it may be possible to introduce a form of therapy based on induction of differentiation (20,57,59,60,74,85,86).
This would include pre-screening in culture to select for the most
effective compounds, and using these compounds for a low-dose chemotherapy protocol aimed at inducing cell diferentiation (59).
Since different myeloid leukemic clones respond differently to
MGI-2 and other compounds, such differences will also occur in
leukemic cells from different patients. Based on these suggestions
(86,87), some encouraging clinical results have been obtained with
the use of low dose cytosin arabinoside (3,34,68).

Alternative Pathways for Differentiation

Some of the compounds that induce differentiation in susceptible clones of MGI^+D^+ leukemic cells, including lipopolysaccharide, phorbol ester tumor promoters such as 12-0-tetra-
decanoyl-phorbol-13-acetate (TPA) and nitrosoguanide, can induce
the production of MGI-2 in these clones. These compounds thus induce differentiation by inducing in the leukemic cells the endogenous production of the normal differentiation-inducing protein
MGI-2 (18,58,103). Other compounds such as the steroid dexamethasone can induce differentiation in MGI^+D^+ clones without
inducing MGI-2 (18). This steroid induces differentiation by other
pathways of gene expression than MGI-2 (10,55). The same applies
to dimethylsulfoxide (DMSO).

In a line of human myeloid leukemic cells DMSO induces the
formation of granulocytes (12), whereas MGI-2 (58,59) and the tumor promoting phorbol ester TPA (58,83) which induces the production of MGI-2 (58), induces the formation of macrophages. Studies
on the protein changes induced by these inducers, using two-dimensional gel electrophoresis, showed a similar developmental program
for macrophage differentiation induced by MGI-2 and TPA. This dif-
fered from the beginning from the granulocyte program induced by
DMSO (47). Unlike MGI-2 or DMSO, TPA induces rapid cell attachment
of these myeloid leukemic cells to the Petri dish. Combined treatment with TPA and DMSO showed cell attachment, extensive spreading
of the cells, the regulation of specific proteins and expression
of the macrophage program. The results indicate that cells in suspension can express either the macrophage or granulocyte program

depending on the inducer, and that changes in cell shape associated with cell attachment can regulate specific proteins and restrict the developmental program to macrophages (47). The in vivo environment of cells in relation to the possibilities of cell adhesion may thus play a major role in determining the differentiation program of myeloid and other cell types.

Differentiation by Combined Treatment with Different Compounds

Induction of differentiation in some myeloid leukemic clones requires combined treatment with different compounds (42,56,58,97, 98). In these cases one compound induces changes not induced by the other, so that the combined treatment results in new gene expression. This complementation of gene expression can occur both at the level of mRNA production and mRNA translation (32). With the appropriate combination of compounds, we have been able to induce all our MGI⁻D⁻ leukemic clones to express some differentiation-associated properties (97,98). It will be interesting to determine whether the same applies to differentiation of erythroleukemic cells (24,66). It is possible that all myeloid leukemic cells no longer susceptible to the normal differentiation-inducing protein MGI-2 by itself, can be induced to differentiate by choosing the appropriate combination of compounds to give the required complementation. This can include the use of hormones such as steroids (52,53), or insulin (96,97), and different nonphysiological compounds (86) together with or without MGI-2.

Coupling of Growth and Differentiation in Normal Cells

We have developed a simple procedure for isolating normal myeloid precursor cells from the bone marrow (54). Incubation of isolated normal myeloid precursors with MGI-1, either MGI-IM or MGI-IG (51), induces the viability and growth of these normal precursors, and results in cell differentiation to macrophages or granulocytes even without adding the differentiation-inducing protein MGI-2. The incubation of normal myeloid precursors with MGI-1 also results in the induction of MGI-2 (48,61,62,88). This induction of MGI-2 can be detected already at 6 hours after the addition of MGI-1 (62). This induction of MGI-2 by MGI-1 can thus account for the induction of differentiation after adding MGI-1 to the normal cells. The induction of differentiation-inducing protein MGI-2 by growth-inducing protein MGI-1, thus appears to be an effective control mechanism for coupling growth and differentiation in the normal cells.

It has been shown that the receptor for epidermal growth factor has tyrosine specific protein kinase activity (99). This has also been found for receptors for other growth factors such as insulin (39) and presumably also applies to the receptor for the myeloid cell growth-inducing protein MGI-1. The myeloid differentiation-inducing protein MGI-2, but not MGI-1, can bind to cellular DNA (102). This shows that growth and differentiation in normal myeloid cells are coupled by induction of a differentiation-inducing DNA-binding protein by a growth-inducing protein. This mechanism for coupling growth and differentiation may also apply to other types of cells. Differences in the time of the switch-on of the differentiation inducer would produce differences in the amount of multiplication before differentiation. The platelet-derived growth factor is structurally related to the product of the simian sarcoma virus oncogene sis (17,100). It will be interesting to determine whether MGI-1 and MGI-2 genes are structurally related to any of the known oncogenes.

The multiplication of normal cells is regulated at two control points. The first control is that which requires MGI-1 to produce more cells that can then differentiate by the MGI-2 induced by MGI-1. The second control is the cessation of cell multiplication that occurs as part of the program of terminal differentiation to mature cells induced by MGI-2. There is thus a coupling of growth and differentiation in normal cells at both these points. Mature cells can also produce feedback inhibitors that interfere with the induction of growth of the normal precursors by MGI-1 (6,7,38,73).

Uncoupling of Growth and Differentiation in Leukemia

As pointed out above, there are MGI^+D^+ clones of myeloid leukemic cells that no longer require MGI-1 for growth but can still be induced to differentiate normally by MGI-2. These leukemic cells have thus uncoupled the normal requirement for growth from the normal requirement for differentiation. Experiments on the properties of these cells after induction of differentiation by MGI-2 have shown, that the normal requirement of MGI-1 for cell viability and growth is restored in the differentiating leukemic cells (23,61,62). MGI-1 added to normal myeloid precursors induces the production of MGI-2, so that the cells can then differentiate by the endogenously produced MGI-2. However, in these leukemic cells, MGI-1 did not induce the production of MGI-2 even though, like normal cells, they again required MGI-1 for viability and growth. There was therefore no induction of differentiation after adding MGI-1 (61,62). There is another type of leukemic cell that constitutively produces its own MGI-1 and can also show this lack of induction of MGI-2 by MGI-1, so that the cells do not differentiate (95). The absence of induction of MGI-2 by MGI-1 therefore uncouples growth and differentiation in these leukemic cells. The lack of requirement of MGI-1 for growth and the absence of induction of the differentiation-inducing protein MGI-2 by the growth-inducing protein MGI-1, are thus mechanisms that uncouple growth and differentiation in MGI^+D^+ leukemic cells (61,62,88,95).

In leukemic cells with constitutive production of MGI-1, changes in specific components of the culture medium can result in an autoinduction of differentiation due to the restoration of the induction of MGI-2 by MGI-1, which then restores the normal coupling of growth and differentiation (Fig. 7). These changes in the culture medium include the use of mouse or rat serum instead of horse or calf serum, serum-free medium, and removal of transferrin from serum-free medium (95). Autoinduction of differentiation in this type of leukemic cell may also occur under certain conditions in vivo.

MGI-1 AND MGI-2 IN GROWTH AND DIFFERENTIAION

Type of myeloid cells	Requirement of MGI-1 for growth	Induction of MGI-2 by MGI-1	Differentiation
Normal	+	Production of MGI-2 ⟶	+
Leukemic	+ or −	No production of MGI-2	−
	Constitutive production MGI-1	Production of MGI-2 ⟶	+ *

*Autoinduction of differentiation under specific conditions

Fig.7. Differences in induction of MGI-2 by MGI-1 in normal and leukemic myeloid cells.

The coupling of growth and differentiation in normal cells is regulated at two control points. The uncoupling of growth and differentiation in MGI$^+$D$^+$ leukemic cells is at the first control point, but the coupling at the second control in normal cells, between the induction of differentiation by MGI-2 and the cessation of multiplication in the mature cells, is maintained. There are differentiation-defective MGI$^+$D$^-$leukemic cells, that like the MGI$^+$D$^+$leukemic cells, no longer require addition of MGI-1 for growth. However, in these cells MGI-2 induces only a partial differentiation, mature cells are not produced and the cells do not stop multiplying. In addition to uncoupling growth and differentiation at the first control point, MGI$^+$D$^-$ leukemic cells thus show a second uncoupling between the initiation of differentiation by MGI-2 and the interruption of cell multiplication that occurs as part of the normal program of terminal differentiation. It has been suggested that leukemia originates by uncoupling the first control and that uncoupling of the second control then results in a further evolution of leukemia (86,88).

Chromosome Changes and Retroviruses in the Leukemic Cells

None of the clones of myeloid leukemic cells studied has a completely normal diploid chromosome banding pattern. There are also specific chromosome differences between the normal and leukemic cells and between MGI^+D^+ , MGI^+D^- and MGI^-D^- clones (2,28). Chromosome studies on normal sarcomas and revertants from sarcomas which have regained a non-malignant phenotype have indicated, that the difference between malignant and non-malignant cells is controlled by the balance between genes for expression (E) and suppression (S) of malignancy. When there is enough S to neutralize E, malignancy is suppressed, and when the amount of S is not sufficient to neutralize E, malignancy is expressed (Fig.1) (30,79, 80,85,105). Studies on the chromosomes of the myeloid leukemic clones suggest that this balance between different genes also applies to the origin of malignancy in these leukemias and that the ability of the leukemic cells to be induced to differentiate by MGI-2 is also dependent on the balance between different genes. It has been shown that MGI^-D^- cells can give rise to MGI^+D^+ progeny by segregation of appropriate chromosomes, and that these chromosome changes then restore the appropriate gene balance required for the induction of differentiation by MGI-2 (Table 4) (2). Changes in the balance of specific genes due to changes in gene dosage is thus a mechanism that could produce the uncoupling of growth and differentiation in myeloid leukemia. Specific changes in gene dosage have also been found in lymphoid leukemia (16,40).

We have suggested from our chromosome data on these mouse myeloid leukemias, that inducibility for differentiation by MGI-2 is controlled by the balance between genes on chromosome 2 and on chromosome 12, and that these chromosomes also carry genes that control the malignancy of these cells (2). There were also in the leukemic cells deletions of chromosome 2 and re-arrangements with chromosome 12 (2). It has been found since then, that the immunoglobulin heavy chain gene is on mouse chromosome 12 (14), that the c-abl gene is on mouse chromosome 2 (26) and that in human chronic myelocytic leukemia c-abl is involved (13) in the translocation of the Philadelphia chromosome (84). The origin and further evolution of malignancy can involve, in different cases, changes in gene dosage, deletions, re-arrangements, or mutation. Genetic changes in the regulation or structure of the normal genes that control growth and differentiation, can produce the uncoupling required for the origin and further evolution of malignancy.

Normal myeloblasts and the different types of myeloid leukemic cells from mice contain endogenous retroviruses (46,49). Superinfection of normal myeloblasts with endogenous ecotropic virus from normal myeloblasts or MGI^+D^+ leukemic cells induces viability and multiplication of these normal cells when MGI-1 is not added, without blocking the ability of these cells to be induced to differentiate by MGI-2. It has been suggested that this promotion of cell multiplication is due to integration of proviral sequences near regulatory sites that control cell growth (46,49). The promotion of growth induced by the virus from normal or MGI^+D^+ leukemic

TABLE 4

Chromosomes of MGI⁺D⁺ and MGI⁻D⁻ Clones

Cell type	Clone no.	No. of chromosomes in chromosome groups*												Modal chromosome No.
		2	3	6	7	12	14	X	T(3;6)	T(3;12)	T(7;15)	T(12;15)	U	
MGI⁺D⁺	11	2	2	2	2	2	1+B	2	0	0	0	0	0	40
MGI⁺D⁺	7-M9	1+F	1	1	1	0	1	1	1	1	1	1	1	38
MGI⁺D⁺	7-M11	1+F	1	1	1	0	1	1	1	1	1	1	1	38
MGI⁺D⁺	7-M16	1+F	1	1	1	0	1	1	1	1	1	1	1	38
MGI⁺D⁺	7-M4	1+F	1	1	1	1	1	1	1	0	1	1	1	38
MGI⁺D⁺	7-M5	1+F	1	1	1	1	1	1	1	0	1	1	1	38
MGI⁻D⁻	7	1+F	1	1	1	1	1	1	1	1	1	1	1	39

*All other chromosome groups had the normal diploid pattern. Translocation (T), deletion (F), insertion (B), unknown (U) (2).

cells is not accompanied by differentiation of the cells unless MGI is added. The integration of proviral sequences near growth regulatory sites can thus uncouple growth and differentiation. However, the cells do not continue to grow for long periods as in the case of leukemic cells. If this stage is followed by the appropriate chromosome changes, this could then produce the more complete uncoupling found in the leukemic cells. Endogenous ecotropic virus from MGI⁻D⁻leukemic cells did not promote growth of the normal myeloblasts, and it has been suggested that this provirus is not integrated near growth regulatory sites (Fig. 8) (49). The promotion of growth induced by the virus from normal or MGI⁺D⁺leukemic cells may increase the probability of these chromosome changes. In human cells which may not have such virus, the chromosome changes could produce this uncoupling without the presence of the virus (90). Studies with avian leukosis virus have provided direct evidence that provirus can be integrated near growth regulatory genes and that this can activate these cellular genes (29,75).

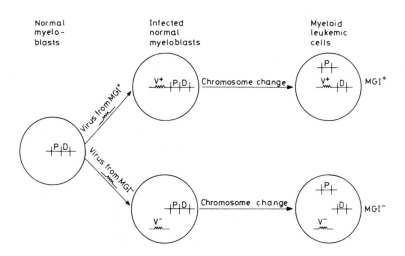

Fig. 8. Model of integration sites for endogenous retrovirus from normal and MGI⁺D⁺ leukemic cells (V⁺) and from MGI⁻D⁻ leukemic cells (V⁻), in relation to the genes for cell viability and growth (proliferation, P) and differentiation (D) (49).

Constitutive Gene Expression in Malignancy

Since there are leukemic cells which, unlike normal myeloblasts, no longer require MGI-1 for cell viability and growth, the molecular changes required for viability and growth that have to be induced in the normal cells are constitutive in these leukemic cells. This also applies to leukemic cells that constitutively produce their own MGI-1. This suggests that the origin of myeloid leukemia can be due to a change from an induced to a constitutive expression of genes that control cell viability and growth (86,88)

Studies on changes in the synthesis of specific proteins in normal myeloblasts, MGI^+D^+, MGI^+D^- and MGI^-D^- leukemic clones at different times after adding MGI-1 and MGI-2, using two dimensional gel electrophoresis (45), have directly shown that there have been changes from inducible to constitutive gene expression in the leukemic cells. The results also indicate a relationship between constitutive gene expression and uncoupling of the induction of differentiation by MGI-2 and the interruption of multiplication in the mature cells. The leukemic cells were found to be constitutive for changes in the synthesis of specific proteins that were only induced in the normal cells after treatment with MGI-1. These protein changes, which included the appearance of some proteins and disappearance of other proteins, were constitutive in all the leukemic clones studied derived from different tumors. These have been called C_{leuk}, meaning constitutive for leukemia. There were other protein changes that were induced by MGI-2 in normal and MGI^+D^+ leukemic cells, and were constitutive in MGI^+D^- and MGI^-D^- leukemic cells. There were more of these constitutive changes in MGI^-D^- than in MGI^+D^- leukemic cells. These have been called C meaning constitutive for differentiation defective (Fig. 9) (45).

These results thus indicate that changes from an induced to a constitutive expression of certain genes is associated with the uncoupling of growth and differentiation, both at the control which requires MGI-1 to produce more cells and at the control of the cessation of cell multiplication that occurs in the formation of mature cells.

The protein changes during the growth and differentiation of normal myeloblasts seem to be induced by MGI-1 and MGI-2 as a series of parallel multiple pathways of gene expression (45). It can be assumed, that the normal developmental program that couples growth and differentiation in normal cells requires synchronous initiation and progression of these multiple parallel pathways. The presence of constitutive gene expression for some pathways can be expected to produce asynchrony in the co-ordination required for the normal developmental program. Depending on the pathways involved, this asynchrony could then result in an uncoupling of the controls for growth and differentiation and produce different blocks in the ability to be induced for and to terminate the differentiation process.

We have been able to treat MGI^-D^- leukemic cells so as to induce the reversion of specific C_{def} proteins from the constitutive to the non-constitutive state. This reversion was then associated with a gain of inducibility by MGI-2 for various differentiation-associated properties. Reversion from the constitutive to the non-constitutive state in these cells thus restored the synchrony required for induction of differentiation (98).

The suggestion derived from these results (45,86,88) is, therefore, that myeloid leukemia originates by a change that produces certain constitutive pathways of gene expression, so that

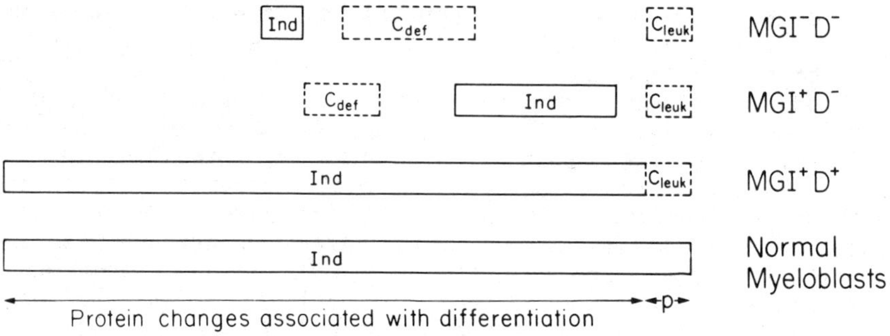

Fig. 9. Schematic summary of protein changes associated with growth (proliferation) and differentiation in normal myeloid precursor cells (myeloblasts) and different types of myeloid leukemic cells. C_{leuk}; constitutive expression of changes in leukemic compared to normal myeloblasts. C_{def}; constitutive expression of changes in the differentiation defective MGI$^+$D$^-$ and MGI$^-$D$^-$ clones compared to MGI$^+$D$^+$ clones. Ind; MGI induced changes and p; protein changes associated with proliferation to produce more cells before differentiation (45).

cells no longer require MGI-1 for growth or constitutively produce MGI-1 without inducing MGI-2. These leukemic cells can, however, still be induced to differentiate normally by MGI-2 added exogenously or induced in the cells in other ways. The differentiation program induced by MGI-2 can thus proceed normally when it is uncoupled from the growth program induced by MGI-1. This can be followed by constitutive expression of other pathways resulting in the uncoupling of other controls and an asynchrony that interferes with the normal program of terminal differentiation. These second changes then result in the further evolution of leukemia (88).

The MGI-1 independent growth of myeloid leukemic cells seems to proceed through stages (11) probably starting from a small decrease in MGI-1 requirement to ending, finally, in complete independence of MGI-1. There are presumably also stages in the amount of constitutively produced MGI-1 and the degree of lack of inducibility of MGI-2 by MGI-1. These stages would produce different degrees of asynchrony resulting in differences in the degree of hematological abnormality, the final stages of asynchrony then resulting in leukemia.

Development Programs, and Reversion of Malignancy by Induction
of Differentiation, in Different Types of Tumors

These conclusions on the origin and evolution of myeloid leukemia may be applicable to malignant tumors derived from other types of cells whose viability, growth and differentiation are induced by other physiological inducers. Identification of the physiological inducers of growth and differentiation for different cell types would be a crucial requirement in extending these conclusions to those other tumors. However, even in the absence of such identification, it appears likely that teratocarcinoma cells (15,69) may be comparable to MGI^+D^+ myeloid leukemic cells. The presence of fetal proteins in certain tumors, may also be due to constitutive gene expression in the tumor of a protein that is induced by the physiological inducer during the developmental program in the normal fetus (88). There are probably a variety of tumors in which (A) the original malignancy has a normal differentiation program and the cells are malignant because of uncoupling of the requirement for growth from the requirement for differentiation by changing the gene expression required for growth from inducible to constitutive; and (B) where the further evolution of the tumor results from changes from inducible to constitutive of other pathways of gene expression that produce asynchrony in the normal differentiation program, so that mature non-dividing cells are not formed by the physiological inducer of differentiation. However even these tumors may still be induced to differentiate to form non-malignant cells, by treatment with compounds that can reverse the constitutive to the non-constitutive state or induce the differentiation program by other pathways. The stopping of cell division in mature cells by inducing differentiation can by-pass the genetic changes that produce the malignant phenotype.

New Forms of Therapy

Our results suggested some novel possibilities for the therapy of myeloid leukemia (86,87). The finding of MGI^+D^+ myeloid leukemic cells that can be induced to differentiate normally by MGI-2 suggests the use of MGI-2 injection, stimulation of the production of MGI-2 in vivo, or grafting of MGI-2 producing cells, to induce the normal differentiation of these leukemic cells in patients with myeloid leukemia. This would be an alternative to cytotoxic agents, which kill normal cells as well as tumor cells. There are membrane differences between the cells which differ in their response to MGI-2 that may be useful markers to predict the response of the leukemic cells to MGI-2 in vivo. MGI^+D^+ leukemic cells can be induced by MGI-2 to again require MGI-1 for cell viability and growth. This suggests that induction of differentiation of the leukemic cells to this stage may also result in the loss of viability and growth of the induced MGI^+D^+ leukemic cells in vivo if there is not enough MGI-1.

The induction of growth of the normal myeloid precursors by MGI-1 and their differentiation to macrophages or granulocytes by MGI-2, also suggests that injected MGI or MGI induced in vivo might be used to restore the normal macrophage and granulocyte population after cytotoxic therapy. MGI therapy may also be useful for treatment of non-malignant macrophage or granulocyte diseases.

Our results can also help to explain the response of some, but not all patients, to chemical and irradiation cytotoxic therapy. We have shown that chemicals and irradiation used in therapy can at low doses induce differentiation in clones of myeloid leukemic cells with the appropriate genotype, and that clonal differences in inducibility for differentiation are not necessarily associated with differences in the response of these clones to the cytotoxic effect of these compounds. The growth in vivo of leukemic cells with the appropriate genotype may thus be controlled by the therapeutic agents used not only for their cytotoxic effect, but because they induce differentiation. Differences in the competence of cells to be induced by these agents may thus explain differences in response to therapy in different individuals. The possible induction of MGI-2 by these compounds may also play a role in the therapeutic effects obtained in vivo.

These studies therefore suggest new forms of therapy of leukemia based on the use of a normal regulatory protein such as MGI-2 to induce differentiation in malignant cells, and of MGI-1 and MGI-2 to induce a more rapid recovery of the normal cell population after the present forms of therapy. In addition, it is possible to use other compounds that induce MGI-1 or MGI-2 in vivo, or can affect mutant malignant cells at differentiation sites that are no longer susceptible to the normal regulator. The malignant cells of each patient should be pre-screened for the compounds to which they are susceptible. These possibilities should also be applicable to diseases in other types of cells whose growth and differentiation are controlled by other normal regulators (86).

REFERENCES

1. Austin, P.E., McCulloch, E.A. and Till, J.E. (1971) J.Cell. Physiol., 77:121-134.

2. Azumi, J. and Sachs, L. (1977) Proc. Natl. Acad. Sci. USA., 74:253-257.

3. Baccarani, M. and Tura, S. (1979) Brit. J. Haematol., 42:485-487.

4. Bishop, J.M. (1983) Ann. Rev. Biochem. 52:301-354.

5. Bradley, T.R. and Metcalf, D. (1966) Aust. J. Exp. Biol. Med. Sci., 44:287-300.

6. Broxmeyer, H.E., de Sousa, M., Smithyman, A., Ralph, P., Hamilton, J., Kurland, J.I. and Bognacki, J. (1980) Blood, 55:324-333.

7. Broxmeyer, H.E., Smithyman, A., Eger, R.R., Myers, P.A. and de Sousa, M. (1978) J. Exp. Med., 148:1052-1067.

8. Burgess, A.W., Camakaris, J. and Metcalf, D. (1977) J. Biol. Chem., 252:1998-2003.

9. Burgess, A.W. and Metcalf, D. (1980) Int. J. Cancer, 26:647-654.

10. Cohen, L. and Sachs, L. (1981) Proc. Natl. Acad. Sci. USA, 78:353-357.

11. Collins, S.J., Gallo, R.C. and Gallagher, R.E. (1977) Nature, 270:347-349.

12. Collins, S.J., Ruscetti, F.W., Gallagher, R.E. and Gallo, R.C. (1978) Proc. Natl. Acad. Sci. USA, 75:2458-2462.

13. De Klein, A., Van Kessel, A.D., Grosveld, G., Bartman, C.R., Hagemeijer, A., Bootsma, D., Spurr, N.K., Heisterkamp, N., Groffen, J. and Stephenson, J.R. (1982) Nature, 300:765-767.

14. D'Eustachio, P., Pravtcheva, D., Marcu, K. and Ruddle, F.H. (1980) J. Exp. Med., 151:1545-1550.

15. Dewey, M.J., Martin, D.W. Jr., Martin, G.R. and Mintz, B. (1977) Proc. Natl. Acad. Sci. USA, 74:5564-5568.

16. Dofuku, R., Biedler, J.L., Sprengler, B.A. and Old, L.J. (1975) Proc. Natl. Acad. Sci. USA, 72:1515-1517.

17. Doolittle, R.F., Hunkapiller, M.W., Hood, L.E., Devare, S.G., Robbins, K.C., Aaronson, S.A. and Antoniades, H.N. (1983) Science, 221:275-277.

18. Falk, A and Sachs, L. (1980) Int. J. Cancer, 26:595-601.

19. Fibach, E., Hayashi, M. and Sachs, L. (1973) Proc. Natl. Acad. Sci. USA 70:343-346.

20. Fibach, E., Landau, T. and Sachs, L. (1972) Nature New Biol., 237:276-278.

21. Fibach, E. and Sachs, L. (1974) J. Cell. Physiol., 83:177-185.

22. Fibach, E. and Sachs, L. (1975) J. Cell. Physiol., 86:221-230.

23. Fibach, E. and Sachs, L. (1976) J. Cell. Physiol., 89:259-266.

24. Friend, C. (1978) Harvey Lectures 72:253-281, New York: Academic Press.

25. Ginsburg, H. and Sachs, L. (1963) J. Natl. Cancer Inst., 31:1-40.

26. Goff, S.P., D'Eustachio, P., Ruddle, F.H. and Baltimore, D. (1982) Science, 218:1317-1319.

27. Gootwine, E., Webb, C.G. and Sachs, L. (1982) Nature, 299: 63-65.

28. Hayashi, M., Fibach, E. and Sachs, L. (1974) Int. J. Cancer, 14:40-48.

29. Hayward, W.S., Neel, B.G. and Astrin, S.M. (1981) Nature, 290:475-479.

30. Hitosumachi, S., Rabinowitz, Z. and Sachs, L. (1971) Nature, 231:511-514.

31. Hoffman-Liebermann, B., Liebermann, D. and Sachs, L. (1981) Dev. Biol., 81:255-265.

32. Hoffman-Liebermann, B., Liebermann, D. and Sachs, L. (1981) Int. J. Cancer, 28:615-620.

33. Hoffman-Liebermann, B. and Sachs, L. (1978) Cell, 14:825-834.

34. Housset, M., Daniel, M.T. and Degos, L. (1982) Brit. J. Haematol., 51:125-129.

35. Ichikawa, Y. (1969) J. Cell. Physiol. 74:223-234.

36. Ichikawa, Y., Maeda, N. and Horiuchi, M. (1976) Int. J. Cancer, 17:789-797.

37. Ichikawa, Y., Pluznik, D.H. and Sachs, L. (1966) Proc. Natl. Acad. Sci. USA, 56:488-495.

38. Ichikawa, Y., Pluznik, D.H. and Sachs, L. (1967) Proc. Natl. Acad. Sci. USA, 58:1480-1486.

39. Kasuga, M., Fujita-Yamaguchi, Y., Blithe, D.L. and Kahn, C.R. (1983) Proc. Natl. Acad. Sci. USA, 80:2137-2141.

40. Klein, G. (1979) Proc. Natl. Acad. Sci. USA, 76:2442-2446.

41. Klein, G., Friberg, S., Wiener, F. and Harris, H. (1973) J. Natl. Cancer Inst., 50:1259-1268.

42. Krystosek, A. and Sachs, L. (1976) Cell, 9:675-684.

43. Land, H., Parada, L.F. and Weinberg, R.A. (1983) Science, 222:771-778.

44. Landau, T. and Sachs, L. (1971) Proc. Natl. Acad. Sci. USA, 68:2540-2544.

45. Liebermann, D., Hoffman-Liebermann, B. and Sachs, L. (1980) Dev. Biol., 79:46-63.

46. Liebermann, D., Hoffman-Liebermann, B. and Sachs, L. (1980) Virology, 107:121-134.

47. Liebermann, D., Hoffman-Liebermann, B. and Sachs, L. (1981) Int. J. Cancer, 28:285-291.

48. Liebermann, D., Hoffman-Liebermann, B. and Sachs, L. (1982) Int. J. Cancer, 29:159-161.

49. Liebermann, D., Hoffman-Liebermann, B. and Sachs, L. (1979) Proc. Natl. Acad. Sci. USA, 76:3353-3357.

50. Lipton, J. and Sachs, L. (1981) Biochim. Biophys. Acta, 676:552-569.

51. Lotem, J., Lipton, J. and Sachs, L. (1980) Int. J. Cancer, 25:763-771.

52. Lotem, J. and Sachs, L. (1974) Proc. Natl. Acad. Sci. USA, 71:3507-3511.

53. Lotem, J. and Sachs, L. (1975) Int. J. Cancer, 15:731-740.

54. Lotem, J. and Sachs, L. (1977) J. Cell. Physiol., 92:97-108.

55. Lotem, J. and Sachs, L. (1977) Proc. Natl. Acad. Sci. USA, 74:5554-5558.

56. Lotem, J. and Sachs, L. (1978) Int. J. Cancer, 22:214-220.

57. Lotem, J. and Sachs, L. (1978) Proc. Natl. Acad. Sci. USA, 75:3781-3785.

58. Lotem, J. and Sachs, L. (1979) Proc. Natl. Acad. Sci. USA, 76:5158-5162.

59. Lotem, J. and Sachs, L. (1980) Int. J. Cancer, 25:561-564.

60. Lotem, J. and Sachs, L. (1981) Int. J. Cancer, 28:375-386.

61. Lotem, J. and Sachs, L. (1982) Proc. Natl. Acad. Sci. USA, 79:4347-4351.

62. Lotem, J. and Sachs, L. (1983) Int. J. Cancer, 32:127-134.

63. Lotem, J. and Sachs, L. (1983) Int. J. Cancer, 32:781-791.
64. Lotem, J. and Sachs, L. (1984) Int. J. Cancer, 33:147-154.
65. Maeda, M., Horiuchi, M., Numa, S. and Ichikawa, Y. (1977) Gann, 68:435-447.
66. Marks, P. and Rifkind, R.A. (1978) Ann. Rev. Biochem. 47: 419-448.
67. Metcalf, D. (1969) J. Cell. Physiol., 74:323-332.
68. Michalewicz, R., Lotem, J. and Sachs, L. (In press) Leukemia Res.
69. Mintz, B. and Illmensee, K. (1975) Proc. Natl. Acad. Sci. USA, 72:3585-3589.
70. Moore, M.A.S. (1982) J. Cell. Physiol. Suppl., 1:53-64.
71. Nicola, N.A., Burgess, A.W. and Metcalf, D. (1979) J.Biol. Chem., 24:5290-5299.
72. Paran, M., Ichikawa, Y. and Sachs, L. (1968) J. Cell. Physiol., 72:251-254.
73. Paran, M., Ichikawa, Y. and Sachs, L. (1969) Proc. Natl. Acad. Sci. USA, 62:81-87.
74. Paran, M., Sachs, L., Barak, Y. and Resnitzky, P. (1970) Proc. Natl. Acad. Sci. USA, 67:1542-1549.
75. Payne, G.S., Bishop, J.M. and Varmus, H.E. (1982) Nature, 295:209-214.
76. Pike, B. and Robinson, W.A. (1970) J. Cell. Physiol., 76: 77-84.
77. Pluznik, D.H. and Sachs, L. (1965) J. Cell. Comp. Physiol. 66:319-324.
78. Pluznik, D.H. and Sachs, L. (1966) Exp. Cell. Res., 43: 553-563.
79. Rabinowitz, Z. and Sachs, L. (1968) Nature, 220:1203-1206.
80. Rabinowitz, Z. and Sachs, L. (1970) Nature, 225:136-139.
81. Rabinowitz, Z. and Sachs, L. (1970) J. Cancer, 6:388-398.
82. Ringertz, N.R. and Savage, R.E. (1976) Cell Hybrids, Academic Press, New York.
83. Rovera, G., Santoli, D. and Damsky, C. (1979) Proc. Natl. Acad. Sci. USA, 76:2779-2783.
84. Rowley, J.D. (1977) Proc. Natl. Acad. Sci. USA, 74:5729-5733.
85. Sachs, L. (1974) Harvey Lectures, 68:1-35, New York: Academic Press.
86. Sachs, L. (1978) Nature, 274:535-539.
87. Sachs, L. (1978) Brit. J. Haematol., 40:509-517.
88. Sachs, L. (1980) Proc. Natl. Acad. Sci. USA, 77:6152-6156.
89. Sachs, L. (1982) J. Cell. Physiol. Suppl., 1:151-164.
90. Sachs, L. (1982) Cancer Surveys, 1:321-342.
91. Simatov, R. and Sachs, L. (1978) Proc. Natl. Acad. Sci. USA, 75:1805-1809.
92. Simatov, R., Shkolnik, T. and Sachs, L. (1980) Proc, Natl. Acad. Sci. USA, 77:4798-4802.
93. Stanley, E.R. and Heard, P.M. J. Biol. Cheml., 252:4305-4312.
94. Symonds, G. and Sachs, L. (1979) Somat. Cell. Genet., 5: 931-944.

95. Symonds, G. and Sachs, L. (1982) EMBO J., 1:1343-1346.

96. Symonds, G. and Sachs, L. (1982) Blood, 60:208-212.

97. Symonds, G. and Sachs, L. (1982) J. Cell. Physiol., 111:9-14.

98. Symonds, G. and Sachs, L. (1983) EMBO J., 2:663-667.

99. Ushiro, H. and Cohen, S. (1980) J. Biol. Chem., 225:8363-8365.

100. Waterfield, M.D., Scrace, G.T., Whittle, N., Stroobant, P., Johnsson, A., Wasteson, A., Westermark, B., Heldin, C.H., Huang, J.S. and Deuel, T.F. (1983) Nature, 304:35-39.

101. Webb, C.G., Gootwine, E. and Sachs, L. (1984) Develop. Biol., 101:221-224.

102. Weisinger, G. and Sachs, L. (1983) EMBO J., 2:2103-2107.

103. Weiss, B. and Sachs, L. Proc. Natl. Acad. Sci. USA, 75:1374-1378.

104. Wiener, F., Klein, G. and Harris, H. (1974) J. Cell. Sci. 15:177-183.

105. Yamamoto, T., Rabinowitz, Z. and Sachs, L. (1973) Nature (New Biol.), 243:247-250.

106. Yamamoto, Y., Tomida, M. and Hozumi, M. (1980) Cancer Res., 40:4804-4809.

Subject Index

A

A431 cells, EGF receptor, 76
Abelson MuLV, localization, 109–110,112
abl gene
  myelocytic leukemia, 270
  and myoblast differentiation,
    expression, 243–248
  and tx-1 gene, transformation, 6
O-Acetylation, 174–178
Acquired immune deficiency disease, *see*
  AIDS
Activation, lymphoma cells, 251–255
Acute myeloid leukemia, 221–222,
  227,229
Acute retroviruses, 184–185
Adenocarcinomas, antigens, GI tract, 132
Adenovirus Ela oncogene, 40
Adhesion plaques
  onc gene proteins, 109–110
  pp60ˢʳᶜ localization, 108–110,113
Adriamycin, differentiation induction,
  266
Adult T-cell leukemia, 183,187,192,194–
  197,202
AIDS
  and HTLV-III, 183,188–190,195
    seroepidemiology, 199–200
  infected lymphocytes, HTLV-III, 203–
    204
AIDS-related complex, 195
"Allosteric regulator model," 151–153
Ama 420 myoblasts, 243–248
Anhydrodebromoaplysiatoxin, 58
Anti-beta2-microglobulin, 252
Antibodies, *see* Monoclonal antibodies
Antigen p97, 157–165
Antigens
  expression, tumors, glycolipids, 148–
    150
  gastrointestinal cancer, 132–133
  glycolipid changes, oncogenesis, 145–
    148
  human melanoma cells, 123–125,129
Aplysiatoxin
  protein kinase C activation, 58–59
  receptor effects, 60

"Autocrine" mechanism
  and automomy, 42
  leukemia cells, 222
  platelet derived growth factor, 74–76
Avian erythroblastosis virus, 80–82

B

B-cell chronic lymphocytic leukemia, 45–
  52
B-cell differentiation factor, 238
B-cell lymphomas, 5–6
B-cell prolymphocytic leukemia, 254
B-cells
  activation, 251–252
  surface immunoglobulins, 45–50
  TPA differentiation effects, CLL, 233–
    240
B lymphoid neoplasias, 21,24–25
B61B10 cell line, 172
B77 virus, 114–117
BALB/c spleen cells
  c-*myc* cDNA clone, 21
  c-*myc* promoter activity, 24
Benzo(a)pyrene, viral synergy, 56
Beta-glucuronidase, 236
BglII site, c-*myc* gene, 31
Blym gene, 1–6
Blym-1 gene
  Burkitt's lymphoma DNA homology, 4
  chicken and humans, similarity, 4
  and *myc* gene, transformation, 5–6
  and transferrin, 4–5
BPDE, viral synergy, 56
Burkitt's lymphoma
  Blym-1 and *myc* gene, 5
  DNA homology, *Blym-1*, 4
  c-*myc* oncogene expression, 29–37
  myc sequence changes, 33–37
Bursal lymphocytes, 6

C

C kinase, *see* Protein kinase C
C127 murine cells, 97–100
Calcium, protein kinase C action, 57–58
Carcinoembryonic antigen, 132

Carcinogenesis, *see* Chemical
carcinogenesis
Caribbean immigrants, 196–197
cDNA clone, 21–22,33–37,157–165,203
CEA *see* Carcinoembryonic antigen
Cell adhesiveness, glycolipids, 150
Cell-cell junctions, 108
Cell differentiation
B-type CLLs, TPA, 233–240
cancer therapy drugs, 266
cell growth coupling, 268–269,272–274
human lymphoma cells, 251–255
leukemia cells, regulators, 224–227,
257–276
Cell-free systems, 158–165
Cell growth
differentiation coupling, 268–269
glycolipid effects, 150–153
regulators, leukemia, 257–276
Cellular genes, and carcinogenesis, 62–65
Centrocytic lymphoma, 51
Ceramide composition, 149
C3H 10T1/2 cells, 62–63
Chemical carcinogenesis, 55–65
cellular gene involvement, 62–65
molecular mechanisms, 55–65
oncogene synergism, 62–63
retrovirus analogy, 63–64
Chemotaxis, myeloid leukemia cells, 261–
262
Chemotherapy, differentiation induction,
265–266,276
Chicken embryo fibroblasts, 95–104
Chondroitin sulfate proteoglycan antigen,
169–178
Chromosome 1, melanoma, 125
Chromosome 2, myeloid leukemia, 229,
270–271
Chromosome 3, lymphocytic leukemia,
50
Chromosome 6, lymphocytic leukemia,
50
Chromosome 7
epidermal growth factor receptor, 127–
128
melanoma, 125
Chromosome 8, 30–33
Chromosome 11
GM-CSF gene, 229
lymphocytic leukemia, 50
Chromosome 12
chronic lymphocytic leukemia, 45–52
lymphoma cells, 253

mouse myeloid leukemia, 270–271
prognostic aspects, abnormalities, 51–
52
Chromosome 14, 30–33
Chromosome segregation, 258
Chromosome translocation
Burkitt's lymphoma, c-*myc*, 29–37
c-*myc*, reciprocal exchange, 13–17
Chromosomes
in chronic lymphocytic leukemia, 45–
52
leukemia cells, 270–272
lymphoma cells, 253
melanomas, abnormalities, 125
Chronic lymphocytic leukemia
chromosomal aberrations, 45–52
and lymphocytic malignancies, 253–
255
prognosis, 51–52
T-cell effects, 239–240
TPA effects, differentiation, 233–240
Chronic myeloid leukemia cells, 221–
222,227,229
Chronic retroviruses, 184–185
Chymotryptic S6-phosphopeptides, 99–
101
Colony stimulating factors; *see also* G-
CSF; GM-CSF; Multi-CSF
cell division control, 221–223
characterization, 216–218
leukemia cell line production, 222–223
macrophage and granulocyte regulation,
215–220
cloning, 260
myeloid leukemia cells, 215–230
receptors, 218–220
Complimentary DNA, *see* cDNA clone
Cowan staphylococci, 254
Creatine kinase assay, 245
CU12 mutant, 113–117
Cytoplasm, onc proteins, 112–113
Cytosine arabinoside, 266
Cytotoxic T cells, HTLV effect, 192
Cytotoxic therapy, 265–266,276

D
D factor, 260–266
Daudi cell line
c-*myc* sequence changes, 33
c-*myc* translocation position, 30–33
Debromoaplysiatoxin, 58
Dexamethasone, 266

Dextran sulphate, 252–253
Diacylglycerol
S6 phosphorylation, 99
and tumor promotion, 60–61,96–104
Differentiation, *see* Cell differentiation
Difucosylated type 2 chain, 146–147
Dihydroteleocidin B, 59
Dimethylsulfoxide, 266
Dioleoylglycerol, 102–103
Disialoganglioside GD$_3$, *see* GD$_3$
ganglioside
cDNA clone
antigen p 97, 157–165
HTLV-III, 203
myc, 21–22,33–37
Dot blot hybridization, 160

E
E1a oncogene, 40
EcoR1 site, 31–32
ELISA system, HTLV-III, 198
Embryonic development, leukemic cells,
140–143
Endogenous retroviruses, 184
env gene
chronic leukemia viruses, 185
p28^{sis}, 90
Epidemiology, HTLV-I, 196–198
Epidermal growth factor receptor
amino acid sequence, 80
biosynthesis, 76–77
erbB oncogene homology, 41–42
and *erbB* protein, sequences, 79–81
melanoma cells, 127–130
oncogene effects, 71–82
purification, 77–78
structural analysis, 78–80
TPA effects, phosphorylation, 61
Epstein-Barr virus
B-cell immunoglobin stimulation, 46
malignant lymphocyte response, 252
tumor promoter synergy, 56
erb oncogene, 243–248
erbB oncogene
EGFr gene homology, 41–42,79–81
p185 encoding, 42
protein product localization, 112–113
Erythroid burst forming unit, 227
Esh sarcoma virus, 109–110
Exogenous retroviruses, 184
Extracellular growth factors, 40–41

F
Fc receptor
monoclonal antibody binding, 133–134
TPA effects, B-CLL cells, 236
fes oncogene
and myoblast differentiation,
expression, 243–248
protein product localization, 112
FH4 monoclonal antibody, 146–148
FH6 monoclonal antibody, 148
Fibronectin
onc proteins, 114–116
and pp60^{src}, 113–114
FMC7, 254
fms protein, localization, 109–112
Focal adhesion plaques, *see* Adhesion
plaques
fps oncogene, 109–110,112
Fucogangliosides, 148
Fucosylated type 2 chain, 147
Fusiform morphology, 113–118

G
G-CSF
anti-leukemia effects, 229
characterization, 216–217
differentiation induction, 224–227
myeloid leukemia cells, 215–230
binding, 225–226
receptors, 218–220
stem cell suppression, 224–227
gag gene
chronic leukemia viruses, 185
HTLV genome, 200–201
Ganglioside D$_2$, 176–177
Ganglioside D$_3$, *see* GD$_3$ ganglioside
Ganglioside GM$_1$, 150–153
Ganglioside GM$_3$, 150–153
Gangliosides
"allosteric regulator" model, 151–152
cell adhesiveness regulation, 150
cell growth and proliferation effects,
150–153
in embryogenesis, 143–144
monoclonal antibodies, 147
PGDF receptor modulation, 151–152
Gangliotriaosylceramide, 143–145
Gastrointestinal cancer
antigens, 132
therapy, 133–134
Gastrointestinal cancer antigen, 132
GD$_2$ ganglioside, 176–177

GD₃ ganglioside
  melanoma antigen, 169–178
    O-acetylation, 174–178
  monoclonal antibodies, 147,174–175
Gene amplification, 55–56
GICA, *see* Gastrointestinal cancer antigen
Globotriaosylceramide, 147
β-Glucuronidase, 236
Glycerolphosphate, 102
Glycolipids
  "allosteric regulator" model, 151–153
  antigen expression, tumors, 148–150
    markers, 148–150
  biological significance, tumors, 150–
    153
  in embryonic development, 140–145
  monoclonal antibody definition, 146–
    148
  and oncogenic transformation, 145–148
  TPA effects, CLL cells, 235–236
Glycoproteins, TPA effects, 235–236
Glycosphingolipids, 139–153
Glycosylation, 139–141
GM-CSF
  anti-leukemic potential, 229
  characterization, 216–217
  chromosomal location, 229
  granulocyte and macrophage regulation,
    219
  p21 phosphorylation, 220
  receptors, 218–220
GM₁ ganglioside
  cell growth effects, 150–153
  PGDF receptor modulation, 151–152
GM₃ ganglioside, 150–153
Golgi vesicles, 169–170
gp28ˢⁱˢ, localization, 112–113
gp75ᵉʳᵇ⁻ᴮ, localization, 112–113
gp120ᶠᵐˢ, localization, 110–111
gp140ᶠᵐˢ, localization, 110–111
gp180ᵍᵃᵍ⁻ᶠᵐˢ, localization, 110–111
gpt colonies, 62–63
Granulocyte inducers, 259–276
  differentiation control, 266–274
  growth control, leukemia, 261–269
  therapeutic possibilities, 275–276
Granulocytes; *see also* Granulocyte
    inducers
  clone formation, inducers, 259–260
  colony stimulating factor regulation,
    215–220
  differentiation, G-CSF, 224–227

Growth factors; *see also specific factors*
  ganglioside interactions, 151
  and melanomas, 125–128
  oncogene production, 40–42
  oncogene transduction subversion, 71–
    82
Guanine nucleotide, 3

H

H9 cells, 203
Hairy cell leukemia, 188
Helper T-cell phenotype, 191
Helper T-cells, 195
Hematopoiesis, regulators, 257–276
Hemophiliacs, HTLV-III isolation, 190
HHPA, 57–58
HHPA 13,20-diacetate, 58
HindIII site, c-*myc* gene, 31–32
HL-60 cells, 264
HLA-A locus, 191
HLA-B locus, 191
HLA-DR markers
  HTLV-infected cells, 191
  TPA effects, B-CLL cells, 236
Homosexuals
  HTLV-III antibodies, 199–200
  HTLV-III isolation, 190
HTLV-I
  antigenic properties, 205–206
  associated diseases, 194–195
  genome, 200–201
    genetic structure, 185
  human T lymphocyte transformation,
    190–191
  immune system effects, 191–193
  isolation, 187
  long terminal repeats, 200–201
  molecular epidemiology, 198
  morphology, 187
  seroepidemiology, 196–197
  transformation and leukemogenesis,
    202
HTLV-II
  antigenic properties, 205–206
  genome, 200–201
    genetic structure, 185
  HTLV-III homology, genome, 203
  isolation, 188
  long terminal repeats, 201
  T lymphocyte effects, immunity, 191–
    193
  transformation and leukemogenesis,
    202

HTLV-II$_{MO}$, 188
HTLV-III
  and AIDS, 188–190,195
  antigenic properties, 205–206
  biological properties, 193–194
  clones, mapping, 204–205
  genome, 203–205
  isolation, 188–189
  seroepidemiology, 198–200
HTLV "family"
  biological effects, 190–194
  epidemiology, 196–200
  features, 183–184
  isolation, 186–190
Human T-cell leukemia virus, *see* HTLV
  "family"
Human T lymphocytes, 190–191
Hybridization, p97 mRNA analysis, 157–
  165

I

IB9 monoclonal antibody, 148
Ig binding, macrophages, 133–134
Ig production, TPA, CLL cells, 236–237
IgD, TPA, CLL cells, 236
IgG, Cowan staphylococci effect, 254
IgG2a, 133–134
IgM
  Cowan staphylococci effect, 254
  TPA effects, CLL cells, 236–237
Immune deficiency, HTLV effect, 192
Immunocytoma
  chromosome abnormalities, 48
  lymphocytic malignancy comparison,
    253–255
Insulin receptors, TPA, phosphorylation,
  61
Insulin-like growth factor, 72–74
INT 1 oncogene, 49–50
Interleukin-2, *see* T-cell growth factor
Interleukin-3, *see* Multi-CSF
Intracisternal sequences, 63–64
Ion fluxes, 72

J

J774 macrophage cell line, 226
Japanese, HTLV-I seroepidemiology,
  196–197
JI cell line, 30–33,35–37

K

Kaposi tumor tissue, HTLV-III, 205
KpnI site, 32

L

L6 rat myoblasts, 243–248
Lactofucopentaosyl(III) di-lysine, 144
Lacto-*nor*octaosylceramide, 143–144
Lactoseries synthesis, 143–145
Lactosylceramide, 149
Lactotetraosylceramide, 132
Leukemia cells
  chromosome changes, 270–272
  CSF production, 222–223
  G-CSF effects, 224–227
  growth and differentiation contol, 224–
    227,261–266,272–274
  and retroviruses, 270–272
  therapy, 275–276
Lipids
  glycosylation significance, 141
  pp60^{v-src}, phosphorylation, 101–103
Lipopolysaccharide
  B-cell immunoglobins, 46
  malignant lymphocyte response, 252–
    253
  myeloid leukemia cells, differentiation,
    266
Long open reading frame, 201–202
Long terminal repeat sequences
  carcinogenesis analogy, 63–64
  chronic leukemia viruses, 185
  HTLV-I and HTLV-II genomes, 200–
    201
  HTLV-I molecular epidemiology, 198
LY67 cell line
  c-*myc* sequence changes, 33–37
  c-*myc* translocation position, 30–33
LY91 cell line, 30–33
Lymph node cells, 48–49
Lymphadenopathy syndrome
  AIDS sign, 195
  HTLV antibodies, 199
  and HTLV-III, 194
  lymphocyte infection, HTLV-III, 204–
    205
Lymphokines, 238
Lymphoma cells, 251–255
Lymphosarcomas, 24
Lyngbyatoxin A, 58

M

M-CSF
  characterization, 216–217
  receptors, 218–220
M1 cells, G-CSF effect, 224–227
M21 melanoma cells, 172

Mab 3.6, 174–177
Mab 9.2.27, 169–178
Mab D1.1, 174–177
Mab R24, 174–177
Macrophage inducers, 259–276
    cloning, 259–260
    differentiation control, 266–274
    growth control, leukemia, 261–269
    therapeutic possibilities, 275–276
Macrophages; *see also* Macrophage
        inducers
    clone formation, inducers, 259–260
    colony stimulating factor regulation,
        215–220
    monoclonal antibody action, 133
MAKU, 30–33
Markers, glycolipids, tumors, 148–150
Mashran gm, 260
MC29 protein, 111–112
ME492 antibody, 126
Melanoma cells
    antigens, 123–125,157–165,169–178
    chromosomal abnormalities, 125
    in culture, characteristics, 130–132
    and growth factors, 125–129
    monoclonal antibody eradication, 170–
        173
    p97 antigen, cDNA clone, 157–165
Metaphase characteristics, B-CLLs, 48–
        49
Methotrexate, differentiation induction,
        266
Mezerein
    protein kinase C activation, 57–58
    receptor effects, 60
Mitomycin C, 266
Monoclonal antibodies
    adenocarcinomas, 132
    antigen p97 cDNA probe, 162–165
    gastrointestinal cancer, 132–133
        destruction of, 133–135
    glycolipid definition, 146–148
    melanoma antigen characterization,
        123–125,169–178
Monocytes
    C3F production, 222
    differentiation, G-CSF, 224–227
mos gene
    and myoblast differentiation,
        expression, 243–248
    protein product localization, 112
Mouse myelogeneous leukemia M1 cells,
        140–143

Mouse myeloid leukemia models, 229–
        230
MPC-11 tumor, 13–17
Multi-CSF
    characterization, 216–217
    granulocyte regulation, 219
    leukemogenesis, 228
    receptors, 220
Murine plasmacytomas, 11–25
myb gene, protein product localization,
        112
myc gene
    and *Blym-1* gene, 5–6
    interactions, oncogenesis, 40
    murine plasmacytomas, activation, 11–
        25
    and myoblast differentiation,
        expression, 243–248
    protein product localization, 111–112
    reciprocal exchanges, 13–17
    translocation mechanism, 13–17
c-*myc* gene
    Burkitt's lymphoma, 29–37
    murine plasmacytomas, activation, 11–
        25
    in myoblasts, expression, 248
c-*myc* cDNA clone
    Burkitt's lymphoma, 33–37
    plasmacytomas, 21–22
c-*myc* exons, 19–23,30–33
c-*myc* introns, 18–20
myc RNA
    Burkitt's lymphoma cell lines, 31–32
    lymphoid tumor cells, 13
Myeloid leukemia cells, 215–230,257–276
    colony stimulating factors, 215–230
    growth control, 215–230,261–266,272–
        274
    malignancy reversion mechanism, 258–
        259
    therapy, 275–276
Myoblasts
    inducing factor effects, 273
    oncogene expression, differentiation,
        243–248
Myotubes, 243–244

N
Natural killer cells, *see* NK cells
Neoceramide, 149
Neoglycolipids
    glycolipid expression, 149
    monoclonal antibodies, 146

Nerve growth factor, 125–129
neu oncogene, 41–42
Neuroblastoma, *neu* oncogene, 41–42
Nitrosoguanide, 266
Nevus-associated antigen, 129–130
NK cells
  melanoma eradication, 170–173
  and TPA B-cell effects, 235
Nucleus, *onc* proteins, 111–112
NZB plasmacytomas, 20,24–25

O

OKT4/leu 3, 191,193
1-Oleoyl-2-acetylglycerol, 97–99
Oncogenes; *see also specific oncogenes*
  human melanoma, 128–130
  interactions, 39–42
  tumor promoter synergy, 61–62
Oocytes, 158–165
Osteosarcoma cell line, 91–92

P

P_1 promoter
  Burkitt's lymphoma, *myc*, 30–33,35
  murine plasmacytomas, *myc*, 11–25
P_2 promoter, 11–25,30–33,35
p21
  GM-CSF phosphorylation, 220
  and transferrin receptor, 3–4
  transforming activity, biochemistry, 2–4
p24 antigen, 205–206
p28[sis]
  and *env*, 90
  PDGF homology, 88–91
  in SSV transformed cells, 90
p97 antigen, 157–165
p185 protein, 42
Paragloboside, 132
PC 10916, 18–19
Peripheral blood cells, 48–49
pH, proteoglycan biosynthesis, antigen, 170
PHA, *see* Phytohemagglutinin
Phorbol
  protein kinase C activation, 57–58
  S6 phosphorylation effect, 97–98
Phorbol dibutyrate
  protein kinase C activation, 57–58
  receptor effects, 60
4α-Phorbol-12,13-didecanoate, 57–58
Phosphatidic acid, 102–103

Phosphatidylinositol
  pp60[v-src] phosphorylation, 102–104
  tumor promoters, phosphorylation, 60
Phosphatidylinositol 4-phosphate, 96,102
Phosphoamino acids, 97–98
Phospholipids
  growth factor effect, 73
  and protein kinase C activation, 57–58
Phosphorylation
  GM-CSF, p21, 220
  growth factor receptors, 72–73
  pp60[v-src] stimulation, 95–104
  protein kinase C, proteins, 60–61
  Rous sarcoma virus transformed cells, 95–104
  serine residues, RSV, 95–104
  tumor promoters, 60
Phytohemagglutinin, 234–235
Placental EGF receptor, 77–78
Plasma membrane
  onc proteins, 108–112
  pp60[src] localization, 108,112
Plasmacytomas, c-*myc* activation, 11–25
Platelet-derived growth factor
  "allosteric regulator" model, 153
  amino acid sequence, 88
  autocrine growth regulator, 74–76
  and gangliosides, 150–153
  melanoma cells, 128
  oncogene effects, 71–82
  receptor interaction, biochemistry, 72–74
  and simian sarcoma virus protein, 87–92
Pokeweed mitogen, 252,254
pol gene
  chronic leukemia viruses, 185
  HTLV genome, 200–201
Polyclonal B cell activators, 251–252
Polynucleated giant cells, 193
Polyoma virus
  and chemicals, synergy, 56
  transfection, oncogenes, 40
Polysome immunopurification, 157–165
Poly-X antigen, 146–148
pp60[v-src]
  cellular adhesion plaques, 113
  functional analysis, 116–118
  localization, 108–109
  metabolism, 108
  S6 phosphorylation, stimulation, 95–104
  and transformed morphology, 116–118

Prague C strain, 116
pre-AIDS syndrome, 195
Prednisolone, 266
Primate T-cell leukemia virus, 183,188
Prolymphocytic leukemia, 48,51
Promoters, c-*myc* activation, 12–25
Promyelocytes, G-CSF binding, 227
Protein kinase C
  TPA action, 97
  tumor promoter action, 56–62,96–104
Proteins
  glycosylation significance, 141
  oncogene interactions, production, 41–42
Proteoglycan melanoma-associated
  antigen, 169–170
PstI, 32
Purified protein derivative, 252
pX sequence, 185,201

Q
Quercetin, 103

R
R sequence, HTLV, 201
RAF 1 oncogene, 50
Raji cells
  c-*myc* sequence changes, 33–37
  c-*myc* translocation position, 30–33
ras gene
  B-cell lymphocytic leukemia, 49–50
  interactions, oncogenesis, 39–42
  molecular and junctional analysis, 1–6
  myc oncogene interaction, 40–41
  and myoblast differentiation,
    expression, 243–248
  p21 encoding, 3
  protein localization, and function, 113
*ras*H gene
  activation and function, 2
  tumor promoter synergism, 62–63
N-*ras* oncogene
  human melanoma, 129
  interactions, transfection, 40
Receptors
  and colony stimulating factor response,
    226–227
  growth factors, biochemistry, 72–74
  and oncogene interaction, 41–42
  tumor promoter effects, 60
Reciprocal exchange, c-*myc*, 13–17
Replication competent retroviruses, 184
Replication defective retroviruses, 184

Retroviruses; *see also specific viruses*
  chemical carcinogen similarity, 63–64
  infection cycle, 184
  onc gene proteins, 107–118
    localization, 107–118
  subdivisions, 184–185
Reversibility, malignancy, 258–259
mRNA, p97 antigen, 157–163
Rous sarcoma virus; *see also* pp60v-src
  gene proteins, 107–118
    localization, 108
  phosphorylation events, 95–104

S
S genes, 258–259,270
S region, *myc* reciprocal exchanges, 13–17
S1 nuclease mapping, 21–25
S6 phosphorylation
  RSV transformed cells, 95–104
  serine stimulation, 97–101
  TPA stimulation, 96–101
SacI site, 31–32
Saliva, pre-AIDS patients, HTLV-III, 195
Sarcomas, malignancy reversion, 258–259
Schmidt-Ruppin strain, 116
Semen, HTLV-III, AIDS, 195
Serine phosphorylation, *see* S6
  phosphorylation
Seroepidemiology
  HTLV-I, 196–197
  HTLV-III, 198–200
Serum, S6 phosphorylation, RSV, 95–104
Sialic acid, TPA effect, CLL cells, 236
Sialosyl-Lea antigen, 146
Simian sarcoma virus, 74,87–92
sis proto-oncogene, 243–248
c-*sis* gene
  in human tumor cells, 91–92
    melanoma, 130
  and myogenic differentiation, 248
  and p28sis, 88–91
  protein products, sequences, 75,88–91
v-*sis* gene
  and p28sis, 88–91
  protein product localization, 112
  protein products, sequences, 75,88–91
Sm-FeSV proteins, localization, 110–111
Spleen cells, 48–49
src oncogene, 116–118,243–248; *see also*
  pp60v-src
Stage-specific embryonic antigens
  embryonic development, 140,142–144

glycolipid expression, 144
structure, 140,143
Stem cell suppression, 224–227
Steroids, differentiation induction, 267
Suppression genes, 258–259,270
SV40 cell line, 74–76
Switch sequence
Burkitt's lymphoma cell lines, 30–33
c-*myc*, 13–17

T

T-cell growth factor
gene activation, production, 202
HTLV, 186,191
T lymphocyte production, HTLV, 192
T lymphocytes
cytotoxicity, and HTLV, 192
HTLV immunological effects, 191–193
lymphokine production, and HTLV,
191–192
TPA B-CLL cell effect mediation,
237–238
TBR-IgC, 103
Teleocidin
oncogene synergy, 62–63
and protein kinase C, 57–58
receptor effects, 60
Teratocarcinoma cells, 275
12-*O*-Tetradecanoyl phorbol 13-acetate,
see TPA
Tlym-I, and tx-4, transformation, 6
TPA
B-cell immunoglobin stimulation, 46
B-type CLL cell differentiation, 233–
240
carcinogenesis mechanism, 56–62
malignant lymphocyte response, 252–
253
myeloid leukemia cells, clones, 266
oncogene synergy, 62–63
phenotypic changes, 235–237
protein kinase C activation, 56–62
S6 phosphorylation, 96–104
trans acting factor, 56
Transfection, 62–63

Transferrin
Blym-1 homology, 4–5
HTLV-transformed T cells, 191
p21 complexing, *ras* gene, 3
and p97 antigen sequence, 165
Transformation mechanisms, 107–118
Translocation, *see* Chromosome
translocation
Transplanted myeloid leukemias, 225
Trifucosylated type 2 chain, 146–147
Tumor promoters, 56–62
tx-1 gene, 6
tx-4 gene, 6
Tyrosine phosphorylation, 151–152
Tyrosine-specific protein kinase
and EGF receptor, 81–82
TPA enhancement, 61

U

U-2 OS cell line, 91–92
U5 sequences, HTLV, 201
Umbilical cord blood leukocytes, 190
United States, HTLV-I seroepidemiology,
196–197

V

Viruses, and chemicals, synergy, 55–56
VL30 sequences, 64

W

WEHI-3B cells, 224–227
Western Blot analysis, HTLV-III, 198–
199
Wild-type transformed morphology, 114–
118

X

X-irradiation
differentiation induction, 266,276
response mechanism, leukemia, 276
Xenopus laevis, 157–165
XhoI site, c-*myc* gene, 31–32

Y

Yamaguchi 73, localization, 109
yes gene, protein, 112